Family matters

Family matters
Designing, analysing and understanding family-based studies in life course epidemiology

Edited by

Debbie A Lawlor
Professor of Epidemiology,
MRC Centre for Causal Analyses in
Translational Epidemiology,
Department of Social Medicine,
University of Bristol, UK

Gita D Mishra
Senior Research Scientist,
MRC Unit for Lifelong Ageing
and Health, Department of
Epidemiology and Public Health,
University College London, UK

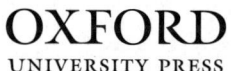

OXFORD
UNIVERSITY PRESS

Great Clarendon Street, Oxford OX2 6DP

Oxford University Press is a department of the University of Oxford.
It furthers the University's objective of excellence in research, scholarship,
and education by publishing worldwide in

Oxford New York

Auckland Cape Town Dar es Salaam Hong Kong Karachi
Kuala Lumpur Madrid Melbourne Mexico City Nairobi
New Delhi Shanghai Taipei Toronto

With offices in

Argentina Austria Brazil Chile Czech Republic France Greece
Guatemala Hungary Italy Japan Poland Portugal Singapore
South Korea Switzerland Thailand Turkey Ukraine Vietnam

Oxford is a registered trade mark of Oxford University Press
in the UK and in certain other countries

Published in the United States
by Oxford University Press Inc., New York

© Oxford University Press 2009

The moral rights of the author have been asserted
Database right Oxford University Press (maker)

First published 2009

All rights reserved. No part of this publication may be reproduced,
stored in a retrieval system, or transmitted, in any form or by any means,
without the prior permission in writing of Oxford University Press,
or as expressly permitted by law, or under terms agreed with the appropriate
reprographics rights organization. Enquiries concerning reproduction
outside the scope of the above should be sent to the Rights Department,
Oxford University Press, at the address above

You must not circulate this book in any other binding or cover
and you must impose this same condition on any acquirer

British Library Cataloguing in Publication Data

Data available

Library of Congress Cataloguing in Publication Data

Typeset by Cepha Imaging Private Ltd., Bangalore, India
Printed and bound in the
United Kingdom
by the MPG Books Group.

ISBN 978–0–19–923103–4

10 9 8 7 6 5 4 3 2 1

Whilst every effort has been made to ensure that the contents of this book are as
complete, accurate and up-to-date as possible at the date of writing, Oxford
University Press is notable to give any guarantee or assurance that such is the case.
Readers are urged to take appropriately qualified medical advice in all cases. The
information in this book is intended to be useful to the general reader, but should
not be used as a means of self-diagnosis or for the prescription of medication.

Contents

Preface *vii*

Contributors *ix*

1 Why family matters: an introduction *1*
  Debbie A Lawlor and Gita D Mishra

Part I **The theoretical underpinning for the use of family-based studies in life course epidemiology**

2 Theoretical underpinning for the use of intergenerational studies in life course epidemiology *13*
  Debbie A Lawlor, Sam Leary and George Davey Smith

3 Theoretical underpinning for the use of sibling studies in life course epidemiology *39*
  Kate W Strully and Gita D Mishra

4 Theoretical underpinning for the use of twin studies in life course epidemiology *57*
  Ruth JF Loos, Charlotte L Ridgway and Ken K Ong

5 Discussant chapter—summary of the theoretical approaches to family-based studies in life course epidemiology *85*
  Hazel M Inskip

Part II **The practicalities of undertaking family-based studies**

6 Birth cohorts: a resource for life course studies *99*
  Anne-Marie Nybo Andersen, Mia Madsen and Debbie A Lawlor

7 Family-based life course studies in low- and middle-income countries *129*
  G David Batty, Cesar G Victora and Debbie A Lawlor

8 Using available family members as proxies to provide information on other family members who are difficult to reach *151*
  Susannah Tomkins

9 Discussant chapter—the practicalities of undertaking family-based studies *181*
  Rebecca Hardy and Diana Kuh

Part III **Statistical methods in family-based studies**

10 Statistical considerations in intergenerational studies *195*
  Dorothea Nitsch and Gita D Mishra

11 Random effects models for sibling and twin-based studies in life course epidemiology *229*
Samuli Ripatti

12 Discussant chapter—statistical considerations in family-based life course studies *251*
Amanda Sacker

Part IV **Some illustrative examples of the use of family-based studies in life course epidemiology**

13 Family-based studies applied to the influence of early life factors on cardiovascular disease *263*
Debbie A Lawlor and David A Leon

14 How family-based studies have added to the understanding of life course epidemiology of mental health *279*
Stephani L Hatch and Gita D Mishra

15 How family-based studies have added to understanding the life course epidemiology of reproductive health *295*
Susan MB Morton and Janet Rich Edwards

16 Discussant chapter—using family-based designs in life course epidemiology *317*
John Lynch and Seungmi Yang

17 The future of family-based studies in life course epidemiology: challenges and opportunities *325*
Gita D Mishra and Debbie A Lawlor

Index *335*

Preface

Life-course epidemiology is now well-founded theoretically, and strategies for statistical analysis have been well-rehearsed. The epidemiology of diseases of adult onset, such as coronary heart disease, has tended to concentrate on adult influences – with a passing nod at a measure of the intrauterine environment such as birth weight. The influences of parents and siblings, partners and children have been largely ignored until now.

The overall aim of the book is to provide the knowledge and skills required to design, analyse and correctly interpret family based studies. As the authors acknowledge (Chapter 1) understanding the underlying assumptions of the different types of family study, and the inferences that can be drawn from them, is complex.

Now that this book has been written, one wonders why the topic of the family in epidemiological studies has not been fully addressed before. That is not withstanding the considerable body of research that has been undertaken by psychologists and psychiatrists who have been at the forefront for many years in studying the long-term effects of early family interactions on the mental health of the individual. The approach of this book is broader and in more depth. As well as mental health it considers physical health and features of development including growth.

The structure of the book is unusual in that it is divided into 4 sections of 2-3 chapters, each followed by a summary chapter by a discussant pulling together the various strands of the arguments. There are many examples quoted to illustrate the topic of each chapter, and intriguing suggestions for future studies (e.g. the use of children born to surrogate mothers in unravelling the difference between the in utero environment and the heredity from the biological mother in Chapter 2).

Of course, the major studies involving the family in the past were, and are, the studies of twins set up to distinguish the ball-park estimates of the effects of heredity compared with those of the environment on different outcomes. As with all aspects of family studies, these are viewed critically, and their limitations summarised. Other types of family study are considered, such as the use of siblings, half-siblings, step-families and adoption studies.

Birth cohort studies are recommended as a useful method of collecting detailed data on the family, and ways in which this can be accomplished are described in Chapter 6. Although most of the examples used in the various sections are from studies in developed countries, it is important to repeat such studies in low- and middle-income countries, as there is the perception that results from the developed world (e.g. on the dangers of smoking) are not relevant to cultures elsewhere where the environment and the genetics are quite different (Chapter 7).

This book provides a unique background for investigators who either wish to analyse data that already are available or those who are designing and implementing their own study. It is thought provoking and provides a useful background to a variety of interesting concepts. It has optimistic views of the use of family based studies – as Mishra and Lawlor say: 'In many ways the future of family-based studies represent new territory in scientific terms, for instance by using observational studies to establish causal pathways' (Chapter 17) and Lynch and Yang say 'If we know how families transmit different diseases across generations then it may elucidate novel …. avenues for prevention' (Chapter 16).

'Family Matters' is a useful pun to aid the memory. Not only does the family matter in all aspects of health and development (from conception to old age), but there are many details (matters) to consider in analysing data related to the family. This volume provides an erudite and thorough approach to many relevant issues, with a star-studded list of authors.

Jean Golding
Centre for Child and Adolescent Health,
Department of Community Based Medicine,
University of Bristol,
UK

Contributors

G David Batty
Wellcome Trust fellow, Medical Research Council Social and Public Health Sciences Unit; University of Glasgow, Glasgow, UK

George Davey Smith
Professor of Clinical Epidemiology, MRC Centre for Causal Analyses in Translational Epidemiology, Department of Social Medicine, University of Bristol, UK

Rebecca Hardy
Senior Research Scientist, MRC Unit for Lifelong Health and Ageing; Reader in Epidemiology and Medical Statistics, Department of Epidemiology and Public Health, University College London, UK

Stephani L Hatch
Lecturer in Social Epidemiology, Department of Psychological Medicine, Institute of Psychiatry, King's College London, London, UK

Hazel M Inskip
Professor of Statistical Epidemiology; Deputy Director, MRC Epidemiology Resource Centre, Southampton General Hospital, UK

Diana Kuh
Director, MRC Unit for Lifelong Health and Ageing; Professor of Life Course, Department of Epidemiology and Public Health, University College London, UK

Debbie A Lawlor
Professor of Epidemiology, MRC Centre for Causal Analyses in Translational Epidemiology, Department of Social Medicine, University of Bristol, UK

Sam Leary
Lecturer in Statistics, Department of Oral and Dental Science, University of Bristol Dental School, UK

David A Leon
Professor of Epidemiology, Non-communicable Diseases Epidemiology Unit, London School of Hygiene & Tropical Medicine, London, UK

Ruth JF Loos
MRC Group Leader, MRC Epidemiology Unit, Institute of Metabolic Science, Addenbrooke's Hospital, Cambridge, UK

John Lynch
Professor of Epidemiology, Division of Health Sciences, University of South Australia, Australia; Department of Social Medicine, University of Bristol, UK

Mia Madsen
Research fellow, Epidemiology, University of Southern Denmark, Odense, Denmark

Gita D Mishra
Senior Research Scientist, MRC Unit for Lifelong Ageing and Health, Department of Epidemiology and Public Health, University College London, UK

Susan MB Morton
Senior Lecturer, The Liggins Institute, The University of Auckland, New Zealand

Dorothea Nitsch
Clinical Lecturer in Genetic Epidemiology, Non-communicable Disease Epidemiology Unit, London School of Hygiene & Tropical Medicine, London, UK

Anne-Marie Nybo Andersen
Professor of Epidemiology, University of Southern Denmark, Odense, Denmark

Ken K Ong
MRC Group Leader, MRC Epidemiology Unit, Institute of Metabolic Science, Addenbrooke's Hospital Cambridge, UK

Janet Rich Edwards
Director of Developmental Epidemiology,
Connors Center for Women's Health and
Gender Biology Brigham and Women's
Hospital, Boston, USA

Charlotte L Ridgway
PhD student, MRC Epidemiology Unit,
Institute of Metabolic Science, Addenbrooke's
Hospital, UK

Samuli Ripatti
Researcher, FIMM Institute for Molecular
Medicine Finland;
Department of Medical Epidemiology and
Biostatistics, Karolinska Institutet,
Sweden

Amanda Sacker
Research Professor, Institute for Social and
Economic Research, University of Essex, UK

Kate W Strully
Assistant Professor, Department of Sociology,
State University of New York at Albany, NY,
USA

Susannah Tomkins
Lecturer, Department of Epidemiology and
Population Health,
London School of Hygiene and Tropical
Medicine, London, UK

Cesar G Victora
Professor of Epidemiology,
Post-Graduate Programme in
Epidemiology, Universidade
Federal de Pelotas, Pelotas, Brazil

Seungmi Yang
Research Associate, Department of
Epidemiology, Biostatistics and Occupational
Health, McGill University, Canada

Chapter 1

Why family matters: an introduction

Debbie A Lawlor and Gita D Mishra

I

Baked the day she suddenly dropped dead
we chew it slowly that last apple pie.

Shocked into sleeplessness you're scared of bed.
We never could talk much, and now don't try.

You're like book ends, the pair of you, she'd say,
Hog that grate, say nothing, sit, sleep, stare…

The 'scholar' me, you, worn out on poor pay,
only our silence made us seem a pair.

Not as good for staring in, blue gas,
too regular each bud, each yellow spike.

At night you need my company to pass
and she not here to tell us we're alike!

You're life's all shattered into smithereens.

Back in our silences and sullen looks,
for all the Scotch we drink, what's still between 's
not the thirty or so years, but books, books, books

II

The stone's too full. The wording must be terse.
There's scarcely room to carve the FLORENCE on it—

Come on, it's not as if we're wanting verse.
It's not as if we're wanting a whole sonnet!

After tumblers of neat Johnny Walker
(I think that both of us we're on our third)
you said you'd always been a clumsy talker
and couldn't find another, shorter word
for 'beloved' or for 'wife' in the inscription,
but not too clumsy that you can't still cut:

You're supposed to be the bright boy at description
and you can't tell them what the fuck to put!

I've got to find the right words on my own.

I've got the envelope that he'd been scrawling,
mis-spelt, mawkish, stylistically appalling
but I can't squeeze more love into their stone.

Book Ends by Tony Harrison[1]

Not surprisingly, family is central to art and literature as well as science. Tony Harrison's early poems in *The Loiners*[2] (a slang name for someone from Leeds) and *From the School of Eloquence and Other Poems*[1] describe the indelible effects of parents, extended family, social class, and the interrelationships of these, on one's wellbeing.[3] Those anthologies provide a very compelling and vivid image of the many ways in which families matter to all aspects of life. In *Book Ends*, the recently deceased mother recognized the unique bond between father and son, whereas Harrison describes the distance between them resulting from his social mobility and education—*'books, books, books'* – but for all his education and way with words he cannot give the poetry he craves to his father's love for his mother. In a more recent poem—*Rice-Paper Man*[4]—Harrison describes his anguish as he tries to cope with his son's severe mental illness and again the complexity of family relationships and how they influence health and wellbeing of all family members are clear.

The contributors to this book may not have the poetic skills of Tony Harrison, but they do have the knowledge and understanding to describe the requirements to set-up, maintain, analyse, and correctly interpret family-based life course epidemiology studies, which is what we hope the book will provide for its readers.

1.1 Time to raise the bar and push life course epidemiology to provide more causal answers

It is just over one decade since the first edition of the first life course book was published,[5] and since that support for a life course approach to epidemiology has increased considerably. In that original book the editors noted that 'The prevailing aetiological model for adult chronic disease emphasizes adult risk factors.'[5] (page 3) The focus on adult risk factors for chronic complex diseases, such as cardiovascular disease, cancer, and mental health problems, can be thought of as a degenerative aetiological model, since it is, on the whole, identifying factors associated with time and speed of degeneration in structure and function.

This degenerative model pays little attention to processes that lead up to the peak or optimal phenotypic state—usually seen to be a feature of early adulthood, such as the greatest lung volume (usually attained in late adolescence/early adulthood in humans), peak vascular function (usually attained in late adolescence in humans) or peak bone mass (usually attained post-puberty in humans). However, over the last 2–3 decades the degenerative model has been supplemented by approaches that view the development of anatomic, physiological and psychological systems as key to later disease susceptibility. This approach to understanding disease processes recognizes the importance of peak phenotypic states (in addition to how rapidly one degenerates from this peak) as having important relevance to the likelihood of developing complex chronic diseases. These development models of disease causation—that echo, but with increased biological motivation, much earlier discussions of determinants of health[6]—together with the degenerative model are at the heart of life course epidemiology. Over the last decade epidemiology has greatly expanded the evidence for the importance of a developmental approach to understanding the aetiology of chronic complex diseases (see, for example, many of the chapters in the second edition of the first book in the life course series[7-9]). However, very little work has really taken the life course approach to its limit of combining understanding of both development and degeneration of systems and function in order to develop appropriate methods for improving population health.

Life course epidemiology is '*the study of the effects on health and health related outcomes of biological (including genetic), environmental and social exposures during gestation, infancy, childhood, adolescence, adulthood and across generations.*'[10] As Diana Kuh and colleagues have noted,[10] this definition does not mean that all epidemiology can be defined as life course, rather a life course approach aims to understand the relevance of different exposures, occurring at different times in the life course on later health. Thus, explicit in the definition is the need to combine understanding of factors that affect both development and degeneration. Furthermore, understanding different life course models is key to using life course epidemiology to inform public health policy and improve population health.[10] Finally, to improve population health the life course approach also has to go beyond merely describing associations, to determining whether these associations are truly causal and, if so, whether in relation to timing of the exposure it can or should be modified.

For example, a recent large Danish record linkage study demonstrated an association between greater body mass index (BMI) in childhood (measured between ages 7–13 years) and future risk of coronary heart disease (CHD) mortality.[11] The risk was linear across childhood BMI distribution, but the magnitude of the association increased with older age at measurement. In girls there was no association until BMI measured at age 10 or older and in both sexes the association was strongest for BMI measured at age 13 years.[11] The strengthening of the effect with older age at measurement might mean that much of the association of childhood BMI with adult CHD is mediated via adult BMI (with the tracking of childhood BMI into adulthood), but the study was unable to determine whether that was the case. If this were the case then interventions aimed at reducing BMI in adulthood might be equally as beneficial for reducing CHD risk as any interventions aimed at preventing childhood obesity. It is also possible that this association is explained by obesity in childhood causing permanent changes in metabolic and vascular function that do not revert to normal even if weight is lost between childhood and adulthood. If this were the case then clearly interventions aimed at preventing the development of childhood obesity would be paramount. Finally it is possible that the association is not causal but explained by confounding, for example by socioeconomic background. To translate the findings from the Danish record linkage study into relevant public health messages a much fuller picture of the life course epidemiology linking childhood BMI to adult CHD is required:

- To what extent is the association causal or explained by confounding, by for example family socioeconomic background and lifestyle characteristics?
- If causal, to what extent is the association mediated by adult obesity and its associated adverse metabolic and vascular effects?
- If causal, to what extent is the association mediated by changes to metabolism and vasculature in childhood that are permanent even if the child were to lose weight?
- If causal, and importantly mediated by both childhood and adult metabolic and vascular changes, is prevention of obesity easier to achieve by interventions in childhood or adulthood; or is there no difference by age at which one tries to prevent obesity?
- What are the main determinants of greater BMI/obesity in childhood (or adulthood)?
- What are the best ways of preventing obesity in childhood and adulthood; do the methods and their cost-effectiveness differ for children and adults?
- Would family-based interventions, aimed at preventing obesity in all family members (adults and children), provide the most effective and cost-effective means of preventing obesity and hence CHD?

This list of questions is not exhaustive, but they serve to illustrate that the association of an exposure during early life (a period of development) and a disease outcome in later life, whilst illustrating that some of the important concepts of a life course approach, raises many more questions that it can answer. No single study will answer all of these questions but as a number of existing birth cohorts, such as the UK 1946[12] and 1958[13] birth cohorts, Perinatal Collaborative Study from US,[14] the Aberdeen children of the 1950s cohort,[15] and the Danish Metropolit cohort,[16] move into adulthood and have very rich prospectively collected data during periods of development and degeneration, we have to start pushing for investigators to publish papers that do engage with a fuller life course picture. This will require more sophisticated statistical approaches than the multivariable regression models commonly used in associational epidemiology and the correct interpretation of these models. Several of these issues are discussed in the last life course book to be published in this series–*Epidemiological methods in life course research*[17]—and also in Chapters 10–12 in this book. Family-based approaches can help with some issues of causality and possibly with timing of different exposures. These too, require use of appropriate statistical techniques and a clear understanding of the theoretical underpinning of different family studies in order to interpret correctly their results. This book aims to describe the key ways in which family-based studies can enhance life course epidemiology, but also highlight the importance of correctly conducting and interpreting the results from these studies.

1.2 The use of family-based studies in life course epidemiology

Families are at the heart of life course epidemiology. Its very definition necessarily involves mothers, who are clearly central to exposures during gestation and family members (parents/care-givers and siblings) who will influence one's experience of childhood and adolescence. Once one is an adult, partners, pregnancies (for females) and offspring (including whether one does or does not have offspring) will shape health and health related behaviours. Furthermore, the definition explicitly includes genetic factors and the intergenerational transfer of characteristics.

There are three potential ways in which family-based studies (i.e. those in which data are purposefully collected on more than one family member) might contribute to life course epidemiology. First, family will directly affect one's health by determining many of the biological, environmental and social exposures across the life course. Secondly, different family members will exert their impact on one's health by different degrees at different times in the life course, and hence detailed studies of family influences could help to understand the importance of timing of exposures across the life course. Lastly, comparing relationships within and between different family members can help to clarify the mechanisms underlying associations in life course studies and help to determine causality.

1.2.1 Direct influences of family on health across the life course

At all stages of the life course behaviours in family members seem to influence health and health related behaviours in the index individual. This is perhaps most notable during fetal development when maternal behaviours and her health and physiology influence normal fetal growth and development in ways that can have lasting effects. Maternal smoking during pregnancy is one of the main causes of low birth weight in industrialized countries.[18] Maternal use of high doses of diethyl-stilbestrol (DES) during pregnancy (a treatment given to pregnant women from the 1930s to 70s, in the mistaken belief that it would reduce pregnancy loss) is now known to cause menstrual and reproductive disorders and vaginal cancer in daughters,[19–25] and is associated with reproductive disorders in sons,[20] and menstrual and reproductive disorders in grand-daughters.[26]

Maternal pregnancy use of the drug thalidomide, a potent anti-emetic used by pregnant women during the 1950s and 60s to combat morning sickness, provides a further example of the direct effect of maternal exposures on the developing fetus.[27] Thalidomide caused infants to be born with phocomelia and other permanent limb deformities, particularly when mothers had taken the drug during the sensitive period of limb development between days 20–40 of gestation.[27]

Families also affect one's health and behaviours at other times in the life course. A mother's ability and decision to breast feed or not affects morbidity and mortality in infancy and in the longer term having been breast fed is causally related to higher cognitive ability at mean age 6.5 years in a large randomized controlled trial.[28] There is evidence that different family members influence health behaviours and outcomes in later life. Though, interestingly for health behaviours there is some evidence that spouses influence each other more than parents influence children or siblings influences each other. For example, in the National Heart, Lung and Blood Institute Family Heart study familial associations for behaviours—alcohol consumption, exercise and smoking—were strongest for spouses and notably weaker for parent-offspring and sibling correlations.[29] Similarly, in the Avon Longitudinal Study of Parents and Children (ALSPAC) cohort there was only weak associations between parental physical activity and their offspring's physical activity at age 11–12.[30] By contrast familial correlations of high and low density lipoprotein cholesterol were stronger for 'blood relatives' (parent-child and siblings) than they were for spouses in the National Heart, Lung and Blood Institute Family Heart study.[29] This suggests that family correlations of these phenotypes are influenced importantly by genetic factors and less so by shared familial behaviours.

The moderate to strong associations for health related behaviours between spouses have been demonstrated in other studies,[31, 32] and these findings formed the basis of a recently evaluated intervention to reduce cardiovascular disease in high risk individuals that targeted both the high risk adults (those with a previous cardiovascular event or predicted with ≥5% risk during the next 10 years to have an event based on risk factor assessment) and their partners for lifestyle changes.[33] At 1 year follow-up higher proportions of those at high risk in the intervention arm, compared to the standard treatment arm, had met goals for dietary saturated fat intake, oily fish intake, fruit and vegetable intake, physical activity, weight loss, smoking cessation and blood pressure. Differences in lipids, HbA_{1C} and medication use (statins, antiplatelets, beta-blockers, and ACE inhibitors) did not differ markedly between the two groups.[33] The differences in health related behaviours in the patients were matched by similar changes in their partners. The effect of spouses on one's health is also demonstrated by the increased risk of all-cause, cardiovascular, cancer and accident and violent mortality in spouses following the death of their spouse.[34]

Several of the chapters in this book, notably Chapter 14, which describes the relevance of family-based studies to understanding the life course epidemiology of mental health, describe other ways in which family members and family relationships directly affect one's health across the whole life course.

1.2.2 Using family influences to understand the importance of timing in life course epidemiology

As noted above it is important in life course epidemiology to go beyond simple associations to understanding whether or not timing matters with respect to interventions to improve population health. For example, if an exposure during a developmental period in early life is causally related to a later health outcome, but only through strong tracking of that exposure during the life course, one would need to consider when in the life course it is most effective to remove the exposure. If it is easier to effectively remove it in adulthood, than childhood, then interventions in adulthood would be most appropriate.

Since our exposure to different family members changes over the life course family studies could help to understand whether exposures at different stages of the life course are important or not. As described in Chapter 2 this has been most exploited with respect to intrauterine exposures. Thus, maternal behaviours during pregnancy have been used to explore the fetal origins of several disease outcomes (i.e. the intrauterine period as a sensitive or critical period for certain risk factors). However, care is required in correctly interpreting these studies, and several recent examples that have shown, for example, similar magnitudes of association between maternal and paternal smoking at the time of pregnancy and future offspring obesity and blood pressure,[35, 36] and similar magnitudes of association of modest maternal and paternal alcohol consumption at the time of pregnancy and future IQ levels in offspring,[37] illustrate that it can be misleading to assume that a maternal behaviour during pregnancy (particularly one that is unlikely to be solely done in pregnancy) is having an offspring effect via intrauterine mechanisms. These issues are discussed in more detail in Chapter 2.

Changes in levels of familial associations at different times of the life course can also give some clues about aetiological subgroups. For example, the within monozygotic twins association for coronary heart disease weakens considerably with increasing age, such that the relative risk for a co-twin dying of coronary heart disease if the other twin has already died of coronary heart disease before age 65 is 15.0, but decreases monotonically with increasing age of the first heart disease death in a twin pair to being consistent with the null once this occurs at age 80 or older.[38] These findings suggest that premature heart disease is more likely to be related to a genetic aetiology than coronary disease occurring at older ages.

1.2.3 Using family comparisons to understand mechanisms underlying

For a large part this book is concerned with the correct conduct and interpretation of family-based studies—intergenerational studies, sibling studies, and twin studies—to help understand causal mechanisms in life course epidemiology. As will be seen in the subsequent chapters, use of family-based studies for this purpose necessarily requires an understanding of the direct effects of family on health and an understanding of how exposure to different family members changes over the life course. Our hope is that the book will demonstrate the potential of these studies and thus motivate researchers to use them more. It would be nice to write a second edition in 10 years' time and be able to demonstrate that life course epidemiology really has moved on in terms of causal understanding and translation to effective interventions for improving population health, and that family-based studies have made major contributions to this development.

1.3 The aims of this book

Family data and specific family-based studies (intergenerational, sibling, and twin studies) could make important contributions to a full life course understanding of health and disease. However, understanding the underlying assumptions of these studies and hence the inferences that can be drawn from them is complex. Furthermore, there are issues relating to study design, including how to obtain valid and reliable data from family members, ensuring correct linkage between members of the same family and indeed how to define members of the same family, and issues relating to the statistical analysis of family-based studies that are not well understood.

The aim of this book is to provide in one volume the knowledge and skills required to design, analyse, and correctly interpret family-based studies.

Our hope is that this book will explain what family-based studies can tell us about life course epidemiology; provide practical guidance on how to set-up and maintain birth cohorts for completing family-based studies in life course epidemiology; describe how to undertake appropriate statistical analyses of family-based studies and correctly interpret results from these analyses; and provide examples that illustrate the ways in which family-based studies can enhance our understanding life course epidemiology.

The book is divided into four sections that correspond to these aims. **Part I** describes the theoretical underpinning for the use of different family-based studies (including intergenerational, twin, and sibling studies) in life course epidemiology, by detailing the assumptions underlying these studies and the inferences and understanding that can be gained from each type of study. **Part II** describes the practicalities of undertaking family-based studies, including undertaking such studies in low and middle income countries and issues relating to use of proxy informants (e.g. parents providing information on children and vice versa or siblings providing information about each other) in family-based studies. **Part III** describes appropriate statistical approaches for family-based studies. Our aim in this part is to provide statistical guidance in non-technical language as well as providing relevant algebra and programming syntax, so that individuals from different backgrounds will find relevant information for undertaking appropriate analyses, checking model assumptions, and correctly interpreting of the statistical output. Finally, **Part IV** provides examples of how family-based studies have been used in understanding the life course epidemiology of cardiovascular disease, mental health, and reproductive health. These examples are intended to illustrate the relevance of family-based studies, not only to these areas, but also more generally to the whole of life course epidemiology. In our final chapter we discuss ideas for further uses of family-based studies in life course epidemiology.

References

1 **Harrison T.** *From the School of Eloquence and Other Poems.* London: Rex Collins, 1978.
2 **Harrison T.** *The Loiners.* London: London Magazine Editions, 1970.
3 **Byrne S. (ed).** *Tony Harrison: Loiners.* Oxford: Oxford University Press, 1997.
4 **Harrison T.** *Laureate's Block: and Other Poems.* London: Penguin Books, 2000.
5 **Kuh D, Ben-Shlomo Y (eds).** *A Life Course Approach to Chronic Disease Epidemiology.* Oxford: Oxford University Press, 1997.
6 **Kuh D, Davey Smith G.** The life course and adult chronic disease: an historical perspective with particular reference to coronary heart disease. In: Kuh D, Ben-Shlomo Y, eds. *A Life Course Approach to Chronic Disease Epidemiology.* 2nd ed. Oxford: Oxford University Press, 2004: pp. 15–40.
7 **Lawlor DA, Ben-Shlomo Y, Leon DA.** Pre-adult influences on cardiovascular disease. In: Kuh D, Ben-Shlomo Y, eds. *A Life Course Approach to Chronic Disease Epidemiology.* 2nd ed. Oxford: Oxford University Press, 2004: 41–76.
8 **Gillman MW.** A life course approach to obesity. In: Kuh D, Ben-Shlomo Y, eds. *A Life Course Approach to Chronic Disease Epidemiology* (2nd edition). Oxford: Oxford University Press, 2004: 189–217.
9 **Forouhi N, Hall E, McKeigue P.** A life course approach to diabetes. In: Kuh D, Ben-Shlomo Y, eds. *A life course approach to chronic disease epidemiology.* 2nd ed. Oxford: Oxford University Press, 2004: pp. 165–88.
10 **Kuh D, Ben-Shlomo Y, Lynch J, Hallqvist J, Power C.** Life course epidemiology. *J Epidemiol Community Health* 2003; **57**(10):778–83.
11 **Baker JL, Olsen LW, Sorensen TI.** Childhood body-mass index and the risk of coronary heart disease in adulthood. *N Engl J Med* 2007; **357**(23): 2329–37.

12 Wadsworth MEJ, Kuh DJL. Childhood influences on adult health: a review of recent work from the British 1946 national birth cohort study, the MRC National Survey of Health and Development. *Paediatric and Perinatal Epidemiology* 1997; **11**: 2–20.

13 Power C, Elliott J. Cohort profile: 1958 British birth cohort (National Child Development Study). *Int J Epidemiol* 2006; **35**(1): 34–41.

14 *The Collaborative Perinatal Study of the National Institute of Neurological and Communicative Disorders and Stroke. The first year of life.* Baltimore: Johns Hopkins University Press, 1979.

15 Leon DA, Lawlor DA, Clark H, Macintyre S. Cohort profile: the Aberdeen children of the 1950s study. *Int J Epidemiol* 2006; **35**(3):549–52.

16 Osler M, Lund R, Kriegbaum M, Christensen U, Andersen AM. Cohort profile: the Metropolit 1953 Danish male birth cohort. *Int J Epidemiol* 2006; **35**(3): 541–5.

17 Pickles A, Maughan B, Wadsworth M. *Epidemiological Methods in Life Course Research.* 1st ed. Oxford: Oxford University Press, 2007.

18 Kramer MS, Olivier M, McLean FH, Dougherty GE, Willis DM, Usher RH. Determinants of fetal growth and body proportionality. *PEDIATRICS* 1990; **86**(1):18–27.

19 Herbst AL, Ulfelder H, Poskanzer DC. Adenocarcinoma of the vagina. Association of maternal stilbestrol therapy with tumor appearance in young women. *N Engl J Med* 1971; **284**(15): 878–81.

20 Bibbo M, Gill WB, Azizi F, Blough R, Fang VS, Rosenfield RL *et al.* Follow-up study of male and female offspring of DES-exposed mothers. *Obstet Gynecol* 1977; **49**(1):1–8.

21 Kaufman RH, Adam E, Binder GL, Gerthoffer E. Upper genital tract changes and pregnancy outcome in offspring exposed in utero to diethylstilbestrol. *Am J Obstet Gynecol* 1980; **137**(3): 299–308.

22 Senekjian EK, Potkul RK, Frey K, Herbst AL. Infertility among daughters either exposed or not exposed to diethylstilbestrol. *Am J Obstet Gynecol* 1988; **158**(3 Pt 1): 493–8.

23 Goldberg JM, Falcone T. Effect of diethylstilbestrol on reproductive function. *Fertil Steril* 1999; **72**(1): 1–7.

24 Kaufman RH, Adam E, Hatch EE, Noller K, Herbst AL, Palmer JR *et al.* Continued follow-up of pregnancy outcomes in diethylstilbestrol-exposed offspring. *Obstet Gynecol* 2000; **96**(4): 483–9.

25 Palmer JR, Hatch EE, Rao RS, Kaufman RH, Herbst AL, Noller KL *et al.* Infertility among women exposed prenatally to diethylstilbestrol. *Am J Epidemiol* 2001; **154**(4): 316–21.

26 Titus-Ernstoff L, Troisi R, Hatch EE, Wise LA, Palmer J, Hyer M *et al.* Menstrual and reproductive characteristics of women whose mothers were exposed in utero to diethylstilbestrol (DES). *Int J Epidemiol* 2006; **35**(4): 862–8.

27 McBride WG. Thalidomide embryopathy. *Teratology* 1977; **16**: 79–82.

28 Kramer MS, Aboud F, Mironova E, Vanilovich I, Platt RW, Matush L *et al.* Breastfeeding and child cognitive development: new evidence from a large randomized trial. *Arch Gen Psychiatry* 2008; **65**(5): 578–84.

29 Ellison RC, Myers RH, Zhang Y, Djousse L, Knox S, Williams RR *et al.* Effects of similarities in lifestyle habits on familial aggregation of high density lipoprotein and low density lipoprotein cholesterol: the NHLBI Family Heart Study. *Am J Epidemiol* 1999; **150**(9): 910–18.

30 Mattocks C, Ness A, Deere K, Tilling K, Leary S, Blair SN *et al.* Early life determinants of physical activity in 11 to 12 year olds: cohort study. *BMJ* 2008; **336**(7634): 26–9.

31 Pyke SD, Wood DA, Kinmonth AL, Thompson SG. Change in coronary risk and coronary risk factor levels in couples following lifestyle intervention. The British Family Heart Study. *Arch Fam Med* 1997; **6**(4): 354–60.

32 Wood DA, Roberts TL, Campbell M. Women married to men with myocardial infarction are at increased risk of coronary heart disease. *J Cardiovasc Risk* 1997; **4**(1): 7–11.

33 Wood DA, Kotseva K, Connolly S, Jennings C, Mead A, Jones J et al. Nurse-coordinated multidisciplinary, family-based cardiovascular disease prevention programme (EUROACTION) for patients with coronary heart disease and asymptomatic individuals at high risk of cardiovascular disease: a paired, cluster-randomised controlled trial. *Lancet* 2008; **371**(9629):1999–2012.

34 Hart CL, Hole DJ, Lawlor DA, Smith GD, Lever TF. Effect of conjugal bereavement on mortality of the bereaved spouse in participants of the Renfrew/Paisley Study. *J Epidemiol Community Health* 2007; **61**(5):455–60.

35 Leary SD, Davey Smith G, Rogers IS, Reilly JJ, Wells JC, Ness AR. Smoking during Pregnancy and Offspring Fat and Lean Mass in Childhood. *Obesity* 2006; **14**(12): 2284–93.

36 Brion MJ, Leary SD, Smith GD, Ness AR. Similar associations of parental prenatal smoking suggest child blood pressure is not influenced by intrauterine effects. *Hypertension* 2007; **49**(6):1422–8.

37 Alati R, McCleod J, Hickman M, Sayal K, May M, Davey Smith G et al. Is intrauterine exposure to alcohol and tobacco use associated with IQ in childhood? Findings from a parental-offspring comparison within the Avon Longitudinal Study of Parents and Children (ALSPAC). *Pediatric Research* In Press, 2008.

38 Marenberg ME, Risch N, Berkman LF, Floderus B, de FU. Genetic susceptibility to death from coronary heart disease in a study of twins. *N Engl J Med* 1994; **330**(15): 1041–6.

Part I
The theoretical underpinning for the use of family-based studies in life course epidemiology

Chapter 2

Theoretical underpinning for the use of intergenerational studies in life course epidemiology

Debbie A Lawlor, Sam Leary and George Davey Smith

Abstract

Intergenerational studies have been widely used in life course epidemiology both to examine primary research hypotheses and to explore underlying mechanisms for established associations. In this chapter we describe the theoretical underpinning for using different types of intergenerational studies in life course epidemiology and discuss how results from such studies should be interpreted. Specifically we consider: the use and interpretation of cousin, sibling, and twin intergenerational studies; egg donation/surrogate mother intergenerational studies; maternal-paternal comparisons; intergenerational migrant studies and Mendelian randomization in intergenerational studies in life course epidemiology.

2.1 Introduction

Life course epidemiology is concerned with the effects on health and health related outcomes of biological (including genetic), environmental and social exposures during gestation, infancy, childhood, adolescence, adulthood, and across generations.[1] Intergenerational (also known as trans-generational) studies are clearly relevant to understanding the effect of exposures across generations. They are also relevant to understanding the effects of parental (and grandparental) characteristics on a wide range of health related outcomes in their offspring, and vice versa, and they have potential to explore the mechanisms underlying association in life course epidemiology.

Intergenerational studies are by definition studies in which the relationships between characteristics obtained from family members from at least two different generations (e.g. parents and offspring) are explored. They include studies in which the association of the same characteristic across generations is examined, for example looking at the correlation of anthropometric measurements (such as birth weight, height or body mass index) across generations[2-7] or exploring the transfer of socioeconomic or behavioural characteristics (such as smoking, physical activity, and diet) across generations.[8-13] They also include studies in which one characteristic (the risk factor or exposures of interest) in one generation is related to a different characteristic (the outcome) in a different generation.

In studies that compare an exposure in one generation to an outcome in another generation it would seem intuitive that the exposure would be in the earlier generation. Such studies would include, for example, those that have looked at the association of maternal smoking during pregnancy with offspring body mass index (BMI)[14–18] and those examining the association of maternal consumption of diethyl-stilbestrol (DES) during pregnancy with menstrual and reproductive disorders and vaginal cancer in daughters,[19–25] reproductive disorders in sons,[20] and menstrual and reproductive disorders in grand-daughters.[26] There are also examples of intergenerational studies where 'exposure' in a more recent generation is related to 'outcome' in an earlier generation. In some of these studies direct associations might be examined, for example the effect of offspring sleeping patterns on parental health.[27] In other studies the 'exposure' in the more recent generation is acting as a proxy, rather than a direct exposure. For example, several studies have explored the association of offspring birth weight with parental cardiovascular disease risk in order to explore the likely mechanism(s) underlying the inverse association of birth weight with cardiovascular disease within individuals.[28] Clearly, offspring birth weight cannot 'cause' parental cardiovascular disease; in these studies offspring birth weight is acting as a proxy for that part of own birth weight that might be determined by genetic factors.

Intergenerational studies have been widely used in life course epidemiology both to examine primary research hypotheses and to explore underlying mechanisms for established associations. In this chapter we will describe the theoretical underpinning of using different types of intergenerational studies in life course epidemiology and discuss correct ways of interpreting results from such studies. We will provide specific examples in order to emphasize and clarify points, but the chapter is not intended to provide a comprehensive review of all intergenerational studies in life course epidemiology. Chapter 10 in this book provides details of statistical methods that can be appropriately used in intergenerational studies.

2.2 Intergenerational transmission of the same characteristic

There is considerable evidence that not only are genetic variants and their associated phenotypes transferred (inherited) across generations but so too are socioeconomic, environmental and behavioural characteristics.[2, 4–6, 8–13, 29] Acknowledging and understanding this intergenerational transfer of a wide variety of characteristics is important for several reasons. Firstly, observing and understanding the intergenerational transfer of adverse characteristics, such as low birth weight or poverty, is likely to be important for improving public health. Secondly, recognizing the intergenerational transfer of characteristics is likely to be important for understanding results from life course epidemiological studies. For example, the intergenerational associations of birth size might be driven by genetic, social, or behavioural characteristics, or a combination of all of these. Understanding the major drivers of intergenerational associations of the same characteristic (such as birth weight) is important in its own right, but is also important in trying to understand associations of that characteristic with different outcomes. Thirdly, understanding the intergenerational transfer of characteristics is helpful to define deviation from normal. For example, short stature might be considered normal in someone whose parents and grandparents are also short. On the other hand, if we understand the main drivers of the intergeneration associations of stature, then we might consider that this is not 'normal' and that groups where generations have been short might be so because of adverse environmental characteristics that could be modified.

2.2.1 Understanding the intergenerational transfer of characteristics: birth weight as an example

The intergenerational association of birth weight is a useful example for further exploration of different types of intergenerational study aimed at understanding mechanisms that might explain the transfer of a single characteristic from one generation to the next. First, the intergenerational correlation of birth weight down the maternal line has been replicated in a number of independent studies from different populations.[2, 3, 30–35] There are considerably fewer studies examining intergenerational correlations of birth weight down the paternal line, but the association here also appears robust.[36] Secondly, the association is likely to be complex and reflect the intergenerational transfer of a number of characteristics, including genetic, environmental, socioeconomic, and behavioural. Therefore, birth weight is a useful example for exploring different study designs aimed at understanding the mechanisms behind the intergenerational association of a complex trait. Thirdly, birth weight is one of the most commonly used markers for examining the developmental origins of health and disease, and therefore having a better understanding of the determinants of birth weight, including intergenerational influences, is important to much of life course epidemiology.

2.2.1.1 Intergenerational studies with measurements of birth weight and potential explanatory factors across generations

Applying conventional multivariable analyses to intergenerational studies is one way to begin to understand the role of different factors in explaining these associations. For example, Baird showed that a woman's reproductive outcomes, including offspring birth weight, were more closely associated with the social class of her father than to that of her own husband, and suggested that this association might explain some of the association of maternal birth weight with offspring birth weight.[37] Similar results were found in the Aberdeen children of the 1950s cohort study.[38] In the latter, the index population consisted of 3,484 females born between 1950–1956 in Aberdeen, Scotland (referred to by the study authors as G1). Information was available on socioeconomic and behavioural characteristics of the woman (G1) and their parents (G0) and perinatal data were available on their offspring (G2).[38] Only females (grand-mothers (G0), mothers (G1), daughters (G2)) were examined and the authors explored the effect of distal (G0) and proximal (G1) biological and social factors on birth size in G2 females. Consistent with previous studies they found that contemporary socioeconomic differentials in birth size (i.e. lower birth weight in G2 offspring from lower socioeconomic groups at the time of birth, based on the occupational social class of G1) were largely explained by the intergenerational continuity of socioeconomic position and in particular by the effect of grand-maternal (G0) socioeconomic position on maternal (G1) birth size, which affected G2 birth size, irrespective of G1 adult biological or socioeconomic characteristics.[38] Taken together these studies suggest that the intergenerational transfer of socioeconomic position and its effect on maternal lifestyle, such as her diet from conception to adulthood, and hence variation in her physiological traits, such as skeletal growth, across generations are important mechanisms for explaining the intergenerational association of birth weight.

These studies are limited in the extent to which they can assess all possible pathways since some covariables, for example maternal smoking, alcohol, detailed dietary intake during pregnancy, and information on earlier generations, are often unavailable. Furthermore, in correctly interpreting such studies, one needs to be clear about how different characteristics across generations are related to each other. In particular, one needs to be careful when considering whether related intergenerational characteristics are potential confounding or mediating factors in any particular association of interest. This is illustrated in Chapter 10 and also in a previous publication[39] using data from the Aberdeen study described above, which focused on statistical methods in life course epidemiology. To illustrate their point, the authors focused on the associations of a limited number of only biological exposures (birth size in G1; parity and heightin both G0 and G1) with birth size in G2. In a conventional multivariable regression model, which included all potential biological explanatory characteristics, maternal (G1) birth size,adult height and parity each had a positive association with offspring (G2) birth size, whereas grand-maternal (G0) adult height and parity had inverse associations with G2 birth size(i.e. birth weight was on average lower in female infants whose grandmothers had been taller or had had a greater number of pregnancies). In properly interpreting these findings, it is important to consider what the mutually adjusted regression coefficients actually mean. The grandmaternal (G0) and maternal (G1) adult height measures will be closely related to each other and the authors suggested that a clearer interpretation might be obtained from examining their difference. In doing so, the results suggest that '*the taller a G1 woman is relative to her* [G0] *mother, the larger her offspring* [G2 at birth]'.[39] To clarify the relative contributions of grandmaternal and maternal characteristics on offspring birth size the authors conducted a path analysis in which direct effects (i.e. not mediated) and indirect effects (those mediated) could be estimated simultaneously. These analyses revealed a positive indirect effect of grand-maternal G0 height on offspring (G2) birth size that was mediated via maternal G1 height. They demonstrate the care that one needs to take in interpreting multivariable intergenerational associations (see Chapter 10 for more detail).

2.2.1.2 Intergenerational studies that include siblings and cousins

One way in which extended family data can be used to further explore mechanisms underlying the intergenerational associations of birth weight (or other characteristics) is by cousin intergenerational comparisons. The theoretical underpinning of this approach is similar to that of within sibling comparisons, described in Chapter 3. An intergenerational maternal-offspring association of birth weight that is maintained within maternal cousins cannot be explained by fixed maternal grandparent characteristics, including the intergenerational transfer of socioeconomic position and behaviours, such as smoking. This is illustrated in Figure 2.1, which is adapted from Conley et al.[40] For simplicity, in this figure we have only shown female offspring of both the first generation (i.e. sisters 1 and 2) and second generation (cousins 1 and 2), and we have only shown two sisters and two cousins in each generation. However, similar principles could be applied to males and in studies with greater numbers of offspring in eachof the 2nd and 3rd generation. In Figure 2.1 sister 1 has lower birth weight than sister 2, but their parental socioeconomic background and

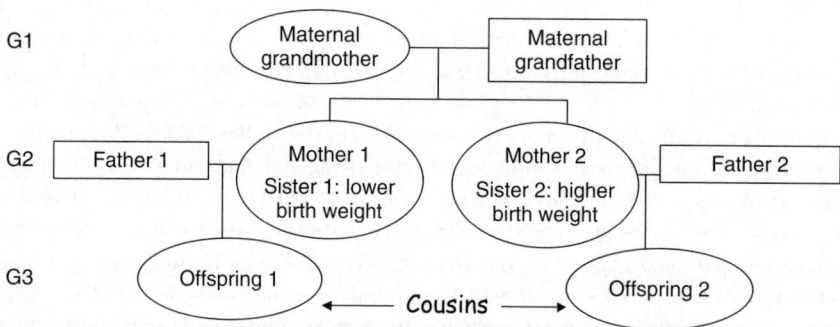

Fig. 2.1 Framework for a within maternal-cousin intergenerational study.

Family intergenerational relations are relative to G3; hence G1 = grand parents. In this framework correlations between the sister's (G2) and cousins (G3) birth weights (or other characteristics) are estimated within family groups (i.e. mother 1-offspring 1 and mother 2-offspring 2). Any positive correlation cannot be explained by the intergenerational transfer of socioeconomic position of behaviours from G1 to G2 since these will not differ for any sisters in G2.

childhood home environment will be the same (under the assumption that they are relatively close in age and both live with their parents in the same home); any association between these two sisters' birth weights and the birth weights of their offspring (cousins 1 and 2), therefore, could not be explained by differences in the mothers (sisters 1 and 2) childhood socioeconomic position or shared environment.

It is conceivable that differences in grand-maternal smoking could explain differences in birth weight between sisters 1 and 2 in Figure 2.1. In particular, if the mother smoked during her pregnancy with sister 1 and was convinced that this child had relatively low birth weight as a result of her smoking, then she might quit smoking before or during the next pregnancy (sister 2). However, this does not matter for in trying to fix the role of the intergenerational transfer of smoking (as a possible explanation for the intergenerational transfer of birth weight), since this depends not only on the association of maternal smoking on offspring birth weight, but also on the relationship between maternal smoking and her daughter's smoking. The effect of parental smoking on the likelihood of offspring smoking is strongest in relation to parental (both mother and father) smoking whilst the offspring is in later childhood/adolescence, rather than in relation to maternal smoking only during pregnancy.[13]

As with other within sibling comparisons (see Chapter 3), the within maternal cousin intergenerational study can be used to control for the effect of any maternal grand-paternal characteristics that are likely to have similar effects on all of their daughters (sisters 1 and 2 in Figure 2.1), even when these grand-parental characteristics are not observed. Thus, these studies are particularly powerful when characteristics of the earlier generation (e.g. maternal grand-parental socioeconomic position and behaviours) have not been measured or there is concern that they have been inaccurately measured. However, they require datasets in which it is possible to link families and that have sufficient numbers of families to obtain precise within maternal-cousin estimates of association.

A final important point that needs to be taken into account when interpreting the within maternal-cousin intergenerational study is that *paternal*-grandparental effects are not fixed. Thus this frame work is specifically fixing factors that might act via intra-uterine mechanisms and is limited in the extent to which it can distinguish a mechanism involving the transfer of genetic variants associated with birth weight from parents to offspring from intrauterine mechanisms (see Section 2.2.1.5 for further discussion of this), unless paternal-cousin comparisons are also made.

In one study that looked at the association of birth weight across various family groups of probands of small for gestational age, average for gestational age, and large for gestational age, there were strong associations of birth weight for maternal-cousins, where the connection was between two aunties (i.e. as shown in Figure 2.1).[41] However, these associations were not present for cousins related on the maternal side through a maternal uncle (the child of the mother compared to the child of the mother's brother), nor were there any within cousin associations on the paternal side. These findings, together with other family associations in this study, led the authors to conclude that '*a maternal regulator controls the growth rate of the mammalian fetus*' and that '*this acts by means of constraint*' of fetal growth.[41] They suggested that this maternal effect could be attributed to the maternal genome, but that epigenetic effects and the mother's own *in utero* environment were also likely to be relevant.

These findings are consistent with those of a second, more recent study, which found strong positive associations of maternal low birth weight with offspring low birth weight in both African-Americans and white Americans within cousins.[40] The authors interpreted these findings as supporting a biological explanation for the intergenerational transmission of birth weight. Such biological explanations would include maternal genetic factors or maternal health (such as her vascular health) that affect the intrauterine environment and that would differ between the pregnancies of sisters. However, unlike the previous study, this study did not have comparative information on paternal cousins.[40]

2.2.1.3 Intergenerational studies that include within twin comparisons

An extension of the within cousin comparison is to compare intergenerational associations within mothers who are twins. The theoretical underpinning of within twin comparisons is described in detail in Chapter 4, and similar principles apply here. Monozygotic twin sisters are genetically identical (with the exception of mitochondrial DNA), whereas dizygotic twins share on average 50% of their genetic variation (the same as non-twin siblings). In addition any set of twins (monozygotic or dizygotic) will have been exposed to the same maternal socioeconomic position, behaviours, health status, and other characteristics during their intrauterine period. Therefore, any positive association of maternal birth weight with offspring birth weight within either monozygotic or dizygotic twin mothers could not be explained by maternal socioeconomic background, behaviours, or their mother's health during their intrauterine gestation. Furthermore, within monozygotic twin mothers a positive association of their birth weight with their offspring birth weight could not be explained by maternal genes, other than mitochondrial DNA.

In three large record linkage studies, two of which examined maternal-offspring associations in maternal monozygotic and dizygotic twins[42, 43] and one of which extended earlier analyses by comparing associations across three generations (i.e. grandmaternal twins—sons and daughters—grand-sons and grand-daughters),[44] it was concluded that fetal genes accounted for a large proportion of the variation (40–69%) in birth weight and that the transmission of genes that influence birth weight explained a substantial part of the intergenerational association of birth weight. Random non-genetic factors, which would include maternal behaviours and health during pregnancy, accounted for 20–30% of the variation, with maternal genotype alone accounting for little (<5%) of the variation.

2.2.1.4 Egg donation / surrogate mother intergenerational studies

A further way of exploring the extent to which the transmission of genes from parents to fetus, rather than intrauterine mechanisms, underlies the intergenerational associations of birth weight would be through egg donation or surrogate mother studies. Such studies would have the same theoretical underpinnings as the use of adoption studies to distinguish genetic from environmental contributions to individual characteristics, but since birth weight is determined during gestation the 'adoption' in these studies is into a non-biological maternal uterus. If offspring birth weight is more strongly related to the birth weight of the mother who carried the pregnancy than it is to the birth weight of the genetic mother (egg donor or biological mother in the case of a surrogate pregnancy), then this suggests that factors that influence the intrauterine environment are more important determinants of intergenerational associations of birth weight than are genetic factors.

In the only study of this nature that we could identify the associations of ovum donor characteristics (age, race, adult height and weight) with birth weight were compared to the association of these characteristics in the ovum recipient with birth weight for 62 live born infants resulting from ovum donation.[45] Data on birth weight for either the maternal ovum donor or maternal ovum recipient were not available and therefore this study did not directly explore factors underlying the intergenerational association of birth weight. The researchers found that (other than infant's gestational age) the only factor that was statistically related to birth weight was the recipient mother's weight at the beginning of pregnancy. They concluded that the intrauterine environment provided by the human mother is a more important determinant of birth weight than her genetic contribution.[45] However, the small sample size, the lack of information on birth weight in donor and recipient mothers, and of paternal information (see below) limit the conclusions that can be drawn from this study.

This design offers a potentially elegant way of separating mechanisms that are transmitted via the intrauterine environment from those that are related to parental to offspring transfer of genetic variants. However, the generalisability of the results may be limited since the uterine environment of the recipient mother may differ importantly from that of women in general. Furthermore, there may be certain fetal genetic factors that increase the likelihood of a donated ovum succeeding to delivery that are also related to birth weight, which make it difficult to extrapolate findings from such studies. Of note in the above study, of 541 ovum donation IVF cycles potentially eligible for study, 101 pregnancies occurred and of these there were 62 live singleton births delivered at or later than 28 weeks.

2.2.1.5 Maternal and paternal intergenerational comparisons

The association of paternal birth weight with offspring birth weight is less likely to act via intrauterine effects, and therefore an association between paternal and offspring birth weight of a similar magnitude to the association between maternal and offspring birth weight is supportive of the transfer of genetic variants associated with birth weight being the most likely underlying mechanism.

It is possible that some parental characteristics might act via intrauterine pathways; in particular passive smoking (the mother inhaling her partner's smoke) could conceivably link fathers' smoking to offspring birth weight via an intrauterine effect. Whilst possible, in reality, passive smoking is unlikely to have a marked effect on intrauterine growth, particularly in comparison to direct (maternal) smoking. This can be seen with data from the Avon Longitudinal Study of Parents and their Children (ALSPAC), a prospective study of over 13,000 families who were recruited in the early 1990s during the mother's index pregnancy (http://www.bristol.ac.uk/alspac). Figure 2.2 demonstrates that in ALSPAC, maternal smoking during pregnancy is associated with lower offspring birth weight (with a magnitude of 162g lower weight in those whose mothers smoked during pregnancy compared to those who did not, that is consistent with other studies), whereas her partner smoking during pregnancy is only weakly associated with offspring birth weight.[46] When both maternal and partner smoking during pregnancy are taken into account in the same multivariable statistical model, the former shows a robust association that is little attenuated, whereas the latter association is essentially abolished. These results suggest that the weak association of paternal smoking with offspring birth weight is explained by the association of paternal smoking with maternal smoking and provides very little evidence of any effect of passive smoking on birth weight.

Fathers' birth weight could be associated with their offspring's birth weight, via an intrauterine mechanism, if there was assortative mating (i.e. that couples self-select each other on the basis of trait/lifestyle similarity) in relation to birth weight (i.e. couples self-selected each other on the basis of having had similar birth weights). The spousal correlation for birth weights is in fact remarkably low (0.02),[47] so that despite the possibility of assortative mating, it is unlikely that any observed association between paternal and offspring birth weight is due to paternal birth weight being a proxy for maternal (their partner's) birth weight. Finally, teratogenesis could provide a link between father's and offspring birth weight. For example, exposure of the father to a toxin whilst he was *in utero* might affect his birth weight and the development of his sperm, which in turn might affect the development and intrauterine growth of his future offspring. As noted in the introduction, in one study DES exposure *in utero* was shown to affect male, as well as female, reproductive function,[20] but there is no evidence that this (or other toxins that we are aware of) result in intergenerational associations of birth weight.

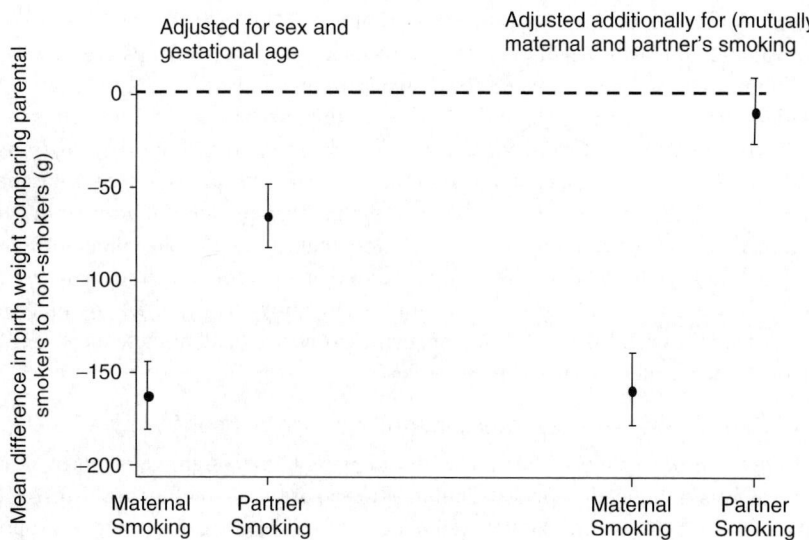

Fig. 2.2 Mean difference in birth weight by mother's and partner's smoking status during pregnancy. The analyses are restricted to singleton births and all results are adjusted for infant sex and gestational age; the results on the right are additionally mutually adjusted for mother's and partner's smoking status during pregnancy. Partner's were described as being biological fathers by the mothers.

Several studies have compared maternal-offspring to paternal-offspring birth weight associations, and found positive associations for both, but with stronger effects for the maternal-offspring association.[2, 4, 36, 47, 48] For example, in a recent large record linkage study that included 101,748 families (mother, father and up to three siblings) from Norway, the maternal-child birth weight correlation was 0.254 (0.249, 0.258), whereas the paternal-child birth weight correlation was 0.161 (0.157, 0.166).[36, 49] Using the logic outlined above, the positive paternal-offspring correlations in these studies have been interpreted as largely reflecting the transfer of genes related to intrauterine growth from either parent to their offspring or the effects of common intergenerational (between spousal) environmental factors. The 'additional' effect in mothers represents intrauterine influences on birth weight resulting from any or several of maternal genes that influence the intrauterine environment or her health, behaviours, and socioeconomic background that influence the intrauterine environment.

In the record linkage study, described above, the authors used extended families that included siblings and maternal half-siblings (same biological mother but different fathers) and concluded that genetic factors transmitted from parents to offspring (i.e. fetal genotype) accounted for 31% of the normal variation in birth weight, with specific maternal factors (non-genetic and genetic) accounting for 22% of this variation.[36] In comparison to the intergenerational twin studies described in Section 2.2.1.3 above, these results suggest a somewhat lower effect of fetal genotype on variation in birth weight. Intergenerational twin studies suggest between 40–69% of the variation in birth weight is related to fetal genotype with maternal genotype accounting for <5% and other non-genetic characteristics (e.g. maternal health and behaviours affecting the intrauterine environment) accounting for 20–30% of the variation.

In contrast to these largely European origin population studies, a small study (468 maternal-offspring pairs and 341 paternal-offspring pairs) from India found no difference in the magnitude of the maternal-offspring birth weight correlation compared to the paternal-offspring birth weight correlation.[50] They did, however, find a stronger association of paternal-offspring birth length than maternal-offspring birth length and a stronger association of maternal adult BMI (at the time of pregnancy) with offspring birth weight than paternal adult BMI. These results cannot be directly compared to those from other studies since there was little overlap between parent-offspring duos with just 57 trios that had complete information on both parents of the same child. However, as noted in Chapter 7, family life course associations are likely to differ in populations from low and middle income countries, to those from high income countries but few studies are available in low and middle income countries to fully exploit this. Thus, this study in India provides an important resource.[51]

2.2.1.6 Intergenerational migrant studies

Mean birth weight is lower and the prevalence of low birth weight is higher in developing compared with developed countries. Infants born in south Asia have particularly low birth weight; the latest UNICEF and WHO report indicated that in the year 2000 south-central Asia had at 27% the highest proportion of low birth weight (< 2500g) neonates of any region of the world (this compares to 6.5% for Northern Europe, 5.9 for Southern Europe and 7.7 for North America).[52] It is generally assumed that this difference between developing and developed countries reflects poor maternal nutrition and health, but it could potentially relate to genetic factors associated with ethnicity and birth size.

Intergenerational migrant studies can help to elucidate the mechanisms that underlie these marked geographic/ethnic differences in birth weight. If poor maternal nutritional and health status during pregnancy is the main driver of these differences, then one would expect infants of 1st generation migrants from south Asia (i.e. those born in the new country but whose parents were born in South Asia) in more prosperous countries to maintain the birth weight difference in comparison to the indigenous population. However, over successive generations this difference would be expected to decrease as maternal health and nutritional status improved in the new country. If differences of the same magnitude persist across many generations, this might imply that genetic differences between ethnic groups explain birth weight differences between these groups. A persistent difference could also be explained by an enduring effect of poor maternal health across many generations (for example, if one's great grand mother was poorly nourished and this resulted in her daughters having low birth weight and a small pelvic size, then their daughters, in turn, might be constrained *in utero* even if she is better nourished than her mother) or by cultural behavioural characteristics that affect birth weight and persist across generations of migrants.

Four UK based studies have compared differences across infants born to 1st and 2nd generation south Asian migrants,[53–56] one of which[53] also had information on infants of 3rd generation migrants. Three of these studies found that UK born south Asian origin babies born to mothers who were themselves born in the UK (2nd generation mothers) had similar birth weights to UK born south Asian origin babies whose mothers had been born in south Asia (1st generation mothers), both of whom had lower birth weights than the indigenous UK population.[53, 55, 56] In the one study with 3rd generation mothers it was also found that the birth weights of south Asian babies born in the UK, whose mothers and grand-mothers had also been born in the UK, were similar to the birth weights of their mother's and grand-mother's cohorts and lower than the indigenous UK population.[53] Thus, these studies suggest factors that endure across at least two generations explain the lower birth weight in south Asian compared to indigenous UK infants. Just one UK study has, to date, found considerable increases in birth weights of infants born to second compared to first generation mothers (second generation weighing on average 249 g more than first generation and with birth weights approaching those of the indigenous UK population).[54] That study included the offspring of just 220 first generation and 111 second generation south Asian women from one city (Bolton) in the North of England and the totality of evidence so far from these four studies tends to suggest that birth weight differences endure across at least two generations. However, further studies with larger sample sizes and with additional generations are important to be confident about the stability or not of ethnic differences in birth weight across generations. Furthermore, studies that include information on fathers, grandfathers, and great-grandfathers, as well as mothers and grandmothers etc. are necessary for examining the influence of ethnicity down paternal lines on offspring birth weight.

2.3 Intergenerational associations of exposures in parents with health related outcomes in their offspring

A large number of studies have related risk factors in parents, particularly mothers, to outcomes in offspring. Many of these have direct relevance to the developmental origins of adult disease hypothesis. Whilst insights might also be gained from exploring the effects of exposures in grand-parents (or even earlier generations), as well as those in parents on offspring outcomes, few studies have the ability to do this and for many hypotheses the interest is in a parental effect.

2.3.1 The developmental origins of adult disease

The developmental origins of adult disease hypothesis suggests that exposure to risk factors during early life developmental periods can have important consequences for adult disease and health. Over the last two to three decades there has been increasing epidemiological interest in this hypothesis. The developmental exposures that have been explored include those acting during (or before) the period of fetal development—such as maternal nutrition, smoking or alcohol use; those acting in infancy—such as breast or bottle feeding; and those acting in childhood—such as passive exposure to parental tobacco smoke. Nearly all domains of later health experience—including cardiovascular disease, various cancers, respiratory disease, cognitive function—have been associated with early-life exposures of one kind or another. In terms of public health policy it is important to separate out causal associations, which offer the possibility of intervention and disease prevention, from non-causal association.

Since many of the exposures implicated in the developmental origins of disease are maternal in origin with the outcomes experienced in her offspring, intergenerational studies are central to exploring the nature of these associations. In this section we describe types of intergenerational study that might enhance understanding of the developmental origins of adult disease.

2.3.1.1 Comparing maternal-offspring associations to paternal-offspring associations

An important aspect of the developmental origins hypothesis is the possibility that maternal exposures during pregnancy have a direct biological effect on offspring outcomes. Thus, maternal smoking during pregnancy may influence offspring obesity in later life,[14–16, 57] or maternal alcohol consumption during pregnancy may lead to impairments in various domains of offspring functioning.[58, 59] However, there are many confounding factors that could generate non-causal (or non intrauterine) links between the smoking and drinking behaviours of mothers during pregnancy and the later health of their offspring. One approach to this issue is to compare the strength of associations between an exposure among mothers and offspring outcomes and the same exposure among fathers and the offspring outcomes. If there were a direct biological effect of intrauterine exposure on offspring health status, then the link with offspring health should be stronger for exposure among mothers than for exposure among fathers. This can be illustrated with respect to birth weight where there is strong evidence of a causal influence of maternal smoking during pregnancy. As discussed in Section 2.2.1.5 and demonstrated in Figure 2.2

maternal smoking during pregnancy is strongly related to offspring birth weight, whereas paternal smoking is not.[46] Since the direct intrauterine link between maternal smoking during pregnancy and reduced offspring birth weight is not controversial, this example provides a proof of principle of this method of maternal-paternal comparison for exploring the possible causal intrauterine effect of maternal behaviours and characteristics on other offspring outcomes.

If we apply this approach to other associations it becomes apparent that some, though not all, previously assumed intrauterine developmental effects might be explained by confounding. Several epidemiological studies have found an association between maternal smoking during pregnancy and greater body mass index in offspring at various ages.[14–16, 57] It has been suggested that exposing the developing fetus to nicotine might adversely affect development of hypothalamic function and through this mechanism impact appetite control over the life course and hence increase the risk of future obesity.[60, 61] In ALSPAC, data show that the average BMI at age 7 of children whose mothers smoked during pregnancy is raised compared to those whose mothers did not smoke, with the magnitude of this effect being similar to findings of previous epidemiological studies.[18] However, a similar sized association is seen with partner smoking (assessed at the same time as the mother's smoking during pregnancy), and including both maternal and partner smoking behaviour in the same multivariable model leaves residual effects of similar magnitude.[18] Furthermore, when a more direct measure of adiposity—DXA scan determined fat mass—was used as the outcome, findings were similar.[18] These results suggest, that in the case of offspring adiposity, maternal smoking during pregnancy does not have a direct intrauterine effect. Rather, confounding factors, such as socioeconomic position and other parental behaviours (diet and physical activity) that are associated with both parental smoking and offspring adiposity generate a similar magnitude of association between both maternal smoking and greater offspring adiposity as that between paternal smoking and greater offspring adiposity. Similar findings are seen with respect to parental smoking and offspring blood pressure.[62] By contrast, for offspring leg length at age 7, maternal smoking shows stronger effects than paternal smoking,[63] suggesting a biological effect of maternal smoking on femur development, as supported by other studies of this issue.[64]

There is particular controversy regarding the potential influence of maternal smoking on cognitive development of offspring.[65–67] Are the associations found in most studies of this issue causal—as some suggest[65]—or do they reflect the considerable confounding that will exist in many databases, given the associations between maternal smoking and a wide variety of parental socioeconomic, cognitive, and behavioural factors?[66, 67] For several studies that have assessed this association, complete data on all potential confounding factors (in particular maternal characteristics such as her educational attainment and cognitive ability) were not available. The comparison of the association of maternal smoking during pregnancy with offspring cognitive ability to that of paternal smoking with this same outcome, provides a useful means of determining the potential effect of unmeasured confounders in this instance. This is illustrated in Figure 2.3, in which we again use data from ALSPAC. In the unadjusted analyses there is a similar inverse association of maternal and partner smoking at the time of pregnancy with offspring IQ assessed at mean age 8 years. These findings suggest that any association is unlikely to be explained by specific intrauterine effects and are likely to be explained by factors, such as family socioeconomic background and parental education and cognition, which would have a similar effect in relating either maternal or paternal smoking to offspring IQ. It is possible to make this conclusion with no available data on potential confounding factors. As it happens, in ALSPAC we do have extensive information on characteristics that might confound this association. The right hand results in Figure 2.3 demonstrate that adjustment for these characteristics attenuates to the null both associations of maternal smoking and paternal smoking with offspring IQ, supporting our earlier

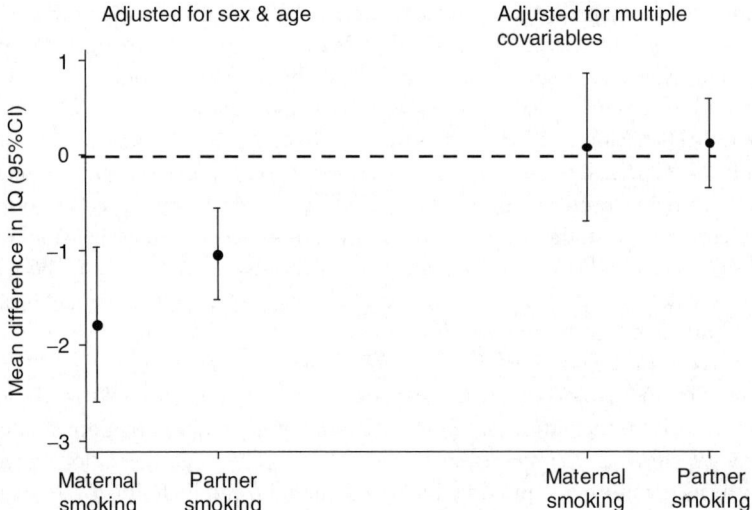

Fig. 2.3 Mean difference in childhood IQ at age 8 by mother's and partner's smoking status during pregnancy.

All results are adjusted for child's sex and exact age at time of IQ test; the results on the right are additionally mutually adjusted for mother's and partner's smoking status during pregnancy, social class, parity, ethnicity, house ownership, crowding, maternal and partner education, maternal and paternal alcohol consumption during pregnancy. The Weschler Intelligence Scale for Children (WISC-III^{UK}) was used to assess intelligence. Partner's were described as being biological fathers by the mothers.

conclusion (based on parental comparisions of the association) that the maternal association was unlikely to be explained by specific intrauterine mechanisms and demonstrating the potential use of this approach in studies with limited data on potential confounding factors.

In our view the strong implication of seeing that maternal and paternal characteristics during pregnancy are associated in similar ways with offspring outcomes suggests that these associations are largely explained by shared familial lifestyles rather than a direct intrauterine causal effect. The appropriate public health response in our view would therefore be to develop interventions that promote healthier lifestyles in all family members, rather than, for example suggest that women should behave in certain ways specifically whilst they are pregnant. However, Pembrey et al.[68] suggest that the association between paternal smoking and offspring BMI reflects epigenetic influences. While it is possible that male-line epigenetic factors exactly mimic a biological influence of maternal smoking on the intrauterine environment to generate near identical associations, we feel this is unlikely. Informal or formal approaches to comparing explanatory models, which adopt the parsimony principle of Occam's Razor,[69] would suggest that the likelihood of such perfectly mimicked effects, when they are produced by mechanistically completely distinct effects, is very low.

2.3.1.2 Dealing with possible non-paternity in parental-offspring comparisons

Whilst we have confidence in assuming that similar maternal-offspring to paternal-offspring associations reflect a similar mechanism (that of confounding by shared familial socioeconomic position and lifestyles), it does not follow that a stronger maternal-offspring association necessarily implies intrauterine effects. It is possible that weaker associations of father's exposures with offspring outcomes, compared to equivalent associations with mother's exposures, occur as a result of unknown non-paternity, with non-biological fathers, perhaps being more temporary in the child's life and providing a weak proxy for shared familial socioeconomic position and lifestyles. Ideally researchers should ask whether a 'father' is the known biological father and restrict analyses only to those parent-offspring trios where the father is believed to be the biological father. In addition, sensitivity analyses that assume different potential levels of non-paternity can be performed to determine the robustness of any results to adjustment for plausible levels of non-paternity (see also Chapter 10).[70–72]

2.3.1.3 The use of Mendelian randomization studies to make causal inferences about the role of maternal exposures in the developmental origins of offspring health

Mendelian randomization is the term that has been given to studies that use genetic variants in observational epidemiology to make causal inferences about modifiable (non-genetic) risk factors for disease and health related outcomes.[73–75] Such studies exploit what is known as Mendel's second law or the law of independent assortment:

> 'that the behavior of each pair of differentiating characters in hybrid union is independent of the other differences between the two original plants, and, further, that the hybrid produces just so many kinds of egg and pollen cells as there are possible constant combination forms.'[76]

In simple terms this means that the inheritance of one trait is independent of (i.e. randomized with respect to) the inheritance of other traits. The independent distribution of alleles (or blocks of alleles in linkage disequilibrium) from parents to their offspring means that a study relating health outcomes in the offspring to genetic variation transmitted from the parents will not suffer from confounding. This holds true for full-siblings who are not monozygotic twins. Despite the actual random allocation of groups of alleles being at the level of parent to offspring dyads, at a population level—when relating genetic variants to disease outcome—alleles are generally unrelated to those confounding factors (in particular socioeconomic position and lifestyle factors) that distort the interpretations of findings from observational epidemiology.[77, 78] Furthermore, disease processes do not alter germline genotype and therefore associations between genotype and disease outcomes cannot be affected by reverse causality. Finally, for genetic variants that are related to a modifiable exposure this will generally be the case throughout life from birth to adulthood and therefore their use in causal inference can also avoid attenuation by errors (regression dilution bias), and provides an estimate of the effect of a modifiable exposure across the life course on disease outcome.[79] Mendelian randomization studies have being likened to a 'natural' RCT.[80, 81]

Mendelian randomization studies can provide unique insights into the causal nature of maternal exposures on later disease outcomes in her offspring, by using maternal genotype (adjusted for offspring genotype) as an instrument for determining the unconfounded and unbiased effect of a maternal exposure that is influenced by her genotype. The causal effect of maternal folate (via intrauterine mechanisms) on neural tube defects (NTDs) provides a valuable example of this approach. It is now widely accepted that NTDs can in part be prevented by periconceptual maternal folate supplementation. RCTs of folate supplementation have provided the key evidence in this regard.[82, 83] But it is possible that this evidence could have been obtained from observational genetic epidemiology, without the need to conduct these trials. The MTHFR

677C→T polymorphism is a genetic variant that is associated with methyltetrahydrofolate reductase activity and as a consequence circulating folate and homocysteine levels; TT genotype being associated with lower circulating folate levels. A number of separate studies have looked at the association between this MTHFR variant in parents, and in the offspring themselves, in relation to the risk of NTD in the offspring. Reviews of these studies suggest that mothers who have the TT genotype have an increased risk of 2.04 (95% CI 1.49–2.81) of having an offspring with a NTD compared to mothers who have the CC genotype.[84, 85] By contrast there is little association of fathers genotype with offspring risk of NTD (relative risk comparing fathers with TT to all other fathers is 1.18 (95% CI 0.65–2.12).[84] For offspring the relative risk of having a NTD comparing those with TT genotype to CC genotype is 1.75 (95% CI 1.41–2.18).[85] Whilst it would be useful to see combined analyses of maternal-paternal-offspring genotype associations within the same family, the pattern of associations seen across different populations and presented above suggests that it is the intra-uterine environment—influenced by maternal TT genotype—rather than the genotype of offspring that is related to disease risk. The association with offspring's own genotype being explained by the fact that one of the T alleles amongst offspring who are homozygote for this allele (and shown to be at increased risk of NTD) will have come from the mother and one from the father (i.e. for offspring with genotype TT both the mother and father must be TT or TC). Mothers who are TT will, by definition, have exposed their offspring to lower levels of folate *in utero*, whereas father's genotype will not influence exposure *in utero* to folate. Consequently, if in utero exposure to lower folate levels is causally related to NTD, one would expect the association of offspring genotype to NTD to be intermediate in magnitude to that seen for maternal and paternal genotype, which is what the results presented above suggest. This is consistent with the hypothesis that maternal folate intake is the exposure of importance.

In this case the findings from observational studies, genetic associations studies, and RCTs are similar. Had the technology been available, the genetic association studies, with the particular influence of maternal versus paternal genotype on NTD risk, would have provided strong evidence of the beneficial effect of folate supplementation before the results of any RCT had been completed; though trials may still have been necessary to confirm the effect was causal for folate supplementation.

There are an increasing number of examples in which Mendelian randomization can be utilized to understand the causal nature of intrauterine exposures, an important (but diminishing) limitation being the identification of genetic variants that are robustly associated with environmentally-modifiable risk processes. Another challenge is the large samples required to have adequate power to detect the small (but importantly unconfounded) associations. The use of genotype, in Mendelian randomisation studies, to provide causal inference for the effect of a modifiable (non-genetic) exposure on disease outcome is an application of the general theory of *instrumental variables analysis*.[75] An *instrumental variable* (IV) is a variable that is associated with the outcome only through its robust association with the exposure of interest. As such an instrumental variable will not be associated with factors that confound the association of exposure with outcome. The main reason why the Mendelian randomization instrumental variables approach requires very large sample sizes is that one is relating only the proportion of the risk factor of interest (in the above example maternal folate action) that is influenced by the instrument (MTHFR genotype in the above example) to the outcome of interest (NTD).[75] In most Mendelian randomization studies the genotype will only explain a small proportion of the modifiable risk factor of interest (commonly less than 2%), thus the required sample sizes to obtain precise estimates will often prove to be sobering.[86, 87]

2.3.1.4 Combining parental-offspring comparisons and Mendelian randomization approaches

So far we have discussed a number of different approaches to understanding the intergenerational transfer of a single characteristic using birth weight as a specific example (Section 2.2) and different approaches to understanding the association of maternal exposures on offspring outcomes as part of the developmental origins hypothesis. In both of these situations there are clear advantages to be gained from combining two or more of these different methods within the same dataset. If several methods provide the same conclusion (whether supporting or refuting the original hypothesis) one has more faith in the validity of this conclusion. This is because each approach will have different potential sources of bias and it would be unlikely to arrive at exactly the same result through different mechanisms of bias.[69] If different approaches produce different conclusions then one needs to consider the specific biases of each method to try and understand why the results differ. Whilst this might feel like adding more confusion than clarity we believe that ultimately using several different methods to test the same hypothesis (even when different answers are obtained) will provide more valid answers to important public health questions.

In a recent example we combined a comparison of parental-offspring associations with the Mendelian randomization approach to explore the developmental overnutrition hypothesis.[88] The developmental overnutrition hypothesis suggests that greater maternal obesity during pregnancy results in increased offspring adiposity in later life.[89] If true, this would result in the obesity epidemic progressing across generations irrespective of environmental or genetic changes.[90] It is therefore important to robustly test this hypothesis. We compared the associations of maternal and partner pre-pregnancy BMI with offspring DXA determined fat mass measured at 9 and 11 years (4,091 parent-offspring trios) and used maternal *FTO* genotype, controlling for offspring *FTO*, as an instrument for maternal adiposity.[88] *FTO* is a genetic variant that has been shown to be robustly associated with greater BMI and fat mass;[91] though the mechanisms for this association are currently not understood. Figure 2.4 shows the directed acyclic graph (DAG) depicting these two approaches to assessing this hypothesis.

Both maternal and partner BMI were positively associated with offspring fat mass, but the size of the maternal association was larger than that of the partner association in all models: mean difference in offspring sex and age standardized fat mass z-score per 1 SD BMI 0.24 (95% CI: 0.22, 0.26) for maternal BMI vs 0.13 (95% CI: 0.11, 0.15) for partner BMI, p-value for difference in effect < 0.001.[88] The stronger maternal association was robust to sensitivity analyses assuming levels of non-paternity up to 20%. A plausible explanation for the stronger maternal association is provided by the developmental overnutrition hypothesis, which suggests that mothers with greater BMI in pregnancy will tend to expose the developing fetus to higher concentrations of glucose, free fatty acids, and amino acids and that this greater exposure will result in permanent changes in appetite control, neuroendocrine functioning or energy metabolism in the developing fetus and thus lead to greater adiposity and risk of obesity in later life. However, when maternal *FTO*, controlling for offspring *FTO*, was used as an instrument for the effect of maternal adiposity the mean difference in offspring fat mass z-score per 1SD maternal BMI was −0.08 (95% CI: −0.56, 0.41).[88] The point estimate for this instrumental variables analyses suggest that greater maternal adiposity during pregnancy does not result in greater adiposity in later life in her offspring. However, the confidence interval is wide (see above) and statistically this finding is not different from that found for the parental comparison analyses.

In the journal publication of these findings,[88] we concluded that these two sets of results do not suggest a strong specific maternal adiposity-offspring adiposity association. The maternal-paternal difference was small. Assuming no non-paternity in this sample, and that the parental

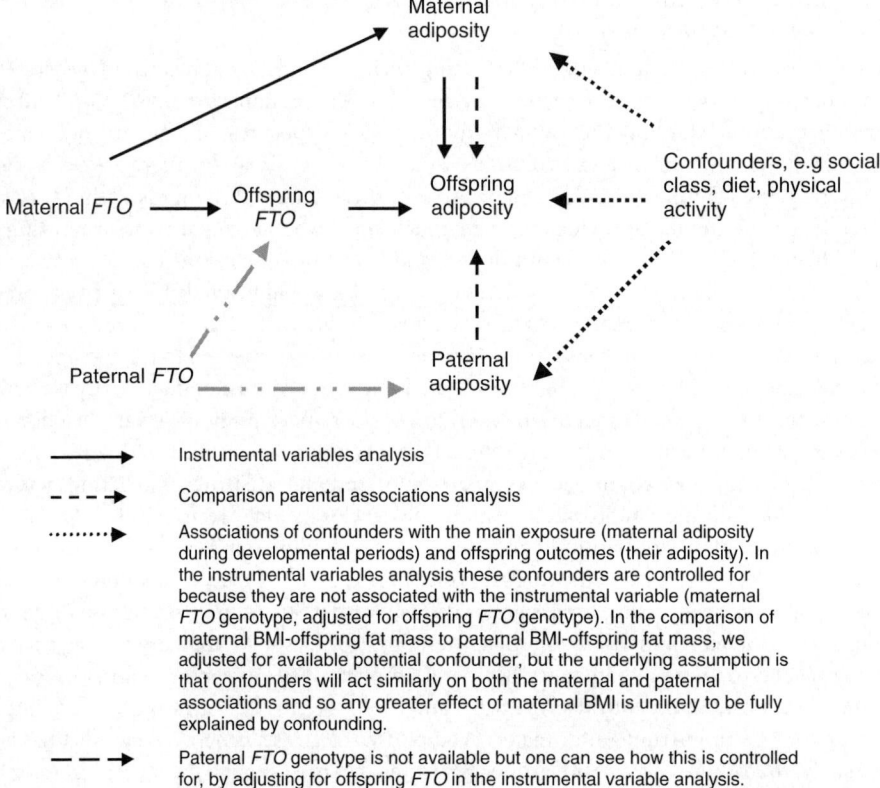

Fig. 2.4 Directed acyclic graph demonstrating the associations used to assess the developmental overnutrition hypothesis in this study.

differences are completely explained by development overnutrition, the findings would suggest that the offspring of mothers who have a pregnancy BMI greater by 1 SD than other mothers will have on average 0.11 SD greater fat mass at age 9 to 11 as a result of developmental overnutrition. Effects of this magnitude across many generations could result in a slow and steady increase in population levels of obesity, something that might have been occurring from the early part of the 20th century. However, the recent obesity epidemic has taken the shape of a major increase in mean BMI and obesity prevalence over a period of 10–15 years. This time period would be the equivalent of one generation and therefore we concluded that the weak specific maternal effect that we found, even if due to developmental overnutrition, is unlikely to have made a major impact on the obesity epidemic.[88]

2.4 The association of exposures in offspring with outcomes in parents

In this section we look at intergenerational studies in which the exposure of interest is assessed in a more recent generation (e.g. offspring), with the outcome examined in a more distal generation (parents or grandparents).

2.4.1 Use of offspring as proxies for parental exposures

A common use of intergenerational studies in life course epidemiology has been to relate early life exposures (most notably birth weight) in offspring to chronic disease outcomes (e.g. cardiovascular disease) in parents in order understand the mechanisms underlying these associations within individuals. If the birth weight-cardiovascular disease association seen within individuals is due to a genetic mechanism from both maternal and paternal genes, then one would predict that offspring birth weight would be inversely associated with cardiovascular disease in both mothers and fathers. Offspring birth weight has been found to be inversely associated with increased risk of parental cardiovascular disease, with a recent meta-analysis of all published studies finding that amongst mothers the pooled confounder adjusted hazard ratio of cardiovascular disease mortality for a one standard deviation increase in offspring birth weight was 0.75 (95% CI: 0.67, 0.84) and among fathers the equivalent association was 0.93 (95% CI: 0.91, 0.95), with statistical evidence of a difference between these two effects p < 0.001 (Figure 2.5).[28, 92–97]

The stronger association with maternal (compared with paternal) cardiovascular disease is generally seen both within each individual study that includes both parents and when the pooled results of all studies are compared. Possible explanations for the stronger association of offspring birth weight with maternal cardiovascular disease than with paternal cardiovascular disease include[98]:

1. 'Fetal programming', whereby fetal undernutrition in the mother programmes her increased cardiovascular disease and also leads to lower birth weight offspring due to a smaller pelvic size.
2. Direct effects of maternal health-related behaviours, such as smoking, heavy alcohol consumption, and poor diet, both on offspring birth weight and on maternal cardiovascular disease risk.

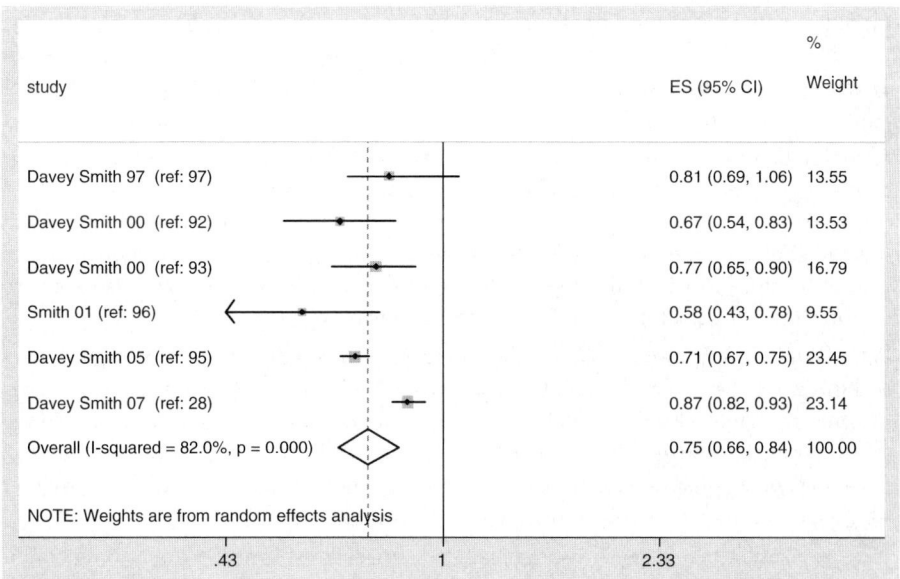

Fig. 2.5a Association of offspring birth weight with mother's cardiovascular disease risk.

ES: Effect Size; CI: Confidence Interval; I-squared is a measure of between study heterogeneity; it is the % of variation in the pooled estimate explained by between study differences. Here there is strong evidence of heterogeneity.

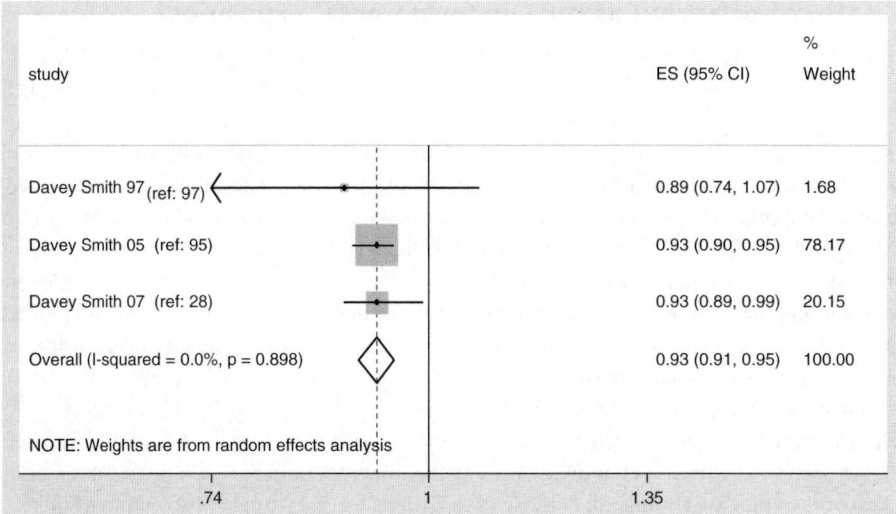

Fig. 2.5b Association of offspring birth weight with father's cardiovascular disease risk.

ES: Effect Size; CI: Confidence Interval; I-squared is a measure of between study heterogeneity; it is the % of variation in the pooled estimate explained by between study differences. Here there is strong evidence of heterogeneity.

3. Maternal imprinting (i.e. the phenotype resulting from a particular gene locus is differentially modified by the sex of the parent contributing that particular allele). In this example a gene with pleiotropic effects resulting in lower birth weight and increased insulin resistance/cardiovascular disease risk would be more likely to be expressed in females compared to males.

4. Other epigenetic effects (i.e. a change in the outcome of a gene that is controlled by non-genetic factors so that the phenotype resulting from a particular gene is modified by environmental exposures). In this example, cardiovascular disease in the mother may result in a different intrauterine environment (than that in women free of cardiovascular disease), for example there might be reduced nutrient transfer to the developing fetus. This in turn may influence gene expression of variants that regulate fetal growth and this result in an association between mothers' cardiovascular disease risk and offspring birth weight.

5. Paternal misclassification, as some fathers in these studies will not be the biological parents and this would be expected to dilute the paternal association, assuming this is largely driven by genetic variants related to both birth size and insulin resistance and hence CVD. However, sensitivity analyses suggest implausible levels of non-paternity—30%—would be required to make the pooled offspring birth weight-maternal cardiovascular disease and offspring birth weight-paternal cardiovascular disease associations consistent.[28]

6. It is also plausible that the weak association in fathers is fully explained by residual confounding, and the non-specificity of the association in fathers suggests that this is possible.[28]

7. Finally, it is possible that some of the offspring birth weight-maternal cardiovascular disease association reflects lower offspring birth weight due to pregnancy related health-compromising factors in some mothers (i.e. reverse causality). In this case the expectation would be that the elevated cardiovascular mortality risk would be greater for periods closer in time to the index

pregnancy and, as with other cases of health-related selection, this effect would reduce over time. For coronary heart disease mortality this was found in analyses of one of the largest studies to date and this time-related effect explains some of the heterogeneity between studies relating offspring birth weight to maternal cardiovascular disease risk (Figure 2.5a).[28]

Of course it is possible that all of the above might contribute to the stronger association seen for mothers compared to fathers. Additional analyses suggested that non-paternity was unlikely, residual confounding in fathers likely, and some reverse causality in mothers possible.[28] Overall, we would conclude that these findings support a specific maternal (intrauterine) effect in the general population for the association between birth size and later cardiovascular disease risk, that is unlikely to be explained primarily by genetic variants with pleiotropic effects. In terms of public health interventions understanding just what the mechanisms are behind this association is important.

2.4.2 Assessing exposures in offspring that directly influence parental health

Whilst in the above example the exposure in the offspring is not believed to directly affect parental health, but is being used as a proxy measure to try and understand the mechanisms of associations that are not necessarily intergenerational (in the above example the association of birth weight with cardiovascular disease in individuals), other intergenerational studies are testing hypotheses that exposures in offspring have a direct effect on their parents health or health related characteristics.

On the whole such studies examine the effect of offspring behaviours, disability, and disease on parental health and socioeconomic outcomes.[27, 99–101] In these examples, as in other types of intergenerational study, careful interpretation is required. These intergenerational associations may be explained by the offspring exposure indeed causing the parental outcomes. However, they could also be explained by parental 'outcome' (for example parental health/disease) causing the offspring 'exposure' (for example offspring disease or behaviour), confounding, or in studies where parents report both on their child's illness/disability and their outcomes, the association could be explained by reporting bias.[101] For example, both maternal and paternal depression are related to offspring behaviour problems and vice versa.[102–105] Understanding the true nature of these studies requires large prospective studies with repeat measurements in both generations and accurate measurement of potential confounding or explanatory factors. Even then investigators should be careful to consider several plausible explanations for any associations noted and the extent to which their data can provide robust evidence for one being more likely than any alternative.

2.5 To what extent can different intergenerational studies distinguish specific mechanisms of association

Broadly speaking, intergenerational studies in life course epidemiology aim to describe associations across generations or to elucidate the mechanisms underlying these associations. In terms of the latter the aim is often to quantify the extent to which different mechanisms explain associations across generations; most commonly to quantify the extent to which genetic or non-genetic (the latter often termed 'environmental') mechanisms underlie the association. As noted above, having consistent results from more than one method (including more than one family-based approach) increases the confidence that one has in the consistent conclusion. Going back to our opening example of birth weight and the mechanisms that might explain its intergenerational association, in his classic paper published in 1955, Newton E Morton concluded that 'the resemblance in birth weight of sibs is largely attributable to the maternal constitution or environment, not to genetic similarity of twins.'[106] This conclusion was based on several different intergenerational and other within family correlations of birth weight, as can be seen in Table 2.1. However, as noted in a recent paper by Gjessing and Lie, different studies over the last five to six decades have estimated the heritability for birth weight (the proportion of total variability that can be explained by (own/fetal) genetic factors) to be between 0–70%.[49] In this chapter you will note that in Section 2.2.1.3 we described a number of large intergenerational twin studies suggesting that heritability was 40–69% for birth weight, in Section 2.2.1.5 we described a large extended family (including sibs and half-sibs) that concluded heritability for birth weight was 31%, and going back to Morton's paper the suggestion is that it is considerably lower than this. Gjessing and Lie note a number of methodological issues that are important, and often neglected, in such studies and that contribute to differences in estimates between studies and that need to be borne in mind when interpreting results from all such studies. They note that the sample size of such studies needs to be much larger than is frequently appreciated or used. Furthermore, whilst on the whole genetic correlations in the statistical models used in these studies can be well specified, for example when random mating is assumed there should be zero genetic correlation between spousal birth weights and 0.5 between mother and offspring and 0.5 between father and offspring, there are no unique rules for predicting environmental correlations, and many 'environmental' exposures can mimic genetic transmission. This is important because the 'genetic' contribution (heritability) is expressed as a proportion of overall variability (i.e. that determined by genetic and non-genetic (environmental exposures)). It is also important to remember that since genetic and non-genetic contributions are determined in these studies as a proportion of overall variability, one would actually expect these to vary between different populations. For example, in a population where no-one smoked the genetic contribution to lung cancer would be greater than in a population where 50% smoked. In the latter population, non-genetic factors (smoking) would make an important contribution to the total variation in lung cancer, whereas in the former smoking (the biggest environmental factor for lung cancer) could not make any contribution. Furthemore, as we understand more about epigenetic effects, imprinting and the role of mitochondrial DNA in human phenotypes and diseases, the notion of being able to simply separate genetic from non-genetic mechanisms in family-based studies is challenged. This highlights the need to use a number of different methods to explore the mechanisms underlying specific associations and consider which of several plausible mechanisms the results from different methods support. We then need to formally test the mechanism with additional support in further studies, again with different methodological approaches.

2.6 Conclusions

Intergenerational studies are central to life course epidemiology, which is itself concerned with transfer of risk and health related outcomes from one generation to the next. As with all observational epidemiology intergenerational associations might not be causal and care is required in correctly analysing and interpreting such studies. We have described how intergenerational studies that include cousins, siblings, and twins; egg donation/surrogate mother intergenerational studies; maternal-paternal comparisons; intergenerational migrant studies; and Mendelian randomization in intergenerational studies might help in understanding the mechanisms underlying intergenerational observations. Triangulation of findings in several different approaches will provide greatest confidence in a particular conclusion, but this must be combined with a full biological understanding of several plausible mechanisms that are not simply reduced to 'genetic' versus 'non-genetic' mechanisms.

Table 2.1 Different within family correlations of birth weight taken from Morton NE[106], together with the author's interpretation of these correlations

Half siblings		Twins*		Siblings with different degrees of separation		Random versus related parents	
Relationship	ICC	Relationship	ICC	Relationship	ICC	Relationship	ICC
Maternal half-sibs	0.581	Like-sexed twins	0.557	Adjacent siblings	0.523	Random parents	0.523
Paternal half-sibs	0.102	Unlike-sexed twins	0.655	One sibling intervening	0.425	First cousin parents	0.481
				Two siblings intervening	0.363		
Author's interpretation: The high level of correlation between maternal half-sibs, with little correlation between paternal half-sibs, supports maternal environmental factors explaining the inheritance of birth weight rather than (fetal) genetic factors		**Author's interpretation:** The similarity of correlation between like-sexed and unlike-sexed twins supports a mechanism shared by all twins and not one only shared by genetically identical twins. This supports maternal intrauterine characteristics as key to the inheritance of birth weight rather than genetic factors		**Author's interpretation:** The declining correlation with greater separation of siblings is consistent with a maternal intrauterine mechanism, since maternal age and parity will de facto increase with greater intervals and are related to important differences in intrauterine environment. Maternal behaviours are also likely to differ with greater separation between pregnancies		**Authors' interpretation:** The similarity in correlation in siblings compared with those whose parents are first cousins argues against an important genetic mechanism since correlations would be expected to be higher for siblings of first cousin parents	

ICC: Intraclass correlation coefficient.

* The author assumed that like-sexed twins were largely monozygotic and unlike-sexed were all dizygotic. The latter is clearly true and some justification for the assumption that all like-sexed twins were monozygotic was provided. Furthermore the author noted that the conclusion would be similar even with a margin of error, since the high correlation in unlike-sexed twins alone provides support for an intrauterine mechanism.

References

1. **Kuh D, Ben-Shlomo Y, Lynch J, Hallqvist J, Power C.** Life course epidemiology. *J Epidemiol Community Health* 2003; **57**: 778–83.
2. **Emanuel I, Filakti H, Alberman E, Evans SJ.** Intergenerational studies of human birthweight from the 1958 birth cohort. 1. Evidence for a multigenerational effect. *Br J Obstet Gynaeco* 1992; **99**: 67–74.
3. **Sanderson M, Emanuel I, Holt VL.** The intergenerational relationship between mother's birthweight, infant birthweight and infant mortality in black and white mothers. *Paediatr Perinat Epidemiol* 1995; **9**: 391–405.
4. **Kivimäki M, Lawlor DA, Davey Smith G, Elovainio M, Jokela M, Keltikangas-Järvinen L et al.** Substantial inter-generational increases in body mass index are not explained by the fetal overnutrition hypothesis, The Cardiovascular Risk in Young Finns. *American Journal of Clinical Nutrition* 2007: **86**: 1509–14.
5. **Lake JK, Power C, Cole TJ.** Child to adult body mass index in the 1958 British birth cohort, associations with parental obesity. *Arch Dis Child, 1997;* **77**: 376–81.
6. **Kuh D, Wadsworth M.** Parental height, childhood environment and subsequent adult height in a national birth cohort. *Int J Epidemiol* 1989; **18**: 663–8.
7. **Galton F.** Family likeness in stature. *Proceedings of the Royal Society* 1886; **40**: 42–73.
8. **Black SE, Devereux PJ, Salvanes KG.** Why the apple doesn't fall far, understanding intergenerational transmission of human capital. *California, California Center for Population Research, University of California. On-Line Working Paper Series* 2004; CCPR-019-04.
9. **Corcoran M.** Rags to rags, poverty and mobility in the United States. *Annual Review of Sociology* 1995; **21**: 237–67.
10. **Kuh D, Head J, Hardy R, Wadsworth M.** The influence of education and family background on women's earnings in midlife, evidence from a British national birth cohort study. *British Journal of Sociology and Education* 1997; **18**: 385–405.
11. **Rossow I, Rise J.** Concordance of parental and adolescent health behaviors. *Soc Sci Med* 1994; **38**: 1299–1305.
12. **Cleland V, Venn A, Fryer J, Dwyer T, Blizzard L.** Parental exercise is associated with Australian children's extracurricular sports participation and cardiorespiratory fitness, A cross-sectional study. *Int J Behav Nutr Phys Act* 2005; **2**: 3.
13. **Farkas AJ, Distefan JM, Choi WS, Gilpin EA, Pierce JP.** Does parental smoking cessation discourage adolescent smoking? *Prev Med* 1999; **28**: 213–18.
14. **Power C, Jefferis BJ.** Fetal environment and subsequent obesity, a study of maternal smoking. *Int J Epidemiol* 2002; **31**: 413–19.
15. **Toschke AM, Montgomery SM, Pfeiffer U, von KR.** Early intrauterine exposure to tobacco-inhaled products and obesity. *Am J Epidemiol* 2003; **158**: 1068–74.
16. **von KR, Toschke AM, Koletzko B, Slikker W, Jr.** Maternal smoking during pregnancy and childhood obesity. *Am J Epidemiol* 2002; **156**: 954–61.
17. **Mamun AA, Lawlor DA, Alati R, O'Callaghan MJ, Williams GM, Najman JM.** Does maternal smoking during pregnancy have a direct effect on future offspring obesity? Evidence from a prospective birth cohort study. *Am J Epidemiol* 2006; **164**: 317–25.
18. **Leary SD, Davey Smith G, Rogers IS, Reilly JJ, Wells JC, Ness AR.** Smoking during Pregnancy and Offspring Fat and Lean Mass in Childhood. *Obesity* 2006; **14**: 2284–93.
19. **Herbst AL, Ulfelder H, Poskanzer DC.** Adenocarcinoma of the vagina. Association of maternal stilbestrol therapy with tumor appearance in young women. *N Engl J Med* 1971; **284**: 878–81.
20. **Bibbo M, Gill WB, Azizi F, Blough R, Fang VS, Rosenfield RL et al.** Follow-up study of male and female offspring of DES-exposed mothers. *Obstet Gynecol* 1977; **49**: 1–8.
21. **Kaufman RH, Adam E, Binder GL, Gerthoffer E.** Upper genital tract changes and pregnancy outcome in offspring exposed in utero to diethylstilbestrol. *Am J Obstet Gynecol* 1980; **137**: 299–308.

22 Senekjian EK, Potkul RK, Frey K, Herbst AL. Infertility among daughters either exposed or not exposed to diethylstilbestrol. *Am J Obstet Gynecol* 1988; **158**: 493–8.

23 Goldberg JM, Falcone T. Effect of diethylstilbestrol on reproductive function. *Fertil Steril* 1999; **72**: 1–7.

24 Kaufman RH, Adam E, Hatch EE, Noller K, Herbst AL, Palmer JR et al. Continued follow-up of pregnancy outcomes in diethylstilbestrol-exposed offspring. *Obstet Gynecol* 2000; **96**: 483–9.

25 Palmer JR, Hatch EE, Rao RS, Kaufman RH, Herbst AL, Noller KL et al. Infertility among women exposed prenatally to diethylstilbestrol. *Am J Epidemiol* 2001; **154**: 316–21.

26 Titus-Ernstoff L, Troisi R, Hatch EE, Wise LA, Palmer J, Hyer M et al. Menstrual and reproductive characteristics of women whose mothers were exposed in utero to diethylstilbestrol (DES). *Int J Epidemiol* 2006; **35**: 862–8.

27 Martin J, Hiscock H, Hardy P, Davey B, Wake M. Adverse associations of infant and child sleep problems and parent health, an Australian population study. *Pediatrics* 2007; **119**: 947–55.

28 Davey Smith G, Hypponen E, Power C, Lawlor DA. Offspring birth weight and parental mortality, prospective observational study and meta-analysis. *Am J Epidemiol* 2007; **166**: 160–9.

29 Sanderson M, Emanuel I, Holt VL. The intergenerational relationship between mother's birthweight, infant birthweight and infant mortality in black and white mothers. *Paediatr Perinat Epidemiol* 1995; **9**: 391–405.

30 Emanuel I, Leisenring W, Williams MA, Kimpo C, Estee S, O'Brien W et al. The Washington State Intergenerational Study of Birth Outcomes, methodology and some comparisons of maternal birthweight and infant birthweight and gestation in four ethnic groups. *Paediatr Perinat Epidemiol* 1999; **13**: 352–69.

31 Emanuel I, Filakti H, Alberman E, Evans SJ. Intergenerational studies of human birthweight from the 1958 birth cohort. II. Do parents who were twins have babies as heavy as those born to singletons? *Br J Obstet Gynaeco* 1992; **99**: 836–40.

32 Alberman E, Emanuel I, Filakti H, Evans SJ. The contrasting effects of parental birthweight and gestational age on the birthweight of offspring. *Paediatr Perinat Epidemiol* 1992; **6**: 134–44.

33 Hackman E, Emanuel I, van BG, Daling J. Maternal birth weight and subsequent pregnancy outcome. *JAMA* 1983; **250**: 2016–19.

34 Klebanoff MA, Graubard BI, Kessel SS, Berendes HW. Low birth weight across generations. *JAMA* 1984; **252**: 2423–7.

35 Wang X, Zuckerman B, Coffman GA, Corwin MJ. Familial aggregation of low birth weight among whites and blacks in the United States. *N Engl J Med* 1995; **333**: 1744–9.

36 Lunde A, Melve KK, Gjessing HK, Skjaerven R, Irgens LM. Genetic and environmental influences on birth weight, birth length, head circumference, and gestational age by use of population-based parent-offspring data. *Am J Epidemiol* 2007; **165**: 734–41.

37 Baird D. The epidemiology of low birth weight changes in incidence in Aberdeen, 1948–72. *J Biosoc Sci* 1974; **6**: 323–41.

38 Morton SMB. *Lifecourse determinants of offspring size at birth, An intergenerational study of Aberdeen women.* PhD thesis, University of London, London UK, 2003.

39 De Stavola BL, Nitsch D, dos Santos Silva I, McCormack V, Hardy R, Mann V et al. Statistical issues in life course epidemiology. *Am J Epidemiol* 2005; **163**: 84–96.

40 Conley D, Strully KW, Bennett NG. The Starting Gate. *Birth weight and life chances*. University of California, Berkeley, USA, 2003.

41 Ounsted M, Scott A, Ounsted C. Transmission through the female line of a mechanism constraining human fetal growth. *Ann Hum Biol* 1986; **13**: 143–51.

42 Magnus P. Causes of variation in birth weight, a study of offspring of twins. *Clin Genet* 1984; **25**: 15–24.

43 Clausson B, Lichtenstein P, Cnattingius S. Genetic influence on birthweight and gestational length determined by studies in offspring of twins. *BGOG* 2000; **107**: 375–81.

44 Magnus P. Further evidence for a significant effect of fetal genes on variation in birth weight. *Clin Genet* 1984; **26**: 289–96.

45 Brooks AA, Johnson MR, Steer PJ, Pawson ME, Abdalla HI. Birth weight, nature or nurture? *Early Hum Dev* 1995; **42**: 29–35.

46 Davey Smith G. Assessing intrauterine influences on offspring health outcomes: can epidemiological findings yield robust results? *Basic and Clinical Pharmacology and Toxicology* 2008; **102**: 245–56.

47 Magnus P, Gjessing HK, Skrondal A, Skjaerven R. Paternal contribution to birth weight. *J Epidemiol Community Health* 2001; **55**: 873–7.

48 Magnus P, Berg K, Bjerkedal T, Nance WE. Parental determinants of birth weight. *Clin Genet* 1984; **26**: 397–405.

49 Gjessing HK, Lie RT. Biometrical modelling in genetics, are complex traits too complex? *Stat Methods Med Res* 2007; doi:10.1177/0962280207081241.

50 Veena SR, Kumaran K, Swarnagowri MN, Jayakumar MN, Leary SD, Stein CE *et al.* Intergenerational effects on size at birth in South India. *Paediatr Perinat Epidemiol* 2004; **18**: 361–70.

51 Batty GD, Alves JG, Correia J, Lawlor DA. Examining lifecourse influences on chronic disease, the importance of birth cohort studies from developing countries. *Brazilian Journal of Medical and Biological Research* 2007; **40**: 1277–86.

52 United Nations Children's Fund and World Health Organisation. *Low birthweight. Country, Regional and Global Estimates*. UNICEF, New York USA, 2004.

53 Draper ES, Abrams KR, Clarke M. Fall in birth weight of third generation Asian infants. *BMJ* 1995; **311**: 876.

54 Dhawan S. Birth weights of infants of first generation Asian women in Britain compared with second generation Asian women. *BMJ* 1995; **311**: 86–8.

55 Margetts BM, Mohd YS, Al DZ, Jackson AA. Persistence of lower birth weight in second generation South Asian babies born in the United Kingdom. *J Epidemiol Community Health* 2002; **56**: 684–7.

56 Harding S, Rosato MG, Cruickshank JK. Lack of change in birthweights of infants by generational status among Indian, Pakistani, Bangladeshi, Black Caribbean, and Black African mothers in a British cohort study. *Int J Epidemiol* 2004; **33**: 1279–85.

57 Mamun AA, Lawlor DA, Alati R, O'Callaghan MJ, Williams GM, Najman JM. Does maternal smoking during pregnancy have a direct effect on future offspring obesity? Evidence from a prospective birth cohort study. *Am J Epidemiol* 2006; **164**: 317–25.

58 Testa M, Quigley BM, Eiden RD. The effects of prenatal alcohol exposure on infant mental development, a meta-analytical review. *Alcohol* 2003; **38**: 295–304.

59 Olson HC, Streissguth AP, Sampson PD, Barr HM, Bookstein FL, Thiede K. Association of prenatal alcohol exposure with behavioral and learning problems in early adolescence. *J Am Acad Child Adolesc Psychiatry* 1997; **36**: 1187–94.

60 Kane JK, Parker SL, Matta SG, Fu Y, Sharp BM, Li MD. Nicotine up-regulates expression of orexin and its receptors in rat brain. *Endocrinology* 2000; **141**: 3623–9.

61 Slotkin TA. Fetal nicotine or cocaine exposure, which one is worse? *J Pharmacol Exp Ther* 1998; **285**: 931–45.

62 Brion MJ, Leary SD, Davey Smith G, Ness AR. Similar associations of parental prenatal smoking suggest child blood pressure is not influenced by intrauterine effects. *Hypertension* 2007; **49**: 1422–8.

63 Leary S, Davey Smith G, Ness A. Smoking during pregnancy and components of stature in offspring. *Am J Hum Biol* 2006; **18**: 502–12.

64 Jaddoe VW, Verburg BO, de Ridder MA, Hofman A, Mackenbach JP, Moll HA *et al.* Maternal smoking and fetal growth characteristics in different periods of pregnancy, the generation R study. *Am J Epidemiol* 2007; **165**: 1207–15.

65 Julvez J, Ribas-Fito N, Torrent M, Forns M, Garcia-Esteban R, Sunyer J. Maternal smoking habits and cognitive development of children at age 4 years in a population-based birth cohort. *Int J Epidemiol* 2007; doi,10.1093/ije/dym107.

66 **Breslau N, Paneth N, Lucia VC, Paneth-Pollak R.** Maternal smoking during pregnancy and offspring IQ. *Int J Epidemiol* 2005; **34**: 1047–53.

67 **Batty GD, Der G, Deary IJ.** Effect of maternal smoking during pregnancy on offspring's cognitive ability, empirical evidence for complete confounding in the US national longitudinal survey of youth. *Pediatrics* 2006; **118**: 943–50.

68 **Pembrey ME, Bygren LO, Kaati G, Edvinsson S, Northstone K, Sjostrom M et al.** Sex-specific, male-line transgenerational responses in humans. *Eur J Hum Genet* 2006; **14**: 159–66.

69 **Mackay DJ.** Model comparison and Occams Razor. In, Mackay DJ, editor. *Information theory, inference and learning algorhythms.* Cambridge University Press, Cambridge UK, 2003.

70 **Clemons T.** A look at the inheritance of height using regression toward the mean. *Hum Biol* 2000; **72**: 447–54.

71 **Davey Smith G, Steer C, Leary S, Ness A.** Is there an intra-uterine influence on obesity? Evidence from parent-child associations in the Avon Longitudinal Study of Parents and Children (ALSPAC). *Archives of Disease in Childhood* 2007; **92**: 876–80.

72 **Lawlor DA, Davey Smith G, O'Callaghan M, Alati R, Mamun AA, Williams GM et al.** Epidemiologic evidence for the fetal overnutrition hypothesis, findings from the mater-university study of pregnancy and its outcomes. *Am J Epidemiol* 2007; **165**: 418–24.

73 **Youngman LD, Keavney BD, Palmer A.** Plasma fibrinogen and fibrinogen genotypes in 4685 cases of myocardial infarction and in 6002 controls, test of causality by 'Mendelian randomization'. *Circulation* 2000; **102**: 31–2.

74 **Davey Smith G, Ebrahim S.** 'Mendelian randomisation', can genetic epidemiology contribute to understanding environmental determinants of disease? *Int J Epidemiol* 2003; **32**: 1–22.

75 **Lawlor DA, Harbord RM, Sterne JAC, Timpson NJ, Davey Smith G.** Mendelian randomization, using genes as instruments for making causal inferences in epidemiology. *Statistic in Medicine* 2007; doi:10.1002/sim.3034.

76 **Mendel G.** *Experiments in Plant Hybridization.* http,//www mendelweb org/archive/Mendel Experiments txt Accessed September 2007, 1865.

77 **Bhatti P, Sigurdson AJ, Wang SS, Chen J, Rothman N, Hartge P et al.** Genetic variation and willingness to participate in epidemiologic research, data from three studies. *Cancer Epidemiol Biomarkers Prev* 2005; **14**: 2449–53.

78 **Davey Smith G, Lawlor DA, Harbord R, Timpson N, Day I, Ebrahim S.** Clustered environments and randomized genes, a fundamental distinction between conventional and genetic epidemiology. *PloS Medicine* 2008; **4**: e352. doi:10.1371/journal.pmed.0040352.

79 **Kivimaki M, Lawlor DA, Davey Smith G, Eklund C, Hurme M, Lehtimaki T et al.** Variants in the CRP Gene as a Measure of Life-long Differences in Average C-reactive Protein Levels, the Cardiovascular Risk in Young Finns Study. *American Journal of Epidemiology* 2007; **166**: 760–4.

80 **Davey Smith G, Ebrahim S.** What can mendelian randomisation tell us about modifiable behavioural and environmental exposures? *BMJ* 2005; **330**: 1076–9.

81 **Hingorani A, Humphries S.** Nature's randomised trials. *Lancet* 2005; **366**: 1906–8.

82 **MRC Vitamin Study Research Group.** Prevention of neural tube defects, Results of the Medical Research Council vitamin Study. *Lancet* 1991; **338**: 131–7.

83 **Czeizel AE, Dubas I.** Prevention of the first occurrence of neural-tube defects by periconceptional vitamin supplementation. *NEJM* 1992; **327**: 1832–5.

84 **Scholl TO, Johnson WG.** Folic acid, influence on the outcome of pregnancy. *Am J Clin Nutr* 2000; **71**: 1295S–1303S.

85 **Botto LD, Yang Q.** 5,10-Methylenetetrahydrofolate reductase gene variants and congenital anomalies, a HuGE review. *Am J Epidemiol* 2000; **151**: 862–77.

86 **Clayton D, McKeigue PM.** Epidemiological methods for studying genes and environmental factors in complex diseases. *Lancet* 2001; **358**: 1356–60.

87 **Davey Smith G, Harbord R, Ebrahim S.** Fibrinogen, C-reactive protein and coronary heart disease, does Mendelian randomization suggest the associations are non-causal? *QJM* 2004; **97**: 163–6.

88 **Lawlor DA, Timpson N, Harbord RM, Leary S, Ness A, McCarthy MI et al.** Exploring the developmental overnutrition hypothesis using parental-offspring associations and the *FTO* gene as an instrumental variable for maternal adiposity. *PloS Medicine* 2008; **5**: e33. doi:101371/journal.pmed0050033.

89 **Gillman MW.** A life course approach to obesity. In, Kuh D, Ben-Shlomo Y, editors. *A life course approach to chronic disease epidemiology* (second edition). Oxford University Press, Oxford: pp. 189–217, 2004.

90 **Ebbeling CB, Pawlak DB, Ludwig DS.** Childhood obesity, public-health crisis, common sense cure. *Lancet* 2002; **360**: 473–82.

91 **Frayling TM, Timpson NJ, Weedon MN, Zeggini E, Freathy RM, Lindgren CM et al.** A Common Variant in the FTO Gene Is Associated with Body Mass Index and Predisposes to Childhood and Adult Obesity. *Science* 2007: **316**: 889–94.

92 **Davey Smith G, Whitley E, Gissler M, Hemminki E.** Birth dimensions of offspring, premature birth, and the mortality of mothers. *Lancet* 2000; **356**: 2066–7.

93 **Davey Smith G, Harding S, Rosato M.** Relation between infants' birth weight and mothers' mortality, prospective observational study. *BMJ* 2000; **320**: 839–40.

94 **Lawlor DA, Davey Smith G, Whincup P, Wannamethee G, Papacosta O, Dhanjil S et al.** The association between offspring birth weight and atherosclerosis in middle aged men and women, British Regional Heart Study. *J Epidemiol Community Health* 2003; **57**: 462–3.

95 **Davey Smith G, Sterne J, Tynelius P, Lawlor DA, Rasmussen.** Birth weight of offspring and subsequent cardiovascular mortality of parents. *Epidemiology* 2005; **16**: 563–9.

96 **Smith GC, Pell JP, Walsh D.** Pregnancy complications and maternal risk of ischaemic heart disease, a retrospective cohort study of 129,290 births. *Lancet* 2001; **357**: 2002–6.

97 **Davey Smith G, Hart C, Ferrell C, Upton M, Hole D, Hawthorne V et al.** Birth weight of offspring and mortality in the Renfrew and Paisley study, prospective observational study. *BMJ* 1997; **315**: 1189–93.

98 **Davey Smith G.** Genetic risk factors in mothers and offspring. *Lancet* 2001; **358**: 1268.

99 **Raina P, O'Donnell M, Rosenbaum P, Brehaut J, Walter SD, Russell D et al.** The health and well-being of caregivers of children with cerebral palsy. *Pediatrics* 2005; **115**: e626-e636.

100 **Smith LA, Hatcher JL, Wertheimer R.** The association of childhood asthma with parental employment and welfare receipt. *J Am Med Womens Assoc* 2002; **57**: 11–15.

101 **Powers ET.** New estimates of the impact of child disability on maternal employment. *The American Economic Review* 2001; **91**: 135–9.

102 **Murray L, Cooper P.** Effects of postnatal depression on infant development. *Arch Dse Child* 1997; **77**: 99–101.

103 **Ramchandani P, Stein A, Evans J, O'Connor TG.** Paternal depression in the postnatal period and child development, a prospective population study. *Lancet* 2005; **365**: 2201–5.

104 **Gartstein MA, Sheeber L.** Child behavior problems and maternal symptoms of depression, a mediational model. *J Child Adolesc Psychiatr Nurs* 2004; **17**: 141-150.

105 **Elgar FJ, McGrath PJ, Waschbusch DA, Stewart SH, Curtis LJ.** Mutual influences on maternal depression and child adjustment problems. *Clin Psychol Rev* 2004; **24**: 441–59.

106 **Morton NE.** The inheritance of human birth weight. *Annals of Human Genetics* 1955; **20**: 125–34.

Chapter 3

Theoretical underpinning for the use of sibling studies in life course epidemiology

Kate W Strully and Gita D Mishra

Abstract

Siblings can have a great deal in common (e.g., parents, genes, early life home environments, etc.), but they are also distinct individuals with unique personalities and physical traits. In this chapter, we discuss how researchers can use similarities and differences across siblings to investigate questions of life course epidemiology. First, we discuss how sibling fixed effects models may help deal with residual confounding from unobserved family-level factors. Second, we discuss how behavioural genetics approaches can help unravel genetic heritability from environmental determinants of health. Finally, we discuss genetic linkage studies in which researchers use siblings' DNA information to learn more about the effects of chromosomal regions and genes. When considering each of these strategies, we review the relevant literature and discuss the strengths and weaknesses of the particular methods.

3.1 **Introduction**

Siblings may have much in common and yet it is surprising how much they can differ. They may share many of their parents' genes and have had many of the same prenatal exposures. They may have grown up in the same house, eating the same meals, playing with the same toys, and attending the same schools. But, siblings' experiences can also differ in important ways, particularly depending on the age gap between them. Family events like job loss and divorce may mean that one sibling spends her early years in poverty, while the other does not. A change in maternal health or behaviour may mean that one sibling benefits from a healthier prenatal environment than the other. Of course, parents may also simply treat their children differently, encouraging different behaviours and attitudes in each child. Furthermore, siblings may be related to each other in different ways (e.g. half siblings, full siblings, adopted siblings, etc.), and the degree of similarity or difference in siblings genes and environments should vary systematically across these different types of relationships.[1-4]

In this chapter, we discuss how one can use sibling similarities and differences to investigate questions of life course epidemiology. We focus on three different strategies for sibling analysis. First, we discuss how sibling fixed effects (FE) models can reduce residual confounding from unobserved family-level factors and move us closer to accurate causal estimates for specific exposures. Second, we present behavioural genetics (BG) approaches to sibling analysis. This work addresses questions of nature and nurture that arise in trying to unravel genetic heritability from environmental determinants. Finally, we consider genetic linkage studies where researchers use siblings' DNA information to identify chromosomal regions and genes that may be related to an outcome.

Each of these strategies has distinct goals and logic. In the FE approach, the goal is to reduce bias from unobserved differences. This means researchers will generally try to analyse siblings who share the most genetic and environmental characteristics (i.e., full singleton siblings or twins). In interpreting results, the central question is whether the within-sibling estimates are significantly different from across-sibling estimates. Within-sibling estimates reflect average differences between siblings, while across-sibling estimates reflect average differences across the entire population. If within- and across-sibling estimates are significantly different, unobserved family-level differences may be biasing our estimates. In the BG approach, the goal is to separate out genetic and environmental inputs. This implies that researchers must examine different types of sibling pairs who have varying amounts of genes and environment in common (e.g., comparing adopted siblings to biologically-related siblings, or comparing monozygotic (MZ) twins to dizygotic (DZ) twins). Here the central question is whether the similarity of siblings' outcomes is related to their degree of genetic or environmental similarity. In genetic linkage studies, the aim is not to identify directly the causal gene, but instead use markers (obtained from siblings' DNA) to localize fairly large regions as containing a potentially causal gene. Research in life course epidemiology has seldom utilized linkage methods, even though these should be able to assist in identifying effect specificity on early and late onset disease or on class defined trajectories across the life course for outcomes such as the alcohol intake or physical activity levels.

Before proceeding further it should be noted that, as randomized controlled trials are absent in most life course research, this chapter adopts a more practical approach in describing relationships as 'causal'.[5] Namely, a causal relationship is more likely if 1) the cause preceded the effect; 2) some sort of relationship can be expected between the cause and effect; and 3) the cause identified is the only logical explanation that we can find for the effect. For psychiatry, Robins and Guze imposed additional requirements, such as biological plausibility and a dose-response gradient.[6]

The following discussion covers a wide range of topics, but a common thread is the problem of how early-life exposures are inherited within families, and how those exposures shape development and later wellbeing. In life course studies of health there is a general acceptance that early life physical and mental development play a part in relation to most if not all outcomes of epidemiological and public health concern.[7] The discussion of literature in this area that follows is far from exhaustive. Rather, we focus on topics where sibling analyses have been used the most effectively and/or where the strengths and weakness of each approach are the most apparent. Some types of sibling analyses (e.g., the fixed effects approach) have been most commonly used outside of epidemiology, and the literature we discuss comes from a variety of disciplines—most notably, sociology, economics, and psychology. As a result, inquiries into the connections between health, socioeconomic status, and child development are well represented below. Finally, we discuss the caveats and limitations of each approach in the hope that readers will take away a sense for the types of research questions that are, and are not, appropriate for each approach.

3.2 Sibling fixed effects (FE) models: the problem of unobserved differences

3.2.1 Theoretical underpinning of sibling studies to deal with residual confounding

Although life course epidemiologists spend much time investigating how early exposures (e.g., birth weight, family poverty, etc.) are related to later-life outcomes, estimates of the causal effects of most early-life factors are unclear.[8–9] Further, intergenerational patterns are repeatedly seen in which parental and family disadvantages are associated with early-life risk factors, but whether these reflect actual determinants of early-life exposures remains uncertain.[10–12] In short, family background predicts early-life exposures, which in turn predict later-life wellbeing, but whether this pattern reflects true causal effects is unclear. These ambiguities arise because most social and health disadvantages tend to accumulate within the same populations, making it difficult sort out any unique effects.[13] Epidemiologists refer to this problem as residual confounding of the unique causal effect one is trying to determine. By comparing exposures and outcomes within sibling pairs, who share many genes and environmental exposures, it is possible to hold constant numerous unmeasured potential confounders and move closer to estimating true causal effects.

Consider, as an example, the positive association between low birth weight (LBW) and adult cardiovascular disease (CVD). One popular explanation for this pattern is that prenatal stressors affect fetal development in ways that have lasting implications on health in later-life.[14] However, there are also several alternative explanations arising from the fact that being born with LBW is associated with a variety of additional risks. LBW children are more likely than their normal birth weight counterparts to face multiple negative early-life exposures—such as, family poverty, second-hand smoke, or poorer diet.[15, 11] Since all of these factors can increase the risk of later-life disease, they may be upwardly biasing our estimates of birth weight effects. Individuals with LBW who suffered childhood disadvantages will also tend to face a disproportionate burden of negative adult exposures—such as, poorer educational outcomes, occupational exposures, obesity, diabetes, etc.[10, 16–18] These adult risk factors can also contribute to disease risk, and so may cause further bias. Finally, genetic explanations are a common alternative. The genes that determine fetal development may also determine (or at least be associated with other genes that determine) CVD.[19]

In short, the various different risk factors across the life course that contribute to an outcome, like CVD, will tend to accumulate among individuals who faced the early life exposure-of-interest (i.e., birth weight), and this makes it difficult to estimate causal effects. In the world of ideal data, we would have information on, and therefore could adjust for, all the many additional risk factors. Unfortunately, in the real world, data are limited and we frequently suffer from incomplete information, so alternative strategies have to be developed, such as sibling FE models. Since most siblings share the same parents and grew up in the same household, many of the unobserved environmental and genetic factors that may be causing bias will be held constant within the sibling set.

Consider the following standard ordinary least squares (OLS) regression model:

$$Y = \alpha + X\beta + \varepsilon \qquad (3.1)$$

where X represents the matrix of variables and observations specified in the model and β represents its associated vector of coefficients. In many cases (e.g., LBW and CVD as discussed above), this model is likely to be inadequate because there are probably lurking variables (e.g., all the potential confounders discussed above: childhood poverty, poor diet, occupational exposures, etc.). That is, there is another matrix of unobserved characteristics that are biasing our estimates of β.

Such unobserved characteristics can be explicitly incorporated into the model, separating them into two parts: the unobserved factors that are common to families and those that are unique to individuals. Consider equation (3.2):

$$Y = \alpha + X\beta + FAM\gamma + IND\delta + \varepsilon' \qquad (3.2)$$

where *FAM* reflects family-level unobservables, *IND* reflects individual-level unobservables, and both are correlated with the set of observed factors (*X*).

If information on multiple siblings within a family is available, then the sibling FE model addresses the problem of unobserved family-level factors (*FAM*), as shown in equation (3.2). By taking difference scores between our *Y* variable (e.g., adult CVD) for each sibling and regressing that against the sibling difference in *X* variables (e.g., LBW), the unobserved family-level characteristics that remain constant across siblings drop out of the model:

$$\Delta Y_{ti,tj} = \alpha + \Delta X_{ti,tj2}\beta + \Delta IND_{ti,tj2}\delta + \Delta \varepsilon'_{ti,tj} \qquad (3.3)$$

where ti and tj refers to the ith and jth sibling.

Most analyses that use sibling FE models will first present the standard OLS regression from equation (3.1) and then present the FE model from equation (3.3). The question is then: by how much has the estimate for the exposure-of-interest changed from one model to the next? If the estimate were to drop dramatically in the sibling FE framework, it would appear that unobserved family-level characteristics were largely responsible for the association and existing estimates may have been upwardly biased. Meanwhile, if the estimate were resilient across the models, it would appear that the exposure 'matters', net of unobserved family characteristics, and provides greater confidence that the estimates reflect a causal effect.[10, 20, 21]

Sibling FE models can be a powerful approach for modelling causal effects. *However, the faith we can place in our interpretation of these models depends on how well we understand what does and does not vary among siblings.* First, a rather obvious point is that a sibling FE model is only appropriate if the exposure-of-interest actually varies across siblings. It may be clear that a sibling FE model is inappropriate for estimating the effect of, say, race or parental education, because these characteristics will generally not vary at all across siblings. But, consider a more subtle point, such as, family income during the prenatal period. A family's income will certainly fluctuate over time, but a significant component of family income will remain stable from year-to-year (e.g., a Chief Executive Officer's income will typically be consistently higher than the income of a gas station attendant). If short-term fluctuations in income are not of great consequence for families' circumstances, and it is really the permanent differences in income that matter, the 'important' parts of income are not varying across each siblings' prenatal period. This can make a null result in a FE model difficult to interpret. If we were to run an OLS model and find a positive association between family income and birth outcomes, but then find no association in the FE model, we might be tempted to assume that income does not 'matter,' and conclude that family-level unobservables are driving the relationship. However, this would not be accurate since income does play a causal role, it is just that the time-invariant aspects of income that actually 'matter' are not varying across the siblings. Rather than interpreting OLS results as 'biased' and FE results as 'causal' (as many authors do), it may be more appropriate to treat OLS estimates as an upper-bound and FE estimates as a lower-bound.

It is also important to highlight that sibling FE models can only adjust for unobserved confounders that remain stable within sibling pairs. With many potential confounders (e.g., parents' genes or parents' education), we can be reasonably confident that there is little-to-no within-sibling variation. However, with some other potential confounders, we may not be so sure. Imagine using sibling models to estimate the effect of maternal alcohol consumption during the prenatal period on offspring adult IQ. Let us return to the problem of prenatal family income, but this time we will treat it as a potential, unobserved confounder, rather than as the exposure-of-interest. Since family income is likely to be associated with both maternal behaviour and offspring adult IQ, unobserved differences in family income may be a significant source of bias.[11, 22]

The question here is: how confident are we that sibling comparisons are factoring out the important variation in the potential confounder, family income? As mentioned above, much of the variation in family income will be stable within the sibling pairs, but some families will experience sizable income shocks (e.g., from parental job loss) and what these unobserved changes mean—in this case, for maternal drinking and offspring IQ—may not be clear. This sort of ambiguity can make it difficult to interpret significant FE results. On the one hand, a significant association between maternal drinking and adult IQ in the FE model will be notable evidence for a causal effect—the estimate has 'held up' even when family-level characteristics were factored out. But, on the other hand, ambiguity over precisely how much of income is family-level (i.e., not varying across the siblings' prenatal periods) and how much is individual-level (i.e., unique to each siblings' prenatal experience) means caution is required in interpreting the results as causal.

Unfortunately, the degree of within-sibling variation is unclear in many different cases. For instance, frequently it is not known the extent to which parents treat siblings differently, and how strongly differential treatment is associated with various characteristics (e.g., birth weight, birth order, IQ, or genes). In other words, we may not know how much of the variation in parental behaviour operates at the family or individual-level and what this means for our estimates. Many environmental exposures raise similar questions. It may not be known, for instance, whether a family relocated to a new neighbourhood and if this then exposed the siblings to different environmental factors at critical stages of development.

When considering the appropriateness of sibling FE models, it is useful to note that there are usually three main sources of bias: first, unobserved prenatal/early-life exposures; second, unobserved later-life exposures; and, finally, unobserved genetic variation.[12, 23] If the research is concerned with whether aspects of family background determine early-life risk factors (e.g., LBW or childhood disease), then the main focus should probably be on bias from the first and third sources—that is, from unobserved differences in prenatal/early-life environment and from the genes that parents pass on to children. Bias from the second source, unobserved late-life exposures, will not be an issue here since the outcome precedes these. On the other hand, if the research question deals with how an early-life risk factor affects a later-life outcome, all three sources of bias will need to be addressed. In addition to being concerned with prenatal/early-life exposures and genetic variation, here it is also important to consider if the early-life risk factor of interest is causing unobserved differences in later-life wellbeing, which ultimately explain the correlation-of-interest.

Siblings share many prenatal/early-life exposures by virtue of (usually) growing up in the same household and having the same parents. With age, however, siblings' paths are likely to diverge as each pursues their individual educational, career, and family goals. Given this, sibling models should be more effective at addressing prenatal/early-life confounders, rather than later-life confounders. If one is primarily concerned with bias from later-life exposures, sibling models may be more limited. It should be noted, though, that many unobserved differences in later-life wellbeing may mediate, rather than confound, the effects of early-life risk factors.

With regard to the possibility of genetic spuriousness, full siblings share approximately 50% of their genes. This means that comparisons within full-sibling pairs encounter significantly reduced genetic variation compared to comparisons in samples of unrelated individuals. However, if bias from genetic variation is a primary concern, one should consider analysing MZ twin pairs since they share 100% of their genes (with the exception of mitochondrial DNA).[23–25] FE analyses of data from MZ twin pairs will provide a very stringent test for causal effects. However, as is discussed in the next section (and in detail in Chapter 4), there may be an issue with the generalisability of estimates from MZ twin studies. From this perspective, even in ordinary sibling studies, it would be best to avoid analysing half siblings, who share only about

25% of their genes. Unfortunately, this information is not always available, and therefore it leaves open questions regarding the degree of genetic confounding addressed by the sibling models.

3.2.2 What have sibling FE models taught us about prenatal and early-life exposures?

With all these points in mind, we can begin to assess what sibling FE models have and have not revealed about early-life exposures. Since many of the existing health-related sibling FE analyses focus on birth weight and gestational age, we begin with the question of whether perinatal health has causal effects on later outcomes. Associations between perinatal conditions and adult health or socioeconomic status have generally been resilient to sibling FE analyses. Working with linked data from various Swedish registers and censuses, Lawlor et al. (2007) found that, within pairs of brothers, gestational age and intrauterine growth were negatively associated with systolic blood pressure.[26] Since Lawlor et al. were able to adjust for both maternal and paternal health characteristics, this analysis provides strong evidence for a causal link between prenatal exposures and adult cardiovascular health. After adjusting for parental health, Lawlor and co-authors found there was no statistically significant difference between the sibling FE and non-sibling models, implying that birth weight-blood pressure associations are probably not being driven by unobserved family-level confounders.

When examining associations between perinatal conditions and later socioeconomic outcomes, sibling models have frequently yielded larger estimates than non-sibling models, suggesting that family-level factors may be causing downward bias. Drawing on a nationally representative sample of U.S. families and adjusting for various demographics and childhood conditions (e.g., family income, maternal age at birth), Conley, Strully, and Bennett (2003) found that, in non-sibling models, an additional pound of birth weight was associated with a 32% reduction in the likelihood of not completing high school on time; but, using a sibling FE model, an additional pound of weight reduced this risk by a much larger 79%.[10] This suggests that standard OLS estimates of birth weight and later SES may be causing us to underestimate the importance of perinatal health.

Since singleton siblings share only 50% of their genes, and maternal behaviours or family circumstances may change between pregnancies, confounding from unobserved within-sibling variation could be an issue for the results of Lawlor et al. and Conley, Strully, and Bennett. However, comparing birth weights within MZ twin pairs, who not only share all of their genes (except for mitochondrial DNA) but also shared the same pregnancy, has confirmed this general pattern for a wider range of outcomes. Behrman and Rosenzweig (2004) have examined female MZ twins from the US Minnesota Twin Registry and found that the heavier twin was more likely to be taller, have greater educational attainment, and higher wages. The FE estimates from this analysis were statistically significantly larger than the OLS estimates. They could not, however, identify significant associations between birth weight and adult body mass index.[24] Black, Devereux, and Salvanes (2005) find parallel results from a nationally representative sample of Norwegian twins.[25]

As an aside, it is interesting to note that twin FE estimates of the effects of birth weight on early-life outcomes—most notably, infant mortality—have been significant, but are generally much smaller than the equivalent OLS estimates. Considering this in light of the above results, it appears that family level factors may play a varying role in birth weight effects across the life course.[10, 24, 25]

Taken as a whole, this literature supports a causal link between perinatal health and later wellbeing—and this raises various questions about possible intervening mechanisms. There have been relatively few sibling analyses directly addressing this question of mechanisms. Haas (2006) has applied sibling models using data from a nationally representative US sample to show that general self-assessed childhood health mediates associations between birth weight and educational and labour market outcomes.[27] Addressing the problem of mechanisms slightly less directly, several authors have tested whether birth weight differences within sibling pairs account for sibling differences in IQ. IQ is an important predictor of educational success and occupational status, and therefore could be an important pathway through which birth weight affects later-life attainment. Overall these studies have come to mixed conclusions. Some have found that sibling differences in birth weight predict sibling differences in child IQ, suggesting that individual differences in prenatal exposures impact cognitive development.[28–30] However, other studies have found that birth weight-IQ associations are not resilient to sibling FE models, and therefore most likely reflect shared family characteristics.[31, 32] Another line of research has considered child behavioural disorders as possible mechanisms. Currie (2007), for instance, has shown that sibling differences in behavioural problems during childhood (most notably, ADHD) are strong predictors of later labour market success.[33] Since perinatal outcomes are associated with behavioural disorders this raises another intriguing potential pathway.

We can now turn to the problem of how family background determines the likelihood of experiencing an early-life risk factor. This raises the more general question of how social and health disadvantages are transmitted across generations. Conley, Strully, and Bennett (2003) have identified a slightly complicated process that operates through biosocial interactions. By comparing within US sibling pairs, they found that increases in family income during the prenatal period significantly reduced the risk of LBW, but only within families where there was a history of LBW (i.e., at least one of the parents was born with LBW).[10] This suggests that the accumulation of disadvantages is particularly important in determining early-life risk factors.

Other authors have tackled similar questions by examining the wellbeing of first cousins (i.e. the children of sisters). Being born to a teenage mother is consistently associated with greater exposure to early-life risk factors (e.g., poorer perinatal and childhood health, not being breastfed, etc.). This may reflect an effect of maternal age on early-life exposures, but it might also be due to the fact that young mothers face multiple disadvantages (e.g., poverty, bad neighbourhood conditions, minority racial statuses, etc.), which can further increase the risk of negative exposures for children. Some authors have found that most of the associations of maternal age and behaviour with offspring outcomes (e.g., birth weight, test scores) are not resilient to first cousin FE models.[34, 35] Thus many of the differences by maternal age are explained by unobserved, family-level differences between older and younger mothers, rather than by a mother's age *per se*. This provides little support for a causal interpretation for the role of maternal age and rather suggests that other, more general family-level disadvantages are shaping early-life risk factors (for a similar analysis of pregnancy intention and child development see reference 36).

In summary, since siblings share many environmental factors and genes, using sibling FE models to compare exposures and outcomes within sibling sets can help reduce confounding and move us closer to accurate causal estimates. However, the strength of the interpretation of these models depends on how well we understand what does and does not vary among siblings. If there is not sufficient sibling variation in the exposure-of-interest, FE models may yield false null results. On the other hand, if there are unobserved differences among siblings, which are correlated with both the exposure and the outcome, FE models may suffer from bias and yield incorrect significant results. Existing sibling FE analyses show that perinatal health is consistently associated with later-life outcomes, net of family-level variations. Siblings FE models investigating the determinants (e.g., biological and social factors) of early-life risk factors yield more mixed results, and suggest that their accumulation and interaction effects might well be important.

3.3 Behavioural genetics analyses of siblings: questions of nature and nurture

3.3.1 Theoretical underpinning of sibling studies of heritability

Behavioural genetic (BG) research seeks to determine the relative contribution of genetic variation to individual-level differences in a characteristic (e.g., height, intelligence, disease, etc.); then, given this knowledge of genetic influences, to refine our understanding of environmental influences. The central strategy of BG research involves comparing familial aggregation patterns across different types of family relationships that have varying degrees of genetic and environmental similarity (e.g., MZ versus DZ twins, or adopted versus biologically-related siblings). This research addresses several issues relevant to life course epidemiology. Below, we discuss work on the heritability of early-life risk factors (primarily low birth weight) and how it explores the different patterns of heritability across the life course. BG research methods provide several intuitive, and sometimes powerful, approaches to sibling analysis that may be of considerable use to life course epidemiologists. However, as will be discussed, this approach also requires strong assumptions about the covariance of genes and environment.

In the terminology of BG, observable characteristics (e.g., behaviours, physical traits, illnesses, etc.) are referred to as phenotypes. These are the actual manifestation of genetic traits and they typically will depend to a large degree on environmental inputs. The goal of BG research is to decompose the genetic and environmental variation that is responsible for individual-level differences in phenotypes. There are generally assumed to be three contributors to phenotypic variation: genetic factors (Vg), shared (i.e., family-level) environmental factors (Vc), and non-shared (i.e., individual-level) environmental factors (Ve). The decomposition of total phenotypic variation can be written as:

$$Vp = Vg + Vc + Ve \tag{3.4}$$

The percentage of total variance due to genetic differences ($h^2=Vg/Vp$) is referred to as heritability. The complement to heritability is the percentage of total variance due to environmental differences. This is sometimes referred to as environmentality and can be separated into its shared ($c^2=Vc/Vp$) and non-shared ($e^2=Ve/Vp$) components.[37, 38] Obviously, if this decomposition were performed with a sample of, say, full-siblings who were all reared together little would be gained since all these siblings would share about half of their genes and several environmental factors. BG analysis, therefore, requires different types of siblings with varying degrees of genetic and environmental similarity, such as adopted and biologically-related siblings, or MZ and DZ twins who were reared both together and apart.

In most BG research, neither genes nor environment are directly observed (for an exception see reference 39). Rather, genetic and environmental inputs are inferred based on the additive assumption that total variation is composed entirely of only two independent components: genetic and environmental variation. Thus typically, once heritability has been estimated any variation that remains is assumed to result from environmental effects that are themselves a combination of individual and shared inputs. Since this approach assumes zero covariance between genetic and environmental similarities that are relevant to the phenotype of interest, it follows that siblings with more genes in common should not experience greater environmental similarity than their counterparts with fewer genes in common. If there is such a positive correlation between genes and environment, heritability may be overestimated and environmental inputs may be underestimated. Conversely, if there is a negative correlation between genes and environment, there is a risk of underestimating heritability and overestimating the importance of environment.[37, 40, 41]

Genes and environment may be correlated with each other in many ways—genetic dispositions may lead one to seek out or create particular environments, and environmental factors may be associated with how genes are expressed.[42] Thus an assumption of zero covariance between genes and environment may be problematic, and in some cases, we may not know which direction bias is going in. As is discussed below, one may obtain more precise estimates by adjusting for gene-environment correlations, but this requires reliable measures of genetic and/or environmental factors, which are frequently unavailable. Nature-nurture questions are central to our understanding of human behaviour and wellbeing, and BG offers some useful tools. Nevertheless this issue of potential correlation of gene-environment factors means it is essential to interpret results with caution.

3.3.2 Adoption studies

The most powerful and intuitive application of the BG method is in adoption studies. Adoption events disentangle genes and environment by separating genetically-related individuals and having them share a home environment with genetically-unrelated individuals. Examining adopted siblings who are genetically unrelated, but were raised together, allows researchers to assess family-level environmental inputs. If adopted siblings are highly similar on some outcome, then family environmental is likely to have an important influence. Conversely, studying genetically-related individuals who were reared apart allows researcher to test genetic influences. In this case, if certain outcomes are highly similar, then genetics are likely to have the primary role.[37, 38]

Adoption studies provide an appealing research design, but a number of issues implicit in the adoption process may lead to problematic gene-environment correlations. The logic of adoption studies assumes that full siblings who were raised apart have similar genes, but uncorrelated environments. However, since these siblings share the same biological mother, there is likely to be significant overlap in their prenatal environmental exposures. This could cause adoption studies to overestimate genetic heritability and underestimate these early life environmental effects. On the other hand, adopted siblings, who are genetically unrelated but raised together, are assumed to have been exposed to similar environments. But, since they have different biological mothers, their prenatal exposures may differ greatly and these may be correlated with the genetic differences. Thus, this may similarly lead to results that overestimate genetic and underestimate environmental effects. Some researchers have tried to assess this bias by comparing correlations between birth mothers and their adopted-away children to correlations between birth fathers and these children.[37] While this is a useful idea that is likely to provide some leverage in affirming the basis of results, it requires the further potentially problematic assumption that paternal behaviours correlated with the phenotype of interest have not also significantly influenced the prenatal environment. Chapter 2 provides a full discussion of the extent to which comparisons of maternal-offspring associations with paternal-offspring associations might provide insights into the effects of prenatal (intrauterine) exposures.

A second concern with adoption studies is selective placement. If adopted children are selectively placed with genetically similar families, there will be a positive association between genes and environment, and we risk overestimating the importance of environment. Given sufficient information on birth and adoptive parents, one may be able to model the bias from such gene-environment correlations.[37, 43] Unfortunately, comprehensive information of this sort is only rarely available, especially on birth fathers.

A third point to note with these studies is with respect to the age at placement of children in adoptive homes. Although children adopted not long after birth experience almost continuous care by their adoptive parents, older placed children experience the disruption of at least one major change of caregiver when they join their adoptive family. In the majority of cases, older placed children have generally suffered a pre-adoption history of abuse, neglect and/or rejection.[44]

Lastly, in life course epidemiology it is important to be aware that the social concept of adoption potentially differs greatly according to time, place, and context. Therefore it cannot be assumed that participants with a wide age span or from different cultures define or implement adoption in the same way.[5]

3.3.3 Twin studies

While adoption studies still provide a strong research design, there are practical difficulties in that adoptions themselves are relatively rare, rendering it somewhat difficult to form a study sample (particularly if the phenotype of interest is also rare). As an alternative, many behavioural geneticists turn to twin studies. Chapter 4 in this book considers twin models in detail. Here, we will simply note that, in twin studies, researchers compare the similarity of outcomes within MZ twin pairs (MZ twins are genetically identical, with the exception of mitochondrial DNA) to the similarity of outcomes within DZ twin pairs (DZ twins share, on average, 50% of their genes, just like singleton siblings). If genetic inputs are important, the correlation for MZ twins should exceed that for DZ twins.[37,38]

Because twins share the same pregnancy, variation in prenatal exposures is less problematic than in other sibling studies, but as detailed in Chapter 4, the assumption that all prenatal exposures are identical in twins is not necessarily true. However, post-natal environment may cause significant bias. Twins studies require the assumption that genetically-similar MZ twins do not experience more similar environments that DZ twins. However, parents are likely to respond to children's endowments, and children may shape their environments based, in part, on their genetic dispositions. It, therefore, seems likely that, in many cases MZ twins will have more similar environments than their DZ counterparts.[39,45,46] If this pattern is associated with the phenotype-of-interest, a twin design may overestimate the importance of genetic heritability.

An additional concern with both twin and adoption studies is whether the results are generalizable to larger populations. The unique circumstances of twinning and adoption offer 'natural experiments' that provide leverage on causal questions about the effects of genes and environment. However, this very uniqueness may also mean that results based on these populations do not extend to other groups. In the case of adoption studies, we may be particularly concerned that the samples are more privileged than the average person. In the United States, for instance, adoption is significantly more common among white, well-educated, and higher-income individuals.[47]

3.3.4 Comparisons of full- and half-siblings

Another BG approach involves comparing full-siblings with half-siblings. Since full and half siblings are far more common than twins or adopted siblings, this strategy does not face the same questions about generalizing results. However, genetic and environmental variation may also be more confounded in these models, making interpretation more difficult. With only one parent in common, half siblings have about 25% of the same genes (compared with 50% in common for full siblings). This could imply that stronger correlations among full siblings, relative to half siblings, point to genetic inheritance of a given phenotype. But, of course, parents do not only contribute genes, they also contribute environmental inputs. Thus, half siblings may also share less of their environments than their full sibling counterparts. Most notably, the older member of a half sibling pair was most likely born into the mother's or father's first marriage, and thus into a separate, perhaps quite different, household than the younger half sibling born into the parent's current marriage.[37,48]

3.3.5 Gene-environment interactions and epigenetic effects

Gene-environment interactions are likely to be an important (but still poorly understood) source of phenotypic variation. Genetic heritability may depend on particular environmental exposures and likewise some environmental exposures may only be consequential for those with certain genetic make-ups. Because genes are sometimes discussed as though they were immutable (for instance when they are referred to as the 'blue print' of life), and heritability involves genetic inheritance, heritability estimates are sometimes interpreted as immutable. This, however, is far from the case. Heritability of many phenotypes (e.g., height, IQ, BMI, health behaviours, etc.) is likely to vary along environmental dimensions across the life course (e.g., food availability, income, educational attainments of parents and offspring, etc.).[49–51] It follows that heritability estimates should be thought of as an estimate of genetic determinants for a given population in a given set of circumstances.[38]

In practice, estimating genetic-environmental interactions can be very tricky. Just as is the case when estimating a first-order genetic or environmental effect, estimating a gene-environment interaction requires independent genetic and environmental variation. Consider twin studies that indicate that verbal IQ is less heritable in poor families, African American families, and families with an unemployed parent, relative to what occurs in wealthier families, white families, and families no unemployed parents.[50, 52] These studies provide intriguing evidence that deprived environments 'constrain' genetic expression. However, as is the case with first-order effects, gene-environment correlations may bias estimates. It may be the case, for instance, that different degrees of assortative mating or fertility patterns limit genotypic variation in IQ among disadvantaged groups, and this downwardly biases the heritability estimates.[49]

Recent and on-going research into epigenetics is providing important insight into how gene-environment interactions may lead to phenotypic variation. Epigenetics refers to all modifications to genes other than changes in the DNA itself and it consists of molecular switches and markers that help control gene regulation. In essence, epigenetics 'turns genes on and off' allowing or preventing the gene from being used to make a protein. Since all cells in the body contain the same DNA sequence, epigenetics is crucial to such basic processes as making a heart cell different from a skin cell or a lung cell. There is also increasing evidence of the importance of epigenetics to the familial patterns of disease.[53] For instance, recent research with MZ twin mice has shown that epigenetic process that can be inherited (e.g., DNA methylation) can alter the regulation of a particular gene (e.g., the agouti gene associated with fur colour) leading to increased risk of obesity, diabetes, and cancer. Whether or not a mouse has an un-methylated agouti gene (i.e., the agouti gene is 'turned on' all the time, which is associated with increased risk of disease) has further been linked to maternal nutrition and exposure to contaminants found in plastics.[54] This type of evidence highlights that genes and environment are inextricably linked and shows that environmental exposures of previous generations can impact the gene regulation of offspring.

Gene-environment interactions are likely to be important to phenotypic variation—one of the main ways that future BG research may contribute to our understanding of human behaviour and wellbeing is by documenting how genes and environmental influences work together. However, the complexity of, typically unobserved, gene-environment correlations makes this a challenging task. Future studies might try to overcome this issue by inducing, or finding naturally occurring, random variation in environmental exposures. If heritability varies across randomized environmental variation, then an interaction can be identified with a fair degree of confidence.

3.3.6 Behavioural genetics literature and life course epidemiology

One of the central contributions of life course epidemiology has been to show that prenatal and early-life exposures have lasting implications across the life-course—but, to what extent do these early-life risk factors result from nature or nurture? This discussion focuses on the heritability of birth weight, specifically, because research strategies in this topic area have been diverse and it is illuminating to compare their various strengths and weaknesses. However, there are also interesting BG analyses of various other early-life risk factors, such as infant blood pressure,[55] childhood eating habits,[56,57] and behavioural disorders.[58]

Clausson, Lichtenstein, and Cnattingius (2000) have investigated the heritability of birth weight by comparing the birth outcomes of singleton offspring born to MZ and DZ twin mothers. With this combined twin-intergenerational strategy, the researchers found that about 37% of the variation in low birth weight was explained by genetic heritability.[59] This result might be best interpreted as an upper-bound estimate since this analysis may suffer from the upward bias that is typical of twin studies. Any environmental inputs into perinatal health are likely to be more similar among the MZ twin mothers than the DZ twin mothers. Another issue is that this study cannot identify unique effects of maternal and foetal genes since maternal twins who share more genes will have children who also share more genes—while the offspring of MZ twins will be half 'siblings' (they share about 25% of their genes), the children of DZ twins will be first cousins. If MZ twin mothers tend to select more similar men to father their offspring than DZ twin mothers (i.e., differences in assortative mating), there may be even more genetic similarity among the offspring of MZ twins.

Using birth certificate data to examine twins' own birth weights, Conley and Strully (2007) found that only about 13% of the variance in birth weight can be attributed to genetic heritability.[49] This suggests a far more modest contribution of genetics to birth weight. However, this estimate might be best considered as a lower-bound. Although most twin studies risk overestimating heritability due to positive correlations between genetic and environmental similarity, comparing twins' own perinatal health may cause an underestimate of heritability. Differences in the placental formation of multiple gestation pregnancies can lead MZ twins to have less similar prenatal environments than their DZ counterparts (see Chapter 4 for a more detailed discussion of this).

However, an interesting twist on an adoption design also reveals only a limited role of genetics in birth weight. Brooks *et al.* (1995) examined cases of ovum donation and finds that the recipient's weight is positively associated with the baby's birth weight. However, the donor's weight and the birth weight of her children are not significantly associated with the baby's birth weight.[60] This suggests that the environment provided by the mother is more important than her 'direct' genetic contributions. Of course, the environment provided by the mother (e.g., her height and weight) may be related to her genes, so this does not imply that genes do not matter. Rather, it suggests that any genetic effects are mediated by environmental factors. Examining such an unusual situation as ovum donation, this study may face problems related to a small sample size (62 cases), and it is not clear yet how far these results can be generalized.

Traditionally, BG researchers have focused on the heritability of a given trait at a single point in time. More recently, researchers have begun exploring how heritability varies across the life course and have generally tried to address three questions: (i) how do the relative contributions of genes and environment vary over time and with age, (ii) do on-going genetic contributions reflect the persistence of earlier genetic variation, or a new, distinct source of genetic variation, and (iii) do the relative contributions of individual and shared environment vary over time and with age?

With regard to the first question of variation in the strength of heritability across age and time, some of the most consistent results involve disease onset. Using sibling, twin, and adoption designs, it has repeatedly been found that genetic inputs are more important among people who developed a condition at a younger age, relative to those who developed it at an older age. This has been found for illnesses such as cardiovascular disease,[61] breast cancer,[62] depression,[63] and alcoholism.[64] For most, the cases with earlier onset also tend to be more severe. These findings frequently lead authors to conclude that complex conditions may have distinct classes or types, and genes or environment may be more or less important across these different types.

Research on psychological outcomes (e.g., IQ or personality traits) has also revealed relatively consistent patterns, but rather than heritability declining with age, it is found to increase. Although scholars from various disciplines have critiqued genetic explanations of human intelligence and personality,[40, 65] these outcomes have been traditional foci for behavioural geneticists and have generated the largest number of studies in this area (twin, adoption, and sibling designs, both longitudinal and cross-section). Generally, these studies find that the heritability of IQ and personality increases and environmental inputs decrease as people get older.[41, 43, 66] These results illustrate that the effects of genes are not set at birth (though the actual genes (i.e. DNA sequence) is fixed at conception). However, we must also keep in mind that positive correlations between genes and environment may increase with age, and (particularly in the case of twin studies) this may lead to overestimates of heritability at older ages.

Life course variation in the heritability of health risks and behaviours is a much newer topic and results in this arena tend to be somewhat more mixed and speculative. Considering several longitudinal and cross-sectional twin and adoption studies, there seems to be very little consensus on whether the heritability of BMI increases or decreases with age—some studies have identified increases,[67] others decreases,[68] and some have been unable to detect any discernable pattern[69] (for a more thorough review see reference 70). When it comes to smoking behaviour, increasing heritability at older ages is observed, but this is intimately linked to smoking trajectories and, most likely, to the addictive nature of nicotine.[71, 72] A substantial amount of variation in smoking initiation, which typically occurs during adolescence, is associated with environmental factors shared by siblings. The persistence of smoking behaviour through older ages appears to depend in large part on genetic variation.[71, 72] This suggests there may be environmental vulnerability toward exposure to tobacco, but the likelihood of addiction and persistence of smoking may be in large part genetic.

With regard to the second question, several studies document dynamic genetic processes over time. Many of the numerous studies on psychological outcomes (IQ and personality) and most of the more recent, sparser studies on BMI suggest that genetic effects at later ages do not reflect the mere persistence of earlier genetic variation, but rather new patterns of genetic variation[41, 43, 69, 73] (for an exception to this pattern in the BMI literature see reference 74). That is, genetic expression of various traits appears to be changing with age. Although studies in this area are relatively new, and results need to be replicated, these findings suggest that the effects of genes on phenotype (e.g., gene expression), as well as the importance of genes relative to environment (i.e., heritability), may vary across the life course.

Finally, many researchers have been puzzled by results related to the third question of individual and shared environment. Studies for most psychological outcomes (e.g., IQ, personality, and behavioural characteristics), and the more limited studies on health risk/behaviours (e.g., BMI) reveal much lower estimates for family-level (i.e., shared) environmental inputs than many would expect; and, in several cases, these inputs appear to decline over time.[41, 43, 70, 75] In other words, for these outcomes, individual-level (i.e., within-sibling) differences in environment appear more important across the life course. These results have been troubling to several scholars who believe that families are important to children's outcomes, and they have led some scholars to question the general assumption that family effects are reflected with sibling similarities (see, e.g. reference 40). These authors point out that several aspects of family environment (e.g., parental treatment) may accentuate, rather than reduce, sibling differences, and this does not imply that families or parents matter any less. Recent sociological work has highlighted that within-family differences in environment and outcomes may be heightened when families have fewer resources.[1] Other authors have emphasized that individual-level environmental effects may reflect a gene-environment interaction as parents respond to differences in their children's attributes.[3]

3.4 Genetic linkage studies

Genetic linkage studies that involve families with more than one member affected by a disease provide a means for locating any predisposing genes on a particular chromosome by following the extent of allelic sharing across genomes of family members with the disease. Specifically, since full siblings share 50% of their alleles on average, pairs of affected siblings can be used to identify chromosomal regions that may contain genes whose variations are related to the disease being studied.[76] There are however three areas of concern that frequently occur in such studies with the research on complex traits leading to disease.[77,78] First, there are issues of lack of statistical power due to relatively small sample sizes used. Second, there may also be a lack of replication in results due to the heterogeneity of the predisposition, i.e. the disease may occur due to distinct rather than shared sets of predisposing genes in related individuals.[77] Last, issues of compatibility and interpretation arise from the use of the various statistical techniques, each with its own relative merits that have been developed for investigating linkage studies. In contrast, the strength of these studies is apparent when investigating susceptibility due to a single allele. If the study spans the life course, then further questions are possible in identifying the specificity of the predisposition with respect to timing of early or late onset disease or to class-defined trajectories across the life course for outcomes such as alcohol intake and physical activity levels.

3.5 Conclusion

Comparing outcomes within full or twin sibling pairs is an effective strategy to reduce bias from residual confounding, and sibling FE models are an important tool in the effort to obtain accurate causal estimates from observational data. Comparing sibling FE estimates to non-FE estimates for a broader population can also yield insight into the relative importance of individual and shared family determinants. However, as discussed, the insight that we can gain from sibling FE models depends on how well we understand what does and does not vary across siblings. If we misunderstand, for instance, the extent to which income varies across siblings' childhoods, we risk significantly misinterpreting sibling FE estimates. Thus far, sibling and twin FE models provide considerable evidence that birth weight impacts later-life health and socioeconomic status, independent of shared family-level characteristics. However, sibling analyses of potential mechanisms linking birth weight to later-life wellbeing are less conclusive, and this is an important problem for future research.

Comparison across different types of siblings (e.g., across different types of twins, or across adopted and biological siblings) is a useful strategy for untangling nature and nurture. However, greater environmental similarity among genetically-related siblings may lead to overestimates of genetic heritability in many cases. Gene-environment interactions are likely an important source of difference across people, but they are also difficult to estimate given the complexity of gene-environment interactions and unobserved correlations. It is likely that the best way to get at gene-environment interactions would be including randomized environmental exposures in future BG studies. As has been discussed, much of the research on how nature and nurture vary across the life course remains relatively new, particularly for health risks and behaviours (e.g., BMI or smoking). The dynamic and complex nature of social context adds further challenges when investigating gene-environment interactions across the life course. Thus far, work in this area points to dynamic processes of genetic expression across the life course, as well as to how the complex and dynamic nature of social context adds further challenges to the identification of gene-environment interactions. It raises several questions about how the family environment leads to sibling differences and similarities that remain to be answered.

References

1 Conley D. *The Pecking Order: a bold new look at how family and society determine who we become.* Vintage Books, New York, 2005.
2 Dunn J, Polmin R. Why are siblings so different? the significance of differences in sibling experiences within the family. *Family Process* 1991; **30**: 271–83.
3 Plomin R, Asbury K, Dunn J. Why are children in the same family so different? nonshared environment a decade later. *Canadian Journal of Psychiatry* 2001; **46**: 225–33.
4 Rowe D, Plomin R. The importance of nonshared (E-sub-1) environmental influences in behavioural development. *Developmental Psychology* 1981; **17**: 517–31.
5 Pickles A, Maughan B, Wadsworth. *Epidemiological methods in life course research.* Oxford University Press, Oxford, 2007.
6 Robins E, Guze SB. Establishment of diagnostic validity in psychiatric illness: its application to schizophrenia. *American Journal of Psychiatry* 1970; **126**: 107–11.
7 Marmot MG, Wadsworth MEJ. Fetal and early childhood environment: long term health implications. *British Medical Bulletin* 1997; **53**: 3–9.
8 Kuh D, Shlomo YB. *A Lifecourse Approach to Chronic Disease Epidemiology.* Oxford University Press, New York, 2004.
9 Lynch J, Davey-Smith G. A life course approach to chronic disease epidemiology. *Annual Review of Public Health* 2004; **26**: 1–35.
10 Conley D, Strully K, Neil B. *The Starting Gate: birth weight and life chances.* University of California Press, Berkeley, CA, 2003.
11 Aber J, Bennett N, Conley D, Li J. The effects of poverty on child health and development. *Annual Review of Public Health* 1997; **18**: 63–83.
12 Davey Smith G. Introduction. In: Davey Smith G, editor. *Health Inequalities: life course approaches,* pp. xii-lix. The Policy Press, Bristol, 2003.
13 Davey Smith G, Lawlor DA, Harbord R, Timpson N, Day INM, Ebrahim S. Clustered environments and randomized genes: a fundamental distinction between conventional and genetic epidemiology. *Plos-Medicine* 2007; **4**: e352.
14 Fall C. Developmental origins of cardiovascular disease, type 2 diabetes and obesity in humans. In: Wintour M, Owens J, editors. *Early life origins of health and disease,* pp. 8–27. Springer Science and Business Media, 2006.
15 Gross R, Spiker D, Haynes C, eds. *Helping Low Birth Weight, premature babies: the infant health and development program.* Stanford University Press, Stanford, CA, 1997.
16 Case A, Fertig A, Paxson C. From cradle to grave: the lasting impact of childhood health and circumstance. *National Bureau of Economic Research Working Paper,* 9788, 2003.
17 Hack M, Flannery D, Schluchter M, Cartar L, Borawski E, Klein N. Outcomes in young adulthood for very low birth weight infants. *The New England Journal of Medicine* 2002; **346**: 149–57.
18 Wintour M, Owens J, eds. *Early Life Origins of Health and Disease.* Springer Science and Business Media, 2006.
19 Hattersley A, Tooke J. The fetal insulin hypothesis: an alternative explanation of the association of low birthweight with diabetes and vascular disease. *The Lancet* 1999; **353**: 1789–92.
20 Woolridge J. *Introductory Econometrics.* South-Western College Publishing, 2003.

21. Duncan G, Brooks-Gunn J, Yeung J, Smith J. How much does childhood poverty affect the life chances of children? *American Sociological Review* 1998; **63**: 406–23.
22. Duncan G, Brooks-Gunn J, eds. *Consequences of Growing Up Poor*. Russell Sage Foundation, New York, 1997.
23. Morley R, Dwyer T, Carlin J. Studies of twins: what can they tell us about the developmental origins of adult health and disease? In: Wintour M, Owens J, eds. *Early Life Origins of Health and Disease*, pp. 29–41. Springer Science and Business Media, 2006.
24. Behrman J, Rosenzweig M. Returns to birthweight. *Review of Economics and Statistics* 2004; **86**: 586–601.
25. Black S, Devereux P, Salvanes K. From the cradle to the labor market? The effect of birth weight on adult outcomes. *Institute for the Study of Labor (IZA) Discussion Paper* **1864**, 2005.
26. Lawlor D, Hübinette A, Tynelius P, Leon D, Smith G, Rasmussen F. Associations of gestational age and intrauterine growth with systolic blood pressure in a family-based study of 386,485 Men in 331,089 families. *Epidemiology* 2007; **115**: 562–68.
27. Haas S. Health selection and the process of social stratification: the effect of childhood health on socioeconomic attainment. *Journal of Health and Social Behavior* 2006; **47**: 339–54.
28. Matte TD, Bresnahan M, Begg MD, Susser E. Influence of variation in birthweight within normal range and within sibships on IQ at age 7 years: cohort study. *BMJ* 2001; **323**(7308): 310–14.
29. Lawlor DA, Bor W, O'Callaghan MJ, Williams GM, Najman JM. Intrauterine growth and intelligence within sibling pairs: findings from the Mater-University study of pregnancy and its outcomes. *J Epidemiol Community Health* 2005; **59**(4): 279–82.
30. Bergvall N, Iliadou A, Tuvemo T, Cnattingius S. Birth Characteristics and Risk of Low Intellectual Performance in Early Adulthood: Are the Associations Confounded by Socioeconomic Factors in Adolescence or Familial Effects? *Pediatrics* 2006; **117**(3): 714–21.
31. Lawlor DA, Clark H, Davey Smith G, Leon DA. Intrauterine growth and intelligence within sibling pairs: findings from the Aberdeen children of the 1950s cohort. *Pediatrics* 2006; **117**(5): 894–902.
32. Record RG, McKeown T, Edwards JH. The relation of measured intelligence to birthweight and duration of gestation. *Ann Hum Genet* 1969; **33**(1): 71–9.
33. Currie J, Stabile M. Mental health in childhood and human capital. *National Bureau of Economic Research Working Paper* **13217**, 2007.
34. Geronimus A, Korenman S. Maternal youth and family background? on the health disadvantages of infants with teenage mothers. *American Journal of Epidemiology* 1993; **137**: 213–25.
35. Geronimus A, Korenman S, Hillemeier M. Does young maternal age adversely affect child development? Evidence from cousin comparisons in the US *Population and Development Review* 1994; **20**: 585–609.
36. Joyce T, Kaestner R, Korenman S. The effect of pregnancy intentions on child development. *Demography* 2000; **37**: 83–94.
37. Plomin R. *Nature and nurture: an introduction to human behavioural genetics*. Wadsworth Publishing Co, Belmont, CA, 2004.
38. Hewitt J, Turner R. Behavior genetic approaches in behavioral medicine: an introduction. In: Turner R, Cardon L, Hewitt J, eds. *Behavior Genetic Approaches in Behavioural Medicine* pp. 3–16. Plenum Press, New York, 1995.
39. Reiss D, Neiderhiser J, Hetherington E, Plomin R. *The Relationship Code: deciphering genetic and social patterns in adolescent development* Harvard University Press, Cambridge, MA, 1999.
40. Maccoby E. Parenting and its effects on children: on reading and misreading behaviour genetics *Annual Review of Psychology* 2000; **51**: 1–27.
41. McGue M, Bouchard T. Genetic and environmental influences on human behavioural differences *Annual Review of Neuroscience* 1998; **21**: 1–24.
42. Lewontin R. *The Triple Helix: gene, organism and environment*. Harvard University Press, Cambridge, MA, 2000.

43 **Loehlin J, Horn J, Willerman L.** Modeling IQ change: evidence from the Texas Adoption Project *Child Development* 1989; **60**: 993–1004.

44 **Howe D.** Age at placement, adoption experience and adult adopted people's contact with their adoptive and birth mothers: an attachment perspective *Attachment and Human Development* 2001; **3**: 222–37.

45 **Dunn J, Plomin R.** Determinants of maternal behaviour toward three-year-old siblings *British Journal of Development Psychology* 1986; **57**: 348–56.

46 **Plomin R, DeFries J, Fulker D.** *Nature and Nurture During Infancy and Early Childhood*. Brooks-Cole, Pacific Grove, CA, 1988.

47 **Fisher A.** Still 'not quite as good as having your own?' Toward a sociology of adoption *Annual Review of Sociology* 2003; **29**: 335–61.

48 **Magnusson P, Rasmussen F.** Familial resemblance of body mass index and familial risk of high and low body mass index: A study of young men in Sweden *International Journal of Obesity*, 2006; **26**: 1225–31.

49 **Conley D, Strully K.** Estimating genetic-environmental interaction effects: The case of race, birth weight and infant mortality, unpublished manuscript, 2007.

50 **Guo G, Stearns E.** The social influences on the realization of genetic potential for intellectual development *Social Forces* 2002; **80**: 881–910.

51 **Sørensen T, Holst C, Stunkard A.** Adoption study of environmental modifications of the genetic influences on obesity *International Journal of Obesity and Related Metabolic Disorders* 1998; **22**: 73–81.

52 **Turkheimer E, Haley A, Waldron M, D'Onofrio B, Gottesman I.** SES modifies heritability of IQ in young children *Psychological Science* 2003: **14**: 623–8.

53 **Liu L, Li Y, Tollefschol T.** Gene-environment interactions and the epigenetic basis of human disease *Current Issues in Molecular Biology* 2008; **10**: 25–36.

54 **Miltenberger R, Mynatt R, Wilkinson J, Woychik R.** The role of the *agouti* gene in the yellow obese syndrome *The Journal of Nutrition* 1997; **127**: 1902S–1907S.

55 **Yu M, Chen C, Wang C, et al.** Chronological change in genetic variance and heritability of systolic and diastolic blood pressure among Chinese twin neonates *Acta Genet Med Gemellol* 1990; **39**: 99–108.

56 **Keller K, Pietrobelli A, Johnson S, Faith M.** Maternal restriction of children's eating and encouragements to eat as the 'non-shared environment': a pilot study using the child feeding questionnaire *International Journal of Obesity* 2006 **30**: 1670–5.

57 **Faith M.** Development and modification of child food preferences and eating patterns: behaviour genetics strategies *International Journal of Obesity* 2005; **29**: 549–56.

58 **Faraone S, Doyle A.** The nature and heritability of attention-deficit/hyperactivity disorder *Child Adolesc Psychiatr Clin N Am* 2001; **10**: 299–316.

59 **Clausson B, Lichtnstein P, Cnattingius S.** Genetic influence on birthweight and gestational length determined by studies in offspring of twins *British Journal of Obstetrics and Gynecology* 2000; **107**: 375–81.

60 **Brooks A, Johnson M, Steer P, Pawon M, Abdalla H.** Birth weight: nature or nurture? *Early Human Development* 1995; **42**: 29–35.

61 **Arnett D, Baird A, Barkley R, et al.** Relevance of genetics and genomics for prevention and treatment of cardiovascular disease: a scientific statement from the American Heart Association Council on Epidemiology and Prevention, the Stroke Council, and the Functional Genomics and Translational Biology Interdisciplinary Working Group *Circulation* 2007: **115**: 2878–901.

62 **King M, Lee G, Spinner N, Thomson G, Wrensch M.** Genetic epidemiology *Annual Review of Public Health* 1984; **5**: 1–52.

63 **Baldwin R, Tomenson B.** Depression in later life: a comparison of symptoms and risk factors in early and late onset causes *British Journal of Psychiatry* 1995; **167**: 649–52.

64 **McCue M.** Mediators and moderators of alcoholism inheritance. In: Turner R, Cardon L, Hewitt J, eds. *Behavior Genetic Approaches in Behavioral Medicine*, pp. 17–44. Plenum Press, New York, 1995.

65 **Fischer C, Hout M, Jankowski M, Lucas S, Swingler A, Voss K.** *Inequality by Design: cracking the bell curve myth.* Princeton University Press, Princeton, NJ, 1996.

66 Plomin R, Nesselroade J. Behavioral genetics and personality change *Journal of Personality* 1990; **58**: 191–220.
67 Stunkard A, Foch T, Hrubec Z. A twin study of human obesity *JAMA* 1986; **256**: 51–54.
68 Korkeila M, Kaprio J, Rissanen A, Koskenvuo M. Consistency and change in body mass index and weight: a study on 5967 adult Finnish twin pairs *International Journal of Obesity* 1995; **19**: 310–17.
69 Cardon L. Genetic influences on body mass index in early childhood. In: Turner R, Cardon L, Hewitt J, eds. *Behavior Genetic Approaches in Behavioral Medicine*, pp. 133–44. Plenum Press, New York, 1995.
70 Maes H, Neale M, Eaves L. Genetic and environmental factors in relative body weight and human adiposity *Behaviour Genetics* 1997; **27**: 325–51.
71 Heath A, Madden P. Genetic influences on smoking behaviour. In: Turner R, Cardon L, Hewitt J, eds. *Behavior Genetic Approaches in Behavioral Medicine*, pp. 45–65. Plenum Press, New York, 1995.
72 Rowe D, Linver M. Smoking and addiction behaviours: epidemiological, individual, and family factors. In: Turner R, Cardon L, Hewitt J, eds. *Behaviour Genetic Approaches in Behavioural Medicine*, pp. 67–86. Plenum Press, New York, 1995.
73 Fabsitz R, Carnelli D, Hewitt J. Evidence for independent genetic influences on obesity in middle age *International Journal of Obesity* 1992; **16**: 657–66.
74 Meyer J, Silberg J, Eaves L, *et al.* Variable age of gene expression: implications for developmental genetic models. In: LaBuda M, Grigorenko E, eds. *On the Way to Individuality: current methodological issues in behavioral genetics*. Moscow: Progress Publishers, 1996.
75 Hewitt J. The genetics of obesity: what have genetic studies told us about the environment *Behavior Genetics* 1997; **27**: 353–58.
76 Hernandez L, Blazer D. *Genes, Behaviour, and the Social Environment: moving beyond the nature/nurture debate*. National Academy of Sciences, Washington, 2006.
77 Greenwood T, Libiger O, Kardia S, Hanis C, Morrison A, Gu C, Rice, T, Miller M, Turner S, Myers R, Grove J, Hsiao C, Weder A, Schork N. Comprehensive linkage and linkage heterogeneity analysis of the 4344 sibling pairs affected with hypertension from the Family Blood Pressure Program. *Genetic Epidemiology*, 2007; **31**: 195–210.
78 Crow T. How and why genetic linkage has not solved the problem of psychosis: review and hypothesis. *American Journal of Psychiatry* 2007; **164**: 13–21.

Chapter 4

Theoretical underpinning for the use of twin studies in life course epidemiology

Ruth J F Loos, Charlotte L Ridgway and Ken K Ong

Abstract

This chapter explores how twin-specific characteristics allow a unique insight into the balance of genetic and environmental influences that underlie early-life associations with later disease risks. However, we also describe how the unique determinants of birth weight in twins necessitate caveats in the interpretation of twin studies in life course epidemiology.

The classical twin design is used in genetic epidemiology to estimate the heritability of a trait or disease. Despite potential biases for certain traits at specific stages during the life course, the classical twin method remains a robust and useful tool in human genetics when interpreted with care.

Twins have also been applied to study the fetal origins of adult disease hypothesis. Twins have unique genetic and prenatal characteristics, which can be modelled to disentangle the complex mechanisms that underlie the 'fetal origins' of later disease risks. However, these models have important caveats. The prenatal and early life of twins is substantially different from that of singletons. At birth twins weigh on average 600 g less than singletons, even when their shorter gestation is taken into account. Although this potentially increases the twins' risk for adult disease compared to singleton there is no conclusive evidence to support this notion. Importantly, average birth weight also differs across the major sub-types of twins: monozygotic twins weigh less than dizygotic twins, and monozygotic monochorionic twins weigh less than monozygotic dichorionic twins. These differences in birth weight can be related to zygosity, chorionicity, and location of umbilical cord insertion in the placenta, and these observations challenge several of the assumptions implicit in the above models.

To date, most twin studies have had limited statistical power to robustly test the complex modelling of inter- and intra-pair associations between prenatal environment and adult disease risk. Current very large studies will provide more robust comparisons between the effects of fetal genes, shared maternal environment and individual fetoplacental environment.

4.1 Introduction

For many centuries and across civilisations twins have captured our curiosity, scientist and lay people alike.

Twins are fairly common, even more so since the introduction of fertility treatments which have caused a dramatic rise in the twinning rate in industrialized countries.[1–3] While the spontaneous twinning rate of monozygotic ('identical') twin births is fairly constant at around 4 per 1,000 deliveries, the prevalence of dizygotic ('non-identical' or 'fraternal') twin births varies across ethnicity. The spontaneous dizygotic twinning rate is twice as high among women of African origin (~16/1,000 deliveries) than among women of European ancestry (8/1,000), while it is low in East Asian women (2/1,000).[4] Furthermore, dizygotic twin births have increased prevalence among women over the age of 35, women of greater parity, and those with a maternal family history of twins.[5] Of concern is the striking impact of fertility treatments on the twinning rate. The increasing use of assisted reproductive technologies since the mid-1970s coupled with a rising maternal age at conception, has and continues to, increase the twinning rate of primarily dizygotic twins, but also monozygotic twins.[6–8] The current twinning rate in industrialized countries is 1.2 to 1.5 fold higher than three decades ago.[1–3, 9]

Because of their unique characteristics, it has long been recognized that twins offer valuable opportunities for clinical, psychosocial, and genetic research. Twin registries have been established around the world. Some registries have existed for decades and have carefully collected longitudinal data on behavioural and metabolic traits, disease outcomes and environmental risk factors in large samples of twins and their families.[10]

Broadly speaking, two types of research directions can be distinguished; (a) the research that studies the biology of twinning, twin-specific pre-natal and neonatal pathology, twin development and behavioural characteristics as the main outcome, and (b) the research that takes advantage of the characteristics of twins to better understand genetic and environmental causes of diseases or traits in the general population. This chapter explores how the twin-specific characteristics influence the generalisability of twin studies in life course epidemiology. We start with a brief overview of the classical twin design used in genetic epidemiology to estimate the heritability of a trait or disease. The main focus of this chapter lies in the second part that explores the use of twins to study the fetal origins of adult disease hypothesis. In light of this hypothesis, the determinants of twin birth weight are discussed. We review the specific advantages of using twins, key assumptions, generalisability, and limitations, illustrated with recent examples.

4.2 The classical twin design—Nature versus nurture

As early as 1875, Galton recognized that twins could contribute to the unravelling of nature and nurture by studying them from childhood into adulthood to observe whether they grew more or less similar.[11] In his article 'The History of Twins',[11] Galton described how 35 pairs were almost identical, while 20 other pairs showed extreme dissimilarity, of whom none grew more similar over time. Although Galton recognized that there were similar and dissimilar pairs, it is doubted that he indeed knew these pairs were biologically two distinct twin types. In the years that followed Galton's observations the biology of twinning confused many and it was only in the early 1900s that the obstetric literature supported the existence of the two types of twins; the one-egg (monozygotic) and two-egg (dizygotic) twins.[12] In 1924, Merriman[13] and Siemens[14] reported for the first time, and independent of each other, the principles that underlie the classical twin study. Merriman, an educational psychologist, found the similarity of intelligence tests in identical twins to be higher than the similarity of the total twin population.[13] Siemens, a dermatologist, studied skin moles in twins and found an intra-pair (or 'within-pair') correlation in mole count of 0.40 in identical and 0.20 in non-identical twins.[14]

4.2.1 Basic principles

The classical twin design relies on the distinct genetic characteristics of monozygotic as compared to dizygotic twins. Monozygotic twins arise from a single fertilized ovum and are therefore genetically identical (with some exceptions—see Section 4.3.3). Dizygotic twins originate from two separately fertilized ova and share on average half of their genes, similar to non-twin siblings. The heritability of a trait or disease, defined as the proportion of the total variance that is explained by genetic factors, is derived from the comparison of the intra-pair similarity (correlation or concordance) in monozygotic twins with the intra-pair similarity in dizygotic twins. A greater similarity between monozygotic than dizygotic pairs is considered evidence of genetic influences. The heritability of a trait can be simply derived by calculating twice the difference between monozygotic and dizygotic intra-pair correlations; $h^2 = 2*(r_{MZ} - r_{DZ})$.[15] For example, the monozygotic and dizygotic intra-pair correlations for adult height are about 0.90 and 0.50 and therefore the heritability estimate is ~80%.[16] For behavioural characteristics, the pattern of intra-pair correlations tends to be different. For example, the intra-pair correlations for taking up smoking during adolescence in monozygotic and dizygotic twins are 0.90 and 0.70 respectively, resulting in an estimated 40% heritability.[17] In this case, the intra-pair correlation in dizygotic twins is more than half that of the monozygotic twins, which suggests that the environment shared by both twin members plays a role. The shared family environment results in higher dizygotic intra-pair correlations than would be expected if taking up smoking were only influenced by genetic factors.

With regard to the proportion of shared genetic factors, dizygotic twins are similar to pairs of ordinary siblings. However, given the potential influences of age and prenatal environment on the outcomes of interest, dizygotic twins have the merit of removing these potential confounders and match monozygotic twins as closely as possible for pre- and post-natal conditions.

The early results of heritability studies resulted in major changes in the way scientists and lay people thought about certain diseases. Traits and diseases such as attention deficit hyperactivity disorder (ADHD), autism, substance abuse, depression, and others were no longer considered solely due to environmental factors, but through twin heritability studies it was recognized that the etiology of these traits also had significant genetic components.[18–21]

4.2.2 Genetic model fitting

Although the simple heritability calculations, described above, provide a quick and easy way to estimate the genetic contribution to a disease or trait, they do not accommodate the estimation of combined effects of genes and environment.

The statistical methodology underlying the classical twin design was revolutionized in the 1970s when genetic modelling was introduced.[22] Genetic modelling is a hypothesis-testing approach that uses structural equation modelling, also known as covariance modelling, and allows more in-depth insights into the genetic and environmental architecture underlying variation in disease or traits.

In brief, hypotheses are translated into mathematical models that assume: (i) perfect intra-pair correlation between the shared environments of both twin members of monozygotic as well as dizygotic pairs, (ii) perfect intra-pair correlation between the genetic components in monozygotic twins, and (iii) an intra-pair correlation of 0.50 for additive (or 0.25 for dominant) genetic components in dizygotic twins (Figure 4.1). Depending on the hypothesis, the model partitions the

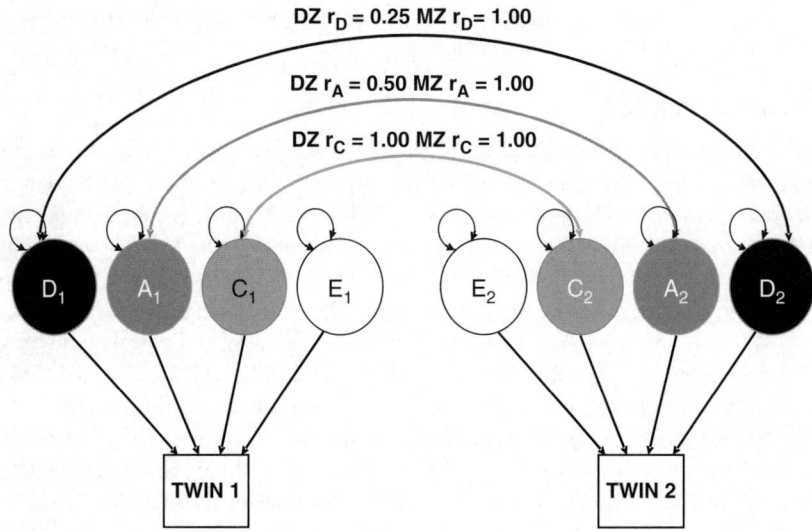

Fig. 4.1 Path diagram for the classical twin study.

D: dominant genetic latent factor; A: Additive genetic factor; C: shared environmental latent factor; E: unique environmental latent factor. DZ: dizygotic twins; MZ: monozygotics twins. (Used with permission from *British Journal of Obstetrics and Gynaecology*: **108**, Loos RJF, 'Birthweight in live-born twins', pgs 943–948. Copyright Elsevier (2001).)

total observed variance of a trait into unmeasured genetic and environmental variances. The genetic variance may be due to additive (A) or dominant (D) genetic influences. The environmental variance can be divided into common environment (C) shared by both twin members (e.g., familial environment), and unique environment (E) specific to each twin member. For example, an ACE-model hypothesises that a trait is influenced by additive genetic (A) as well as shared (C) and unique (E) environmental components, whereas an AE-model assumes that only genes and unique environment contribute to the variance of the trait. To test the hypothesis, data predicted by the model are compared with the observed data; the model is 'fitted', for which a variety of statistical functions such as maximum likelihood and weighted least squares are available. Generally, several models are fitted and the model that fits the observed data best is considered to reflect the true genetic and environmental architecture underlying the total variance most closely.

To assess the complex interplay between genes and environment, genetic modelling allows for testing of a variety of models that can include multiple outcome variables, gene-environment interactions, longitudinal data, age and gender-effects, latent factors, and even data from other siblings and parents. For more complex models, large twin populations are needed to perform meaningful comparisons between different models and to estimate all parameters with sufficient power.

For example, Silventoinen et al.[23] applied a longitudinal twin model to estimate the heritability of growth between age 3y and 12y in 7,755 twin pairs. The heritability estimates ranged from 58% to 91 % for height and from 31% to 82% for BMI. Of interest is that with increasing age the heritability estimates decrease while the contribution of environment become more important for both height and BMI. A more complex model was used in another study to estimate the heritability of age at menarche that included not only twins but also mothers, sisters and female spouses of male twins.[24] A strong genetic component was observed suggesting that at least 70% of variation in age at menarche is heritable.[24]

4.2.3 Assumptions and limitations

The classical twin design aims to estimate the genetic and environmental contributions to a trait or disease in the general population and thus assumes that twins are representative for the general population. However, for traits that relate to prenatal life and early childhood in particular (e.g., birth weight and early growth), this assumption may not be correct and thus the classical twin study may not provide accurate genetic and environmental estimates.[25, 26] Also certain diseases later in life tend to be more common in monozygotic twins than in the general population.[27] However, there is evidence showing that the disadvantaged early environments of twins vanishes by age five years.[28, 29]

Another important assumption to the classical twin design is the equal-environment assumption; i.e. the shared environment between members of a pair is the same for monozygotic and dizygotic twins. This assumption has been debated vigorously as it has been shown repeatedly that monozygotic twins experience more similar environments than dizygotic twins, both in childhood and in later life.[30–34] Parents and teachers may treat monozygotic twins more similarly than dizygotic twins and monozygotic twins might spend more time together and have the same social networks, unlike dizygotic twins. The higher environmental similarity within monozygotic pairs potentially increases the intra-pair correlation for certain traits and would therefore tend to exaggerate the heritability estimates. The validity of the equal-environment assumption has been examined mainly in the context of psychiatric and substance abuse disorders. Some studies showed indeed that for traits like bulimia and initiation of smoking the equal-environment assumption may be violated,[35, 36] whereas for other traits such as major depression, phobia, generalized anxiety disorder, aggression, and alcoholism the assumption was valid.[35, 37–39] It is not known whether the equal-environment- assumption is supported for other lifestyle behaviours (e.g., diet, physical activity and sport participation), physical characteristics and skills, metabolic traits, and diseases, or even intelligence.

The assumption that MZ twin are genetically identical is true in general; MZ twins result from the splitting of one ovum and thus the nuclear DNA at conception is identical. However, the mitochondrial DNA (mtDNA) is not transmitted through the nucleus but passed on separately through the maternal line and not necessarily equally split between the two twin members as nuclear DNA. As variations in mtDNA have been associated to disease and metabolic traits,[40] they could potentially underlie phenotypic differences between MZ twin members.[41, 42] Furthermore, there is growing evidence that also nuclear DNA shows some differences between members of MZ pairs. DNA and chromatin are sensitive to various types of pre- and postnatal environments that might affect members of a MZ twin pair in different ways.[43–46] Examples of genetic differences between MZ twins that resulted in disease discordance have been reported before.[47–49]

Because heritability is the proportion of the total variance that is explained by genetic factors and because the genetic and/or environmental variance can vary across populations, over time, between men and women, etc., heritability represents a relative estimate that is specific to a particular population. Therefore, heritability estimates for one population at a certain time do not necessarily predict heritability for other populations or for the same population at a different time. For example, in a more restrictive or controlled environment (e.g., scarcity of food) the total variation (denominator) for a certain population will be smaller and thus the heritability estimate higher compared to heritability estimates for the same population in an unrestrictive environment.

Despite potential biases for certain traits at specific stages during the life course, the classical twin method remains a useful tool in human genetics when used with care.

4.2.4 Beyond the classical twin design

Although the classical twin study is the most widely used design, other types of twin studies have provided insights in the genetic and environmental contributions to disease and related traits.

The study of twins who were separated early in life and reared apart in different environments from early childhood is considered to be the ideal design to distinguish environmental from genetic influences as similarity within pairs can only be attributed to shared genes. Unfortunately for the genetic epidemiologist, twins reared apart are rare. Furthermore, there are concerns about the representative nature of the reared-apart twins, particularly in the context of behavioural characteristics.[50]

The 'co-twin control' model studies monozygotic twins that are discordant for a trait, disease or experimental intervention. Because monozygotic twins are closely matched for genetic background (see above for how mitochondrial DNA might vary), age and prenatal environment (see later section on zygosity and chorionicity about how there may be some differences in prenatal environment), this design allows us to isolate the postnatal environmental causes of disease or traits with greater accuracy than other study designs. For example, in an observational study of 27 monozygotic twin pairs discordant for the use of oral contraception, the twin member using oral contraception had higher systolic and diastolic blood pressure, heart rate, triglyceride, and total cholesterol levels, than the twin-sister who did not use oral contraception.[51]

Advances in high-throughput genotyping technologies, coupled with the completion of the Human Genome Project and the International HapMap Project, have set the stage for genomewide linkage and association studies. The structural equation modelling technique, used in the classical twin design, has therefore been upgraded to accommodate information on molecular markers to perform genomewide linkage analyses.[52] Also several genomewide association studies using twins are in progress.

4.3 The use of twins in examining determinants of birth weight

The intra-uterine growth and birth weight of twins differs substantially across the different types of twins. Therefore, we will give a brief overview of the twin types and their characteristics, before discussing the determinants of birth weight and birth weight discordance in the different twin types.

4.3.1 Zygosity and chorionicity

Zygosity distinguishes between monozygotic and dizygotic twins based on the number of fertilized eggs (or zygotes) from which the pair arose. Zygosity underlies all genetic twin designs, as described above, and it is the twin feature that is well-known to the general public as it generally results in physical resemblance or not in post-natal life.

Chorionicity or placentation distinguishes between monochorionic and dichorionic twins based on the number of placentas and thus chorionic membranes. Monochorionic fetuses share one placenta, whereas dichorionic fetuses each have their own placenta that sometimes fuses during pregnancy. This feature is generally unknown to the general public as it mainly affects prenatal life. However, chorionicity is of great importance to obstetricians as it is the main determinant of twin and multiple pregnancy outcomes. Monochorionic placentation increases the risk of early pregnancy loss and increases the risk of adverse perinatal outcome and pregnancy complications compared to dichorionic placentation.[3, 53–55] The distinction between monochorionic and dichorionic twins can be made by ultrasound examination in the first and early second trimester. According to the number of amnionic membranes present, monochorionic twins can be divided further into monoamnionic twins and diamnionic twins.

When zygosity, chorionicity, and amniotic membranes are considered together four types of twins can be distinguished; 1) dizygotic twins, 2) monozygotic dichorionic twins, 3) monochorionic diamnionic, and 4) monochorionic monoamnionic. In dizygotic twins, who develop from the fertilization of two eggs, each embryo develops within its own membranes; all dizygotic pairs are therefore dichorionic. Monozygotic twins arise from a single fertilized egg and at some stage between the fertilization and the formation of the embryonic disc, the formative material divides into two parts, each giving rise to a complete embryo. Figure 4.2 shows how the timing of this division determines different sub-groups of monozygotic twin. If the division occurs at an early stage (before the 4th day after the conception[4]), each embryo will have a separate set of membranes (Figure 4.2A). These monozygotic twins are dichorionic and, in this respect, resemble dizygotic twins. If the division of the ovum is delayed until the blastocyst has formed (between day 4 and day 8 after conception[4]), the two embryos will share a single chorionic membrane but develop within two separate amnionic sacs (Figure 4.2B). Such pairs are monochorionic diamnionic. Exceptionally, the division of the formative material may be delayed until the embryonic disc separates from the cavities that will subsequently form the amnionic and chorionic sacs (after implantation into the endometrium).[4] When this happens the embryos will both share a single chorionic and amnionic sac. The twins are monochorionic monoamnionic (Figure 4.2C).

About 70–75% of all monozygotic twins are monochorionic, ~3% of whom are monoamnionic.[3]

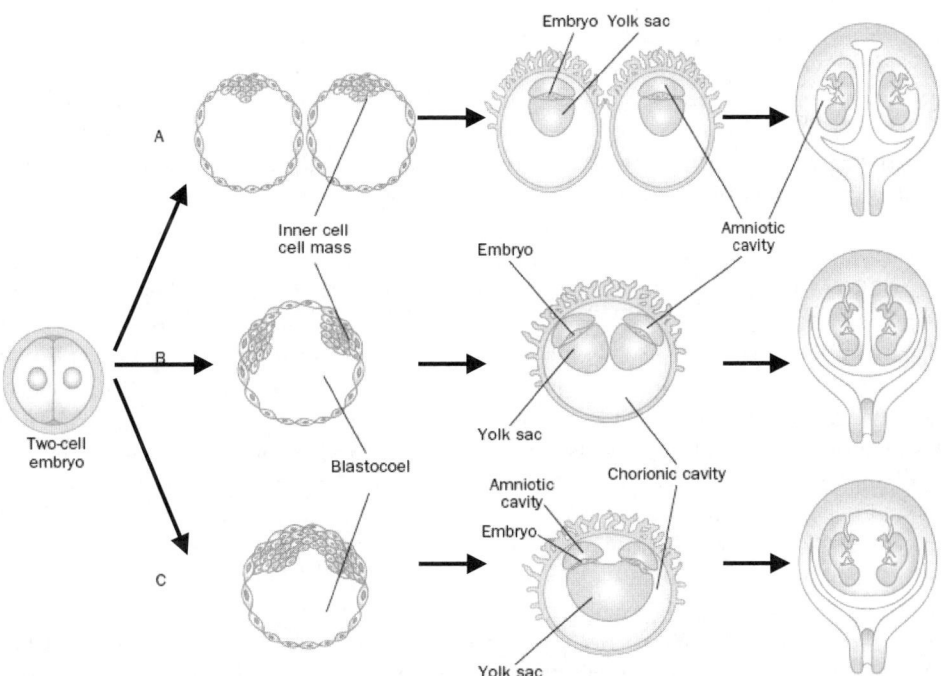

Fig. 4.2 Types of monozygotic twins according to chorionicity and membranes; A dichorionic diamniotic, B monochorionic diamniotic, C monochorionic monoamniotic (reprinted from Hall JG Twinning. 2003; *The Lancet* **362**: 735–43. Copyright (2003), with permission from Elsevier.)

4.3.2 Determinants of birth weight in twins

Birth weight depends on many factors, the most important one being gestational age. In singleton pregnancies fetal growth in the last trimester of pregnancy is linear up to 37 weeks of gestation. A twin fetus grows at the same pace as a singleton up to 32 weeks of gestation, but from then on growth levels off.[56–62] Hence, on average at birth a twin weighs about 600 g less than a singleton; even when allowance is made for the 3 to 4 week shorter gestation.[56–58, 60–62] Limited capacity in maternal-placental nutrient transfer has been suggested as the underlying cause of the birth weight discrepancy between twins and singletons, rather than placental crowding.[63–65]

In addition to the various recognized determinants of birth weight in singletons, such as sex, parity, maternal size, maternal birth weight, smoking in pregnancy, and race, the birth weight of twins is further influenced by zygosity and chorionicity. Monozygotic twins weigh on average 100 g less than dizygotic twins.[3, 59, 63, 66–68] A variety of explanations for this have been proposed, including the effects of events in early embryonic development, when cell mass is reduced by division, the possible beneficial effect that antigenic differences between dizygotic twins may have on intrauterine growth, and maternal factors, such as greater height and higher hormone concentrations in mothers of dizygotic twins.[66, 69]

Furthermore, monozygotic monochorionic twins weigh 70–90 g less than monozygotic dichorionic twins and, despite similar placentation, monozygotic dichorionic twins weigh about 60–75 g less than dizygotic twins.[54, 62, 68] Although these differences are small, they are significant and reflect different prenatal circumstances that are characteristic to each type of twins. In order to identify the prenatal determinants that underlie the birth weight differences between the four types of twins (dizygotic and three types of monozygotic twins), large population-based twin cohorts with detailed information on placentation and zygosity are needed. However, most twin studies that collect placentation data are small and are focussed on abnormal pregnancies. The East Flanders Prospective Twin Survey is unique in that it determines zygosity and collects data on placentation within 24 hours after delivery.[70] This twin cohort was established in 1964, is population-based, and registers all multiple births in the Belgian province of East Flanders of whom at least one infant weighed 500 g or more. In an analysis of 4,529 live born twin pairs they aimed to disentangle the contribution of number and fusion of placentas and site of umbilical cord insertion to the birth weight difference observed between dizygotic, monozygotic dichorionic and monozygotic monochorionic twins (Table 4.1).[71]

Their first observation was that birth weight was significantly lower when the umbilical cord was peripherally inserted on the placenta compared with a central insertion. Similar results have been reported in singletons,[72] suggesting that fetuses with a peripheral cord insertion use their placenta less efficiently. The higher incidence of a central cord insertion in dizygotic than in monozygotic twins might partly explain why dizygotic infants are heavier at birth than monozygotic twins. A second observation was that the two placentas of dichorionic pairs fuse in 50% of the pregnancies, but only in monozygotic twins did the fused dichorionic placentas result in a lower birth weight. Of interest was that when placentas fuse in monozygotic dichorionic twins, 50% of the placentas had peripheral cord insertions, whereas in dizygotic twins with fused placentas only 20% had peripheral cord insertions.

In summary, site of the umbilical cord insertion and number of placentas have independent and additive effects on birth weight of twins. Monozygotic monochorionic twins, who have to share one placenta and often experience peripheral cord insertions, have the lowest birth weights. Dizygotic twins who have two placentas, fused or separate, and mostly with central cord insertion, have the highest birth weights among twins. Monozygotic dichorionic twins are intermediate in birth weight, between monozygotic monochorionic and dizygotic twins. When their placentas fuse,

Table 4.1 Birth weight (g) according to cord insertion and fusion of placentas for dizygotic (DZ), monozygotic dichorionic (MZ DC) and monozygotic monochorionic (MZ MC) in female infants (adapted from Loos RJF, Derom C, Derom R, Vlietinck R Birthweight in liveborn twins: the influence of the umbilical cord insertion and fusion of placentas. 2001; Br J Obstet Gynaecol 108: 943–8)

Cord insertion	DZ				MZ DC				MZ MC	
	Fused placenta		Separate placentas		Fused placenta		Separate placentas		Single placenta	
	mean	(SD)	mean	(SD)	mean	(SD)	mean	(SD)	mean	(SD)
Central	2418	(519.2)	2497	(519.4)	2376	(540.6)	2537	(526.5)	2439	(501.6)
n	978		1112		145		160		583	
Peripheral	2395	(522.9)	2376	(511.6)	2215	(521.5)	2412	(529.4)	2222	(551.2)
n	255		209		139		57		537	
ANOVA										
Cord insertion	0.007				0.006				<0.001	
Number of placentas	0.25				<0.001					
Interaction	0.07				0.730					

monozygotic dichorionic twins resemble monozygotic monochorionic twins; the cord insertions are more often peripheral and birth weights are lower. When their placentas remain separate, monozygotic dichorionic resemble dizygotic twins with more central cord insertions and higher birth weights.

It is not clear why the fusion of dichorionic placentas affects birth weight in monozygotic and not in dizygotic twins. It has been speculated that the placental implantation in monozygotic dichorionic twin pregnancies is at greater proximity than in dizygotic pregnancies.[68, 73] This implies that, if the implantation of one of both fetuses occurs in a site with reduced vascular supply, the placenta will migrate towards the placenta of the other twin, i.e. to a site of better nourishment. Because of the greater proximity, placentas of monozygotic dichorionic pairs will fuse at an earlier stage than those of dizygotic pairs and therefore might hamper placental development. In monochorionic twins, who share only one placenta, unequal sharing of the placenta has been associated with a greater risk for birth weight discordance.[74] Discordant placental location, which can be posterior or anterior, did not seem to affect intra-pair birth weight difference in dichorionic twins.[75]

Analyses considering several potential birth weight determinants together showed that in twins born before 32 weeks of gestation, gestational age and sex of the fetus explained most of the variance in birth weight.[62] It should be noted that at 32 weeks of gestation or earlier, the birth weight of twins is on average less than 1,500g and similar to singleton birth weights. After 32 weeks of gestation, which coincides with a progressive divergence between singleton and twin birth weights, also cord insertion, number of placentas, birth order and maternal parity contribute to birth weight.

4.3.3 Determinants of intra twin-pair differences in birth weight

Birth weight discordance has been associated with increased risk of perinatal mortality and complications and disability in later life in some studies,[76–82] while others found that the actual birth weight of each twin, rather than the difference between the twins, is the more important determinant.[83, 84] However, most of these studies did not take into account the combined effect of zygosity and chorionicity on intra-pair birth weight difference. The intra-pair birth weight difference in dizygotic twins might be due to a different genetic predisposition of each twin member, which is not the case in monozygotic twins who have the same genetic predisposition. Monozygotic monochorionic twins have a less favourable placentation, with only one placenta to share, more frequent peripheral cord insertions and sometimes vascular anastomoses, suggesting that within the group of monozygotic twins monochorionic and dichorionic pairs should be considered separately. Evidently, although sometimes overlooked in previous studies, intra-pair birth weight differences of opposite-sex twins should be considered separately from those of same-sex twins.

Data from the East Flanders Prospective Twin Survey showed that the intra-pair birth weight difference was most pronounced in dizygotic and monozygotic monochorionic twins, and it was significantly lower in monozygotic dichorionic twins (unpublished data, Table 4.2). Consistent findings were observed in a Canadian population-based cohort study that observed a higher prevalence of birth weight discordance of 25% or more in dizygotic and monozygotic monochorionic twins compared to monozygotic dichorionic twins.[54]

The larger intra-pair birth weight difference in dizygotic twins as compared to monozygotic dichorionic twins most likely reflects the influence of genetic factors on birth weight. The reason for the larger intra-pair difference in monozygotic monochorionic twins as compared to monozygotic dichorionic twins is believed to be due to differences in placentation.

Table 4.2 Absolute (gram) and relative (%) birth weight difference (mean, SD) according to zygosity, chorionicity and sex in 4,513 twin pairs from the East Flanders Prospective Twin Survey.

	DZ		MZDC		MZMC		Kruskall-Wallis	
	mean	SD	mean	SD	mean	SD	p	
							All	DZ vs MZDC vs MZ MC
MALE-MALE								
Absolute birth weight difference	316	293	226	222	295	257	<0.0001	DZ, MZ MC > MZ DC
Relative birth weight difference	11.6	10.1	8.7	8.0	11.4	9.5	<0.0001	DZ, MZ MC > MZ DC
N	753		237		531			
FEMALE-FEMALE								
Absolute birth weight difference	299	260	238	222	306	266	0.0014	DZ, MZ MC > MZ DC
Relative birth weight difference	11.3	10.0	9.3	7.7	12.2	10.0	0.0016	DZ, MZ MC > MZ DC
N	681		256		567			
MALE-FEMALE								
Absolute birth weight difference	334	270						
Relative birth weight difference	12.3	9.3						
N	1448							

DZ: dizygotic; MZ DC: monozygotic dichorionic; MZ MC: monozygotic monochorionic.

Monochorionic twins share only one placenta, which not only results in competition for a limited food supply, but also enables vascular anastomoses between the circulations of the two fetuses, and might result in a higher prevalence of peripheral cord insertions and unequal sharing of the placenta. A smaller placenta, vascular anastomoses and unequal degree of placental sharing have been associated with large intra-pair weight differences in monochorionic twins.[74, 82, 85, 86] In addition, velamentous cord insertions and single umbilical arteries, which increase the risk of discordance in birth weight, were more prevalent in monochorionic than in dichorionic twins.[82, 87]

4.4 Twins: a tool to investigate the 'fetal origins' hypothesis

The 'fetal origins' hypothesis suggests that birth weight is inversely associated with risk of metabolic and cardiovascular disease in adult life through a long-term programming effect of suboptimal intra-uterine nutrition on later metabolism.[88] Some have suggested that the association is confounded by socio-economic factors.[89] Others have provided evidence that at least part of the association can by explained by genetic or other intergenerational factors that affect both birth weight and health in adult life.[90–93]

The genetic and prenatal characteristics, typical to the distinct twin types, provide unique opportunities to disentangle the mechanisms that underlie the 'fetal origins' hypothesis. At the same time, because these characteristics are twin-specific, interpretation and generalisation, to the general (non-twin) population, of results of twin studies should be done with care. Twin studies allow researchers to discriminate between the influences of 1) the fetoplacental environment, unique to each fetus, 2) the maternal environment, shared by both fetuses, and 3) fetal genetic influences.

4.4.1 Intra-pair birth weight differences: influence of the individual fetoplacental environment and/or fetal genes

Paired twin analyses in which the intra-pair birth weight difference is regressed against the intra-pair difference in adult health allow estimation of the importance of the individual fetoplacental environment unique to each fetus, while controlling for shared factors, such as maternal environment and genetic influences. Both members of a twin pair share the same maternal environment and, in the case of monozygotic twins, share the same fetal genes. As reflected by the intra-pair birth weight differences, each fetus has its own fetoplacental environment, which may differ substantially from that of its co-twin. In the paired analyses, it is hypothesized that the lighter twin member at birth will have a higher risk of developing cardiovascular and metabolic diseases in adult life, compared to the co-twin, who was heavier at birth (Figure 4.3). Under this hypothesis, the larger the intra-pair difference in birth weight, the larger the intra-pair difference in adult outcome will be. This can be tested by regression of intra-pair birth weight difference as the independent continuous variable and intra-pair difference in adult health outcome (for example blood pressure or BMI) as the dependent continuous variable. A significant inverse association suggests that the fetoplacental environment influences adult health independent from shared twin factors.

Comparison of the slope of the association in monozygotic twins to that observed in dizygotic twins can shed further light on the role of genes (Figure 4.4). As monozygotic twins are genetically identical, the association between the intra-pair differences in birth weight and adult outcome must be due to the individual fetoplacental environment and specifically excludes the influence of genetic factors (other than those related to mitochondrial DNA). In dizygotic twins, genetic influences cannot be excluded; one twin member may have inherited a risk allele that predisposes to both reduced intra-uterine growth and adverse adult health, whereas the co-twin might have received the protective variant. Accordingly, if the association is absent or less pronounced in monozygotic twins, but present or more pronounced in dizygotic twins, the influence of genes is suggested.

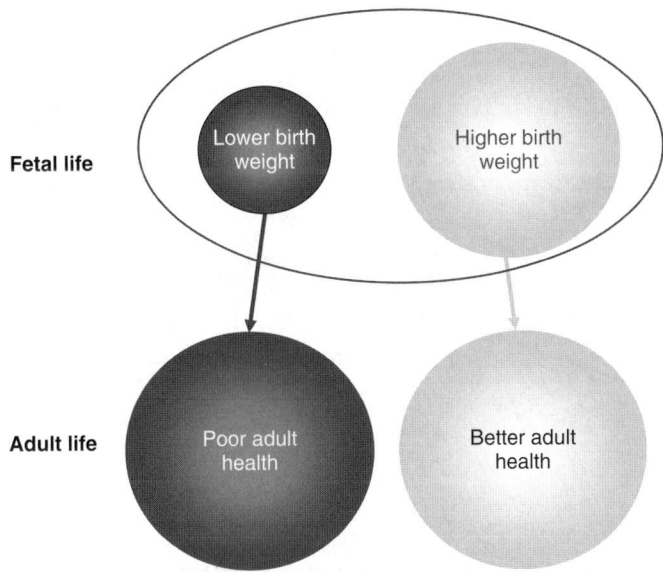

Fig. 4.3 Illustration of the fetal origins hypothesis tested by intra-pair comparison of twins: the lighter twin at birth will have a higher risk of developing adult disease, if the hypothesis is correct.

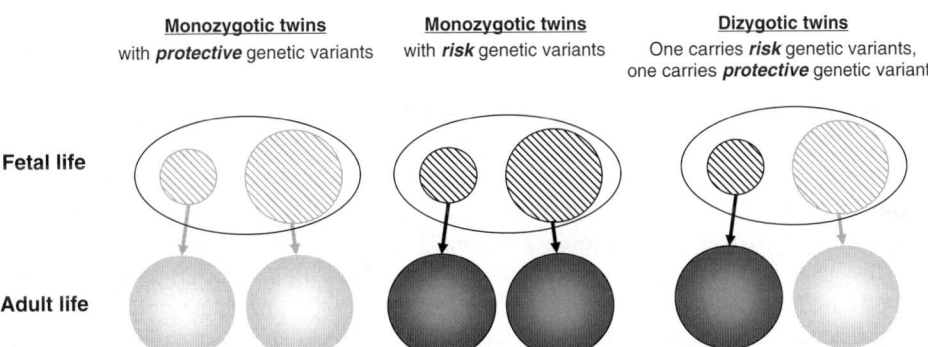

Fig. 4.4 Illustration of the fetal origins hypothesis by comparing the association between intra-pair difference in birth weight and adult outcome of monozygotic and dizygotic twins. A genetic aetiology is deduced if intra-pair differences in birth weight correspond to intra-pair differences in adult outcome only in dizygotic twins, but not in monozygotic twins.

These principles are illustrated with an example of the association between intra-pair difference in birth weight and adult height in 179 male same-sex twin pairs (116 monozygotic and 78 dizygotic pairs) from the East Flanders Prospective Twin Survey (Figure 4.5) (adapted from[94]). A positive association between intra-pair difference in birth weight and adult height was observed, indicating that lower birth weight is associated with shorter stature in adult life. The significant association in monozygotic twins suggest that a sub-optimal fetoplacental environment, reflected by a lower birth weight, has long-term effects on adult height, independent of maternal and even genetic influences. However, fetal genes do seem to play a role as the association was significantly ($p < 0.04$) more pronounced in dizygotic twins. This suggests that fetal genes

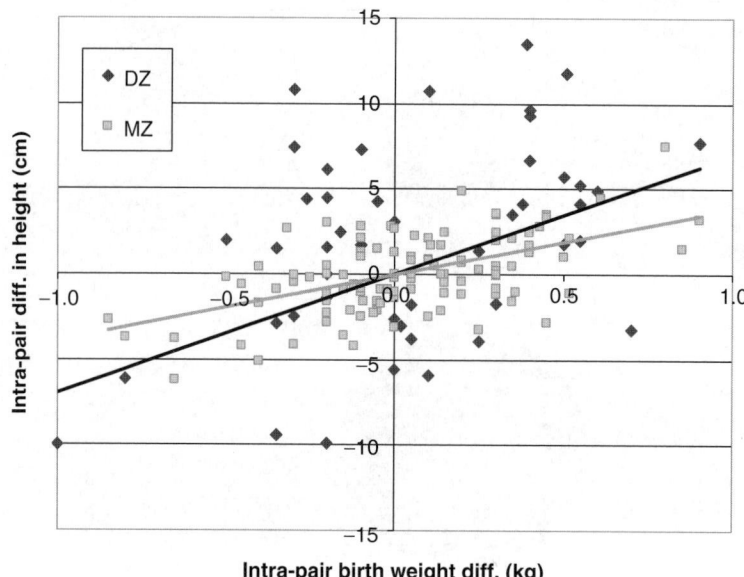

Fig. 4.5 Association between the intra-pair birth weight difference and intra-pair difference in adult height in young adult men (Reproduced with permission from Loos RJF, Beunen G, Fagard R, Derom C, Vlietinck R (2001) Birth weight and body composition in young adult men—a prospective twin study. *International Journal of Obesity*; **25**: 1537–45) MZ: monozygotic twin pairs; DZ: dizygotic twin pairs, BWD: intra-pair difference in birth weight.

that predispose to a higher birth weight may also positively influence adult height. Similar findings were observed in a Dutch study of adolescent twins.[95]

Further examples of the intra-pair twin analyses approach have been reported for body composition,[94, 96] insulin resistance,[97–100] blood pressure,[99,101–105] sympathetic activity,[106] acute myocardial infarction,[107] impaired regulation of muscle glycogen synthesis,[108] and even problem behaviour in children,[109] some of which are discussed in more detail in Chapter 13.

4.4.2 Inter-pair birth weight differences: influence of the shared maternal environment

In contrast to the intra-pair comparisons described above, the study of inter-pair (or 'between-pair') birth weight differences in twins allows us to estimate the influence of the shared maternal environment. Both twins share the same maternal environment, and therefore the influences of maternal factors, such as nutrition, hormones, nicotine, and drugs, will be shared by both twin members. It can therefore be hypothesized that if the fetal origins of cardiovascular and metabolic disease is caused by an adverse maternal environment, then both of the twins in a pair exposed to such an environment will have increased risks of developing such diseases in adult life (Figure 4.6).

For example, in a study of 418 young adult twin pairs, unpaired or 'cohort' analyses, which consider each twin member as an individual observation, showed a significant association between birth weight and adult blood pressure.[105] Fetoplacental influences unique to each twin member were excluded as no association between intra-pair birth weight difference and blood

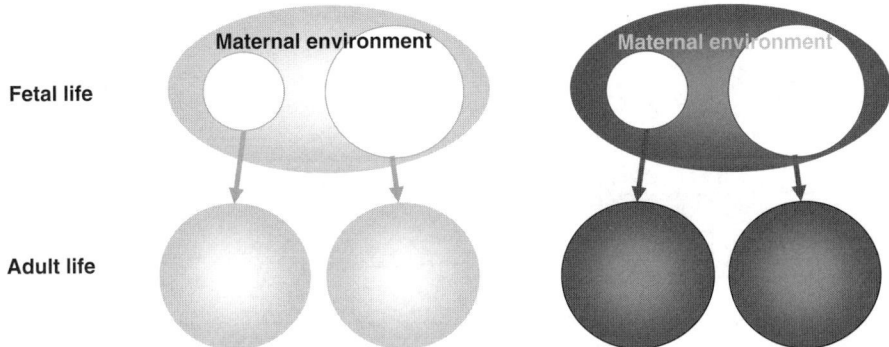

Fig. 4.6 Illustration of the fetal origins hypothesis with twins: an adverse maternal environment programs both twins.

pressure was observed. However, twin pairs of whom both members had a low birth weight both had increased blood pressure in later life, whereas in twin pairs of whom both members had a high birth weight both had lower blood pressure, indicating that the shared maternal factors that restrained the fetal growth of both twins in a pair also contributed to their higher blood pressure in later life (Figure 4.7). The same study observed that prepregnancy BMI and maternal age at delivery were more important determinants for twins' adult insulin sensitivity and β-cell function than was birth weight.[100]

4.4.3 Modelling Intra-pair and Inter-pair differences simultaneously

The individual fetoplacental (intra-pair pair analyses described in 4.5.1.) and shared environmental (between pair analyses described in 4.5.2.) influences on adult health can be modelled simultaneously in one analysis by including regression coefficients to estimate and compare the 'intra-pair' and 'inter-pair' effects. The theoretical principles of this approach have been elegantly outlined by Carlin et al.[110] and applied in relation to the fetal origins of adult blood pressure,[111] body composition,[112] and type 2 diabetes.[113] Random effects statistical models for these studies are described in detail in Chapter 11, and other statistical approaches that have also been used in these studies are noted in Chapter 12.

For example Iliadou et al.[113] used random effects modelling to investigate the relationship between birth weight and the risk of type 2 diabetes in 11,162 adult twins. They observed that between pairs the risk of type 2 diabetes increased more than twofold for every 1 kg decrease in birth weight. Within pairs, the same effect size was observed in monozygotic twins with the lower birth weight twin having an increased risk of type 2 diabetes. However, no association was observed in dizygotic twins. The findings suggest that low birth weight increases the risk of type 2 diabetes despite genetic similarity, providing some support for the hypothesis that non-genetic factors, such as aspects of the intrauterine environment that vary within twin-pairs, explain the association. Nevertheless, in that study the possibility of genetic factors that underlie both birth weight and type 2 diabetes could not be statistically excluded. This highlights the need for very large twin studies to provide robust and precise estimates with this method.

Clearly further studies modelling twin data in this way will be useful for elucidating aetiology of diseases where fetal programming may have an influence, however very large twin cohorts are needed to provide sufficient statistical power to detect and compare the intra-pair and inter-pair effects.

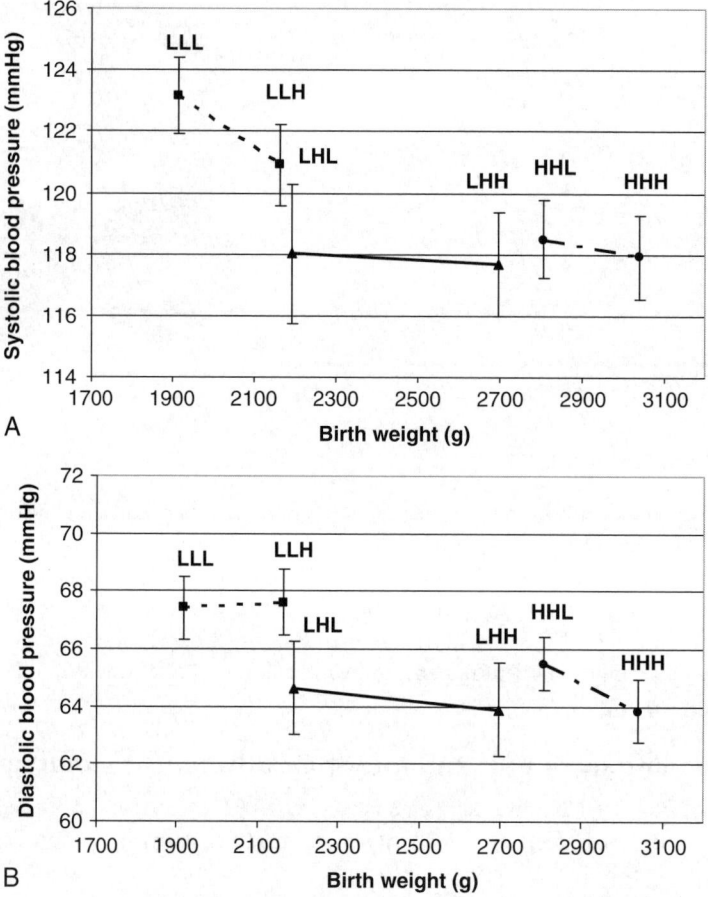

Fig. 4.7 Conventional systolic (A) and diastolic (B) blood pressure (mean and SE), adjusted for adult body mass and age, according to birth weight of female twins that were respectively:
- concordant for low birth weight, LLL and LLH (both < 2500 g)
- discordant for birth weight, LHL and LHH (one < 2500 g, one ≥ 2500 g)
- concordant for high birth weight, HHL and HHH (both ≥ 2500 g)

(Reproduced with permission from Loos RJF, Fagard R, Beunen G, Derom C, Vlietinck R (2001) Birth weight and blood pressure in young adults: a prospective twin study. *Circulation*; **104**: 1633–8).

4.4.4 Influence of zygosity and chorionicity in adult life?

As described above, the prenatal environmental circumstances of dizygotic, monozygotic dichorionic, and monozygotic dichorionic twins (Figure 4.2) differ substantially.[71] Dizygotic twin always have two placentas, and despite the fact that these placentas sometimes fuse, the umbilical cord generally remains inserted centrally to the placenta. Monozygotic dichorionic twins have two placentas, but when they fuse, the umbilical cord insertion often locates to the peripheral site of the placenta, which might impair nutrient supply. Monozygotic monochorionic twins always share one placenta, frequently have umbilical cords inserted at a peripheral site of the placenta and often have vascular anastomoses. In general, they experience the least optimal prenatal conditions.

Therefore, it can be hypothesised that monozygotic twins, the monochorionic ones in particular, are more vulnerable to prenatal programming compared to dizygotic twins and, therefore, they might have an increased risk of adult diseases.

Because only few population-based twin registers collect zygosity and chorionicity data for prospective studies, this hypothesis has not been tested widely. In a study of 424 young adult twin pairs from the East Flanders Twin register, no differences were observed between the three twin types for adult body composition and blood pressure, despite significant differences in birth weight and gestational age.[114, 115] Similarly, IQ at age 7 did not differ between twin types in black or white children from NINCDS Collaborative Perinatal Project (NCPP).[116]

In the absence of data on chorionicity, others have investigated whether monozygotic twins have an increased mortality or higher risk for disease in adult life compared to dizygotic twins. This hypothesis has been extended by comparing the risk of twins to that of singletons, under the assumption that twin pregnancies in general are suboptimal to singleton pregnancies. Reliable incidence data on sufficiently large populations is scarce. Investigators of the Danish Twin Register have had a particular interest in the comparison of twin pairs and singletons, but in general have found no differences.[117] For example, the prevalence of type 1 diabetes was compared between twins, monozygotic and dizygotic, and the general population, and no differences were observed.[118] Overall mortality rates after age 6y did not significantly differ between monozygotic twins, dizygotic twins and the general populations.[28] Likewise, no differences were observed in mortality from coronary heart disease between monozygotic and dizygotic Swedish twins.[119]

4.4.5 Implications for the classic twin studies

The basic assumption of the classical twin design is that monozygotic monochorionic, monozygotic dichorionic and dizygotic twins experience a similar pre- and post-natal environment. This assumption, however, has been questioned in the light of the prenatal programming hypothesis.[27, 120] If the prenatal programming hypothesis is indeed valid for twins, the prenatal differences between the three types of twins may alter the intra-pair concordances or correlations on which the classical twin design is based.

However, it is hard to predict how fetal programming might exert its effects on the intra-pair concordances and correlations, and heritability estimates for different traits. Monozygotic monochorionic twins, representing about 70–75% of all monozygotic twins, generally have larger intra-pair birth weight differences than monozygotic dichorionic twins reflecting their suboptimal prenatal circumstances. In the case of fetal programming, this would result in lower intra-pair correlations for any traits affected by fetal programming, as compared to a situation without fetal programming and, thus, would result in an underestimation of the true relative contribution of genetic variation to the trait. It can however be argued that the lower heritability would be a correct reflection of the truth as it suggests a greater influence of the shared environment; the prenatal environment in this case. But this seems to be a twin-specific result, and is not generalizable to the general population.

Others have hypothesized that because monozygotic monochorionic twins share their circulation through placental anastomoses, the monozygotic intra-pair correlation of a trait may be inflated because of a greater similarity in the prenatal environment on monozygotic monochorionic twins compared to dizygotic twins, resulting in an overestimation of the heritability.[27, 120] As a response to this, it has been suggested to modify the design of the classical twin study by excluding the monozygotic monochorionic pairs,[119] leaving monozygotic dichorionic and dizygotic twins with more similar prenatal environments. However, given that information on chorionicity is lacking in most adult twin studies and, if known it would mean exclusion of two thirds of monozygotic pairs, this modified design might not be the most practical solution.

To date, there is little evidence to support either of these two hypotheses. This is because very few traits have been examined for either hypothesis because few studies are able to examine these hypotheses. It is important to note that any effects are likely to be trait specific, so demonstration that neither hypothesis affects heritability of birth weight, for example, does not mean the same would be true of blood pressure, for example. The National Heart Lung and Blood Institute (NHLBI) Twin Study found that monozygotic monochorionic twins showed greater intra-pair correlations in cholesterol levels in adult life compared to monozygotic dichorionic twins.[121] In contrast, for fibrinogen levels the intra-pair correlation in monozygotic monochorionic twins was less than half that observed in monozygotic dichorionic twins in a young adult population.[122] These findings argue against the prenatal shared-circulation hypothesis, but rather suggest that intra-pair birth weight differences affect intra-pair correlations for these traits. Others found that the intra-pair correlation for adult body composition and blood pressure were not different between monozygotic monochorionic and dichorionic twins.[114, 115]

4.5 Limitations of the twin design

4.5.1 Comparisons of Intra- and Inter-pair birth weight differences: limitations of power

As described in Sections 4.1 and 4.2, comparisons between the birth weight associations with later disease when using the *intra*-pair models in monozygotic versus dizygotic twins, and also *intra*- versus *inter*-pair models, are used to indicate whether the fetal origins of that disease are more likely due to fetal genetic factors, individual fetoplacental environment or shared maternal determinants of fetal growth. For example, a meta-analysis of 10 twin studies on the influence of birth weight on blood pressure showed that in unpaired analyses birth weight was inversely associated with adult blood pressure, which is consistent with the trends observed in singletons.[123] In contrast the association was not confirmed in paired analyses, suggesting that shared maternal environmental factors underlie the association between low birth weight and higher blood pressure.[123] While that study amassed data on over 4,000 twin pairs, it is unclear how birth weights and blood pressures in opposite sex pairs were treated. A very different conclusion was reached in a recent much larger single study of over 16,000 same-sex twin pairs.[124] In the unpaired analysis, the odds ratio for hypertension for each 500-g decrease in birth weight was 1.42 (95% CI, 1.25 to 1.61). This time, the intra-pair analyses showed similar results, with odds ratios of 1.34 (1.07 to 1.69) for dizygotic and 1.74 (1.13 to 2.70) for monozygotic twins, and indicating that the association between birth weight and later hypertension in that study was independent of both shared maternal environment and genetic factors.

A number of factors contribute to reduce the power to detect such crucial associations with intra-pair differences in birth weight. Firstly, it should be recognized that the intra-pair birth weight differences are generally rather small, on average 250–300 g, ranging (95% CI) from 0g to 800g. As a consequence, the statistical power to detect intra-pair differences in the adult health outcome between the members of a pair will be limited. Secondly, in opposite-sex dizygotic pairs it is difficult to assess the degree of concordance in birth weight, despite adjustments for gender. Restriction of the analysis to same-sex pairs essentially removes 50% of dizygotic twin pairs. Further restrictions will occur when further stratifications by gender, zygosity, and chorionicity are performed. Very large twin studies are therefore required to confidently compare or exclude important correlations with intra-pair differences in birth weight. Current examples are the Swedish Twin Registry, which has collected data by telephone interviews in over 11,411 twins,[124] and the UK Adult Twin Registry, which comprises over 10,000 twin pairs most of whom have undergone detailed clinical examinations.[125]

4.5.2 Fetal growth: are twins representative for singletons?

With the increasing number of twin studies that explore the fetal origins of adult disease, the question is being raised whether the results found for twins are representative of singletons.[126–128] For example the above finding that the birth weight link to hypertension in twins is apparently due to individual fetoplacental factors rather than shared maternal environment or genetic factors[124] could possibly reflect a smaller relative contribution of those latter factors on birth weight in twins. While these recent results from the Swedish Twin Registry should certainly focus future research efforts on the fetoplacental transfer of nutrients, they do not necessarily negate the demonstrable role of maternal undernutrition[129] or of potential fetal genetic factors[130] in predicting hypertension risk in the general population.

Furthermore, low birth weight in twins may not have the same significance as in singletons, i.e. twins may be small at birth for different reasons to those of singletons. Fetal growth of twins falls below that of singletons during the third trimester of pregnancy,[57, 131] whereas in singletons growth retardation is likely to occur at any time during gestation.[132] Animal[133, 134] and human[135, 136] studies have shown that the programming effects of fetal growth restriction are dependant on the gestational timing of the insult. As a consequence, fetal undernutrition in twins may programme for different metabolic outcomes than in singletons.

There has been much debate about the underlying factors causing fetal growth retardation in twins and whether these are placental and/or maternal. Five decades ago, McKeown and Record[56, 137] postulated *'crowding in the uterus'* as the main cause of fetal growth retardation, which is more obvious in twin than in singleton pregnancies. More recently, however, a *limited capacity in the maternal/placental supply line* has been proposed as a more likely cause of growth retardation in twins.[58, 63–65, 67] The latter may also restrict fetal growth in singleton pregnancies, but the cause of the limited capacity will probably be different for twins and singletons. In the case of twin pregnancies, the fetal demand for nutrients will easily exceed the 'normal' maternal capacity, especially during the last trimester. In singleton pregnancies, the limited maternal/placental supply will most likely result because of other reasons than excessive fetal demand.

More evidence that prenatal growth retardation of twins differs from that of singletons comes from intergenerational studies in which parental birth weights and offspring birth weights are compared. In singletons, birth weight of the mother is related to that of their children and even their children's children,[138–140] whereas the father's birth weight had no influence on their offspring's birth size.[141] These observations have led to the conclusion that mothers constrain fetal growth and that the degree of constraint they exert is set when they themselves were *in utero*.[142] In twin pregnancies, however, there is no evidence for such an intergenerational constraint. Women, who were born as one of a twin pair and therefore often of low birth weight, had babies with birth weights similar to those of babies of singleton mothers.[140, 143]

4.5.3 Survival of the fittest: selection bias?

Perinatal mortality and morbidity in twins is significantly higher than in singletons.[144] This is not only due to premature delivery and low birth weight, but 'being a twin member' also increases the risk for an adverse outcome.[145]

Furthermore, many twin studies have to rely on volunteer twin registries that are most likely to register healthy twin pairs and twins who have severe morbidity and who are unable to perform the requested tasks will often not be included in the study. As a consequence, twins who have participated in research studies may represent the 'healthy survivors' and, therefore, they may have a lower risk of developing chronic disease in adult life. This 'survival of the fittest' selection bias will decrease the statistical power to detect long-term influences of prenatal programming, and the associations found in twin studies may underestimate the associations for the actual twin population.

4.5.4 Birth weight versus post-natal growth

Several of the original disease associations with birth weight have now been extended by the identification of associations with different patterns of post-natal weight gain.[146] Indeed the 'fetal origins hypothesis' has been succeeded by the 'developmental origins of health and disease' hypothesis, to incorporate the role of growth in early post-natal life and other exposures acting in the developmental period, which for some traits (e.g., lung function) extends to adolescence and early adulthood.[147] As the majority of infants who are growth restrained *in utero* and have lower than average birth weights tend to show rapid catch-up growth during post-natal life,[148] it may be difficult statistically to distinguish between the contributions of antenatal versus post-natal factors.

As described above, birth weight in twins is around 600 g lower than that in singletons, and birth length is also reduced but to a lesser extent, consistent with a marked restriction of fetal growth occurring during later gestation. After birth, much of this deficit in size is rapidly made up by a dramatic recovery in weight occurring particularly during the first three months of life, relative to singleton infants.[149] As children and as adults, twins are therefore broadly similar in height, or only slightly shorter, compared to singletons, and may have only slightly lower levels of BMI or weight for height.[26, 150, 151] It is becoming increasingly recognized that rapid weight gain and growth in the first few weeks and months of life is associated with increased risks for subsequent overweight, obesity and related metabolic traits.[152] As is necessary in studies in the general population, studies of birth weight and life course disease associations in twins need to assess whether apparent associations with differences in birth weight might actually be mediated by differences in their rates of subsequent post-natal catch-up growth and weight gain.

4.6 Conclusions

Twins have unique genetic and prenatal characteristics, which can be modelled to disentangle the complex mechanisms that underlie the 'fetal origins' of later disease risks. The influence of the individual fetoplacental environment, unique to each fetus, can be estimated by associating intra-pair differences in birth weight to intra-pair differences in adult disease risk. Also, the role of fetal genetic influences can be inferred by comparing the intra-pair associations observed in monozygotic twins to those observed in dizygotic twins. Finally, inter-pair comparisons allow estimation of the contribution of the shared maternal environment, common to both fetuses, to adult disease risks.

However, these models have important caveats. The prenatal and early life of twins is substantially different from that of singletons, and therefore generalizing from findings of twin studies to the general population should be done with caution. At birth twins weigh on average 600 g less than singletons, even when their shorter gestation is taken into account. Although this potentially increases the twins' risk for adult disease compared to singleton there is no conclusive evidence to support this notion. Importantly, average birth weight also differs across the major sub-types of twins: monozygotic twins weigh less than dizygotic twins, and furthermore, monozygotic monochorionic twins weigh less than monozygotic dichorionic twins. These differences in birth weight can be related to zygosity, chorionicity, and location of umbilical cord insertion in the placenta, and these observations challenge several of the assumptions implicit in the above models.

To date, most twin studies have had limited statistical power to robustly test the complex modelling of inter- and intra-pair associations between prenatal environment and adult disease risk.

Current very large studies based on national twin registers will certainly help to provide more robust comparisons between the effects of fetal genes, shared maternal environment and individual fetoplacental environment. However, large studies should also ideally collect information on chorionicity and placentation in order to test the basic assumptions used in these twin models.

References

1 **Jones HW.** Multiple births: how are we doing? *Fertil Steril* 2003;**79**: 17–21.
2 **Martin JA and Park MM.** *Trends in Twin and Triplet Births: 1980–97*. National Vital Statistics Reports, **47**(24): 1–16, 1999.
3 **Loos R, Derom C, Vlietinck R, Derom R.** The East Flanders Prospective Twin Survey (Belgium): a population-based register. *Twin Res* 1998; **1**: 167–75.
4 **Bulmer MC.** *The Biology of Twinning*. Oxford University Press, London, 1970.
5 **Nylander PP.** The factors that influence twinning rates. *Acta Genet Med Gemellol (Roma)* 1981; **30**: 189–202.
6 **Derom C, Leroy F, Vlietinck R, Fryns JP, Derom R.** High frequency of iatrogenic monozygotic twins with administration of clomiphene citrate and a change in chorionicity. *Fertil Steril* 2006; **85**: 755–7.
7 **Derom C, Vlietinck R, Derom R, Van den Berghe H.** Increased monozygotic twinning rate after ovulation induction. *Lancet* 1987; **1**: 1236–8.
8 **Edwards RG, Mettler L, Walters DE.** Identical twins and in vitro fertilization. *J Assist Reprod Genet* 1986; **3**: 114–7.
9 **Imaizumi Y.** A comparative study of twinning and triplet rates in 17 countries, 1972-1996. *Acta Genet Med Gemellol (Roma)* 1998; **47**: 101–14.
10 **Boomsma D, Busjahn A, Peltonen L.** Classical twin studies and beyond. *Nat Rev Genet* 2002; **3**: 872–82.
11 **Galton F.** The history of twins, as criterion of the relative powers of nature and nurture. *Fraser's Magazine* 1875; Nov, 576.
12 **Spector TD.** The histroy of twin and sibling-pair studies. In: Spector TD, Snieder H, MacGregor AJ, eds. *Advances in Twin and Sib-pait Analysis*.Greenwich Medical Media, London, pp. 2–9, 2000.
13 **Merriman C.** The intellectual resemblance of twins. *Psychological monographs* 1924; **33**: 1–58.
14 **Siemens HW.** *Zwillingspathologie: Ihre Bedeeutung; ihr Methodik, ihre bisherigen Ergebnisse*. Springer Verlag, Berlin, 1924.
15 **Falconer DS.** *Introduction to Quantitative Genetics*. Longmans Green/John Wiley & Sons, Harlow, 1989.
16 **Silventoinen K, Sammalisto S, Perola M, Boomsma DI, Cornes BK, Davis C, Dunkel L, de Lange M, Harris JR, Hjelmborg JV, Luciano M, Martin NG, Mortensen J, Nistico L, Pedersen NL, Skytthe A, Spector TD, Stazi MA, Willemsen G, Kaprio J.** Heritability of adult body height: a comparative study of twin cohorts in eight countries. *Twin Res* 2003; **6**: 399–408.
17 **Boomsma DI, Koopmans JR, Doornen LJP, Orlebeke JF.** Genetic and social influences on starting to smoke: a study of Dutch adolescent twins and their parents. *Addiction*, 1994; **89**: 219–26.
18 **Bailey A, Le Couteur A, Gottesman I, Bolton P, Simonoff E, yuzda E, Rutter M.** Autism as a strongly genetic disorder: evidence from a British twin study. *Psychol Med* 1995; **25**: 63–77.
19 **Faraone SV, Doyle AE.** The nature and heritability of attention-deficit/hyperactivity disorder. *Child Adolesc Psychiatr Clin N Am* 2001; **10**: 299–316.
20 **Tsuang MT, Bar JL, Harley RM, Lyons MJ.** The Harvard Twin Study of Substance Abuse: what we have learned. *Harv Rev Pshyciatry* 2001; **9**: 267–79.
21 **Kendler KS, Gatz M, Gardner CO, Pedersen NL.** A Swedish National Twin Study of Lifetime Major Depression. *Am J Psychiatry* 2006; **163**: 109–14.
22 **Jinks JL, Fulker DW.** Comparison of the biometrical, MAVA and classical approaches to the analysis of human behavior. *Psychol Bull* 1970; **73**: 311–49.

23 Silventoinen K, Bartels M, Posthuma D, Estourgie-van Burk GF, Willemsen G, van Beijsterveldt TC, Boomsma DI. Genetic regulation of growth in height and weight from 3 to 12 years of age: a longitudinal study of Dutch twin children. *Twin Research and Human Genetics* 2007; **10**: 354–63.

24 Van den Berg SM, Boomsma DI. The familial clustering of age at menarche in extended twin families. *Behav Genet* 2007; **37**: 661–7.

25 Pietilainen KH, Kaprio J, Rissanen A, Winter T, Rimpela A, Viken RJ, Rose RJ. Distribution and heritability of BMI in Finnish adolescents aged 16y and 17y: a study of 4884 twins and 2509 singletons. *Int J Obes Relat Metab Disord* 1999; **23**: 107–15.

26 Estourgie-van Burk GF, Bartels M, van Beijsterveldt TC, Dellemarre-van de Waal HA, Boomsma DI. Body size in five-year-old twins: heritability and comparison to singleton standards. *Twin Research and Human Genetics* 2006; **9**: 646–55.

27 Phillips DIW. Twin studies in medical research: can they tell us whether diseases are genetically determined? *Lancet* 1993; **341**, 1008–9.

28 Christensen K, Vaupel JW, Holm NV, Yashin AI. Mortality among twins after age 6: fetal origins hypothesis versus twin method. *BMJ* 1995; **310**, 432–6.

29 van den Oord EJ, Kooth HM, Boomsma DI, Verhulst FC, Orlebeke JF. A twin-singleton comparison of problem behaviour in 2-3-year-olds. *Journal of child psychology and psychiatry, and allied disciplines* 1995; **36**: 449–58.

30 Pam A, Kemker S, Ross CA, Golden R. The 'equal environments assumption' in MZ-DZ twin comparisons: an untenable premise of psychiatric genetics? *Acta Genet Med Gemellol (Roma)* 1996; **45**: 349–60.

31 Price B. Primary biases in twin studies A review of prenatal and natal difference-producing factors in monozygotic pairs. *Am J Hum Genet* 1950; **2**: 293–352.

32 Joseph J. Twin Studies in Psychiatry and Psychology: Science or Pseudoscience? *Psychiatric Quarterly* 2002; **73**, 71–82.

33 Richardson K, Norgate S. The equal environments assumption of classical twin studies may not hold. *Br J Educ Psychol* 2005; **75**, 339–50.

34 Horwitz AV, Videon TM, Schmitz MF, Davis D. Rethinking twins and environments: possible social sources for assumed genetic influences in twin research. *J Health Soc Behav* 2003; **44**: 111–29.

35 Hettema JM, Neale MC, Kendler KS. Physical similarity and the equal-environment assumption in twin studies of psychiatric disorders. *Behav Genet* 1995; **25**: 327–35.

36 Kendler KS, Gardner CO Jr. Twin studies of adult psychiatric and substance dependence disorders: are they biased by differences in the environmental experiences of monozygotic and dizygotic twins in childhood and adolescence? *Psychol Med* 1998; **28**: 625–33.

37 Xian H, Scherrer JF, Eisen SA, True WR, Heath AC, Goldberg J, Lyons MJ, Tsuang MT. Self-Reported Zygosity and the Equal-Environments Assumption for Psychiatric Disorders in the Vietnam Era Twin Registry. *Behav Genet* 2000; **30**: 303–10.

38 Derks EM, Dolan CV, Boomsma DI. A test of the equal environment assumption (EEA) in multivariate twin studies. *Twin Research and Human Genetics* 2006; **9**: 403–11.

39 Cronk NJ, Slutske WS, Madden PA, Bucholz KK, Reich W, Heath AC. Emotional and behavioral problems among female twins: an evaluation of the equal environments assumption. *Journal of the American Academy of Child and Adolescent Psychiatry* 2002; **41**: 829–37.

40 Taylor RW, Turnbull DM. Mitochondrial DNA mutations in human disease. *Nat Rev Genet* 2005; **6**: 389–402.

41 Blakely EL, He L, Taylor RW, Chinnery PF, Lightowlers RN, Schaefer AM, Turnbull DM. Mitochondrial DNA deletion in 'identical' twin brothers. *J Med Genet* 2004; **41**: e19.

42 Pietiläinen KH, Naukkarinen J, Rissanen A, Saharinen J, Ellonen P, Keränen H, Suomalainen A, Gotz A, Suortti T, Yki-Jarvinen H, Oresic M, Kaprio J, Peltonen L. Global transcript profiles of fat in monozygotic twins discordant for BMI: pathways behind acquired obesity. *PLoS Medicine* 2008; **5**: e51.

43 Gringras P, Chen W. Mechanisms for differences in monozygous twins. *Early Hum Dev* 2001; **64**: 105–17.
44 Petronis A. Epigenetics and twins: three variations on the theme. *TIG* 2006; **22**: 347–50.
45 Bruder CEG, Piotrowski A, Gijsbers AACJ, Andersson R, Erickson S, az de Stahl T, Menzel U, Sandgren J, von Tell D, Poplawski A, Crowley M, Crasto C, Partridge EC, Tiwari H, Allison DB, Komorowski J, van Ommen GJ, Boomsma DI, Pedersen NL, den Dunnen JT, Wirdefeldt K, Dumanski JP. Phenotypically concordant and discordant monozygotic twins display different DNA copy-number-variation profiles. *Am J Hum Genet* 2008; **82**: 763–71.
46 Fraga MF, Ballestar E, Paz MF, Ropero S, Setien F, Ballestar ML, Heine-Suner D, Cigudosa JC, Urioste M, Benitez J, Boix-Chornet M, Sanchez-Aguilera A, Ling C, Carlsson E, Poulsen P, Vaag A, Stephan Z, Spector TD, Wu YZ, Plass C, Esteller M. From the cover: epigenetic differences arise during the lifetime of monozygotic twins. *PNAS* 2005; **102**: 10604–9.
47 Machin G. Some causes of genotypic and phenotypic discordance in monozygotic twin pairs. *Am J Med Genet* 1996; **61**, 216–28.
48 Leonard NJ, Bernier FP, Rudd N, Machin GA, Bamforth F, Grundy P. Two pairs of male monozygotic twins discordant for Wiedemann-Beckwith Syndrome. *Am J Med Genet* 1996; **61**: 253–7.
49 Weksberg R, Shuman C, Caluseriu O, Smith AC, Fei YL, Nishikawa J, Stockley TL, Best L, Chitayat D, Olney A, Ives E, Schneider A, Bestor TH, Li M, Sadowski P, Squire J. Discordant KCNQ1OT1 imprinting in sets of monozygotic twins discordant for Beckwith-Wiedemann syndrome. *Hum Mol Genet* 2002; **11**: 1317–25.
50 Bouchard TJ, McGue M. Genetic and environmental influences on human psychological differences. *J Neurol* 2003; **54**: 4–45.
51 Loos RJF, Verhaeghe J, de Zegher F, Beunen G, Derom C, Fagard R, Mathieu C, Vlietinck R. Markers for cardiovascular disease in monozygotic twins discordant for the use of third-generation oral contraceptives. *J Hum Hypertens* 2003; **17**: 481–5.
52 Martin N, Boomsma D, Machin G. A twin-pronged attack on complex traits. *Nature Genet* 1997; **17**: 387–92.
53 Sato Y, Benirschke K. Increased prevalence of fetal thrombi in monochorionic-twin placentas. *Pediatrics* 2006; **117**: e113–e117.
54 Dube J, Dodds L, Armson BA. Does chorionicity or zygosity predict adverse perinatal outcomes in twins? *Am J Obstet Gynecol* 2002; **186**: 579–83.
55 Sherer DM. Adverse perinatal outcome of twin pregnancies according to chorionicity: review of the literature. *Am J Perinatol* 2001; **18**: 23–37.
56 McKeown T, Record RG. Observation on foetal growth in multiple pregnancy in man. *J Endocrinol* 2001; **8**: 386–401.
57 Naeye RL, Benirschke K, Hagstrom JW, Marcus CC. Intrauterine growth of twins as estimated from liveborn birth-weight data. *Pediatrics* 1966; **37**: 409–16.
58 Bleker OP, Breur W, Huidekoper BL. A study of birth weight, placental weight and mortality of twins as compared to singletons. *Br J Obstet Gynaecol* 1979; **86**: 111–8.
59 Grennert L, Persson P, Gennser G, Gullberg B. Zygosity and intrauterine growth of twins. *Obstet Gynecol*, 1980; **55**: 684–7.
60 Bleker OP, Oosting J, Hemrika DJ. On the cause of the retardation of fetal growth in multiple gestations. *Acta Genet Med Gemellol (Roma)* 1988; **37**: 41–6.
61 Luke B, Minogue J, Witter FR, Keith LG, Johnson TRB. The ideal twin pregnancy: pattern of weight gain, discordancy, and length of gestation. *Am J Obstet Gynecol* 1993; **169**: 588–97.
62 Loos RJF, Derom C, Derom R, Vlietinck R. Determinants of birthweight and intrauterine growth in liveborn twins. *Paediatr Perinat Epidemiol* 2005; **19**: 15–22.
63 Gruenwald P. Environmental influences on twins apparent at birth: a preliminary study. *Biol Neonate*, 1970; **15**: 79–93.

64 Bleker OP, Wolf H, Oosting J. The placental cause of fetal growth retardation in twin gestations. *Acta Genet Med Gemellol (Roma)* 1995; **44**: 103–6.

65 MacGillivray I. Determinants of birthweight in twins. *Acta Genet Med Gemellol (Roma)* 1983; **32**: 151–7.

66 Corney G, Robson EB, Strong SJ. The effect of zygosity on the birth weight of twins. *Ann Hum Genet* 1972; **36**: 45–59.

67 Björo Kjr, Björo K. Disturbed intrauterine growth in twins. *Acta Genet Med Gemellol (Roma)* 1985; **34**: 73–9.

68 Ramos-Arroyo MA, Ulbright TM, Yu P-L, Christian JC. Twin study: relationship between birth weight, zygosity, placentation, and pathologic placental changes. *Acta Genet Med Gemellol (Roma)* 1988; **37**: 229–38.

69 Bryan E. The intrauterine hazards of twins. *Arch Dis Child* 1986; **61**: 1044–5.

70 Derom C, Vlietinck R, Thiery E, Leroy F, Frijns JP, Derom R. The East Flanders Prospective Twin Survey (EFPTS). *Twin Research and Human Genetics* 2006; **9**: 733–8.

71 Loos RJF, Derom C, Derom R, Vlietinck R. Birthweight in liveborn twins: the influence of the umbilical cord insertion and fusion of placentas. *Br J Obstet Gynaecol* 2001; **108**: 943–8.

72 Heinonen S, Ryynänen M, Kirkinen P, Saarkoski S. Perinatal diagnostic evaluation of velamentous umbilical cord insertion: clinical, Doppler, and ultrasonic findings. *Obstet Gynecol* 1996; **87**: 112–7.

73 Corey LA, Nance WE, Kang KW, Christian JC. Effects of type of placentation on birth weight and its variability in monozygotic and dizygotic twins. *Acta Genet Med Gemellol (Roma)* 1979; **28**: 41–50.

74 Fick AL, Feldstein VA, Norton ME, Wassel Fyr C, Caughey AB, Machin GA. Unequal placental sharing and birth weight discordance in monochorionic diamniotic twins. *Am J Obstet Gynecol* 2006; **195**: 178–83.

75 Belogolovkin V, Engel SM, Ferrara L, Eddleman KA, Stone JL. Does sonographic determination of placental location predict fetal birth weight in diamniotic-dichorionic twins? *J Ultrasound Med* 2007; **26**: 187–91.

76 Demissie K, Ananth CV, Martin J, Hanley ML, MacDorman MF, Rhoads GG. Fetal and neonatal mortality among twin gestations in the United States: the role of intrapair birth weight discordance. *Obstet Gynecol* 2002; **100**: 474–80.

77 Hollier LM, McIntire DD, Leveno KJ. Outcome of twin pregnancies according to intrapair birth weight differences. *Obstet Gynecol* 1999; **94**: 1006–10.

78 Armson BA, O'Connell C, Persad V, Joseph KS, Young DC, Baskett TF. Determinants of perinatal mortality and serious neonatal morbidity in the second twin. *Obstet Gynecol* 2001; **108**: 556–64.

79 Amaru RC, Bush MC, Berkowitz RL, Lapinski RH, Gaddipati S. Is discordant growth in twins an independent risk factor for adverse neonatal outcome? *Obstet Gynecol* 2002; **103**: 71–6.

80 Branum AM, Schoendorf KC. The effect of birth weight discordance on twin neonatal mortality. *Obstet Gynecol* 2003; **101**: 570–4.

81 Shi Wu MB, Kee Fung KF, Huang L, Demissie K, Joseph KS, Allen A, Kramer M. Fetal and neonatal mortality among twin gestations in a Canadian population: the effect of intrapair birthweight discordance. *Am J Perinatol* 2005; 279–86.

82 Victoria A, Mora G, Arias F. Perinatal outcome, placental pathology, and severity of discordance in monochorionic and dichorionic twins. *Obstet Gynecol* 2001; **97**: 310–5.

83 Fraser D, Picard R, Picard E, Leiberman JR. Birth weight discordance, intrauterine growth retardation and perinatal outcomes in twins. *J Reprod Med* 1994; **39**: 504–8.

84 Hsieh TT, Chang TC, Chiu TH, Hsu JJ, Chao A. Growth discordancy, birth weight, and neonatal adverse events in third trimester twin gestations. *Gynecol Obstet Invest*,1994; **38**: 36–40.

85 Denbow ML, Cox P, Taylor M, Hammal DM, Fisk NM. Placental angioarchitecture in monochorionic twin pregnancies: relationship to fetal growth, fetofetal transfusion syndrome, and pregnancy outcome. *Am J Obstet Gynecol* 2000; **182**: 417–26.

86 Machin GA. Velamentous cord insertion in monochorionic twin gestation: an added risk factor. *J Reprod Med* 1997; **42**: 785–9.

87 Hanley ML, Ananth CV, Shen-Schwarz S, Smulian JC, Lai YL, Vintzileos AM. Placental cord insertion and birth weight discordancy in twin gestations. *Obstet Gynecol* 2002; **99**: 477–82.

88 Barker DJP, Gluckman PD, Godfrey KM, Harding JE, Owens JA, Robinson JS. Fetal nutrition and cardiovascular disease in adult life. *Lancet* 1993; **341**: 938–41.

89 Kramer MS, Joseph KS. Enigma of fetal/infant-origins hypothesis. *Lancet* 1996; **348**: 1254–7.

90 Hattersley AT, Beards F, Ballantyne E, Appleton M, Harvey R, Ellard S. Mutations in the glucokinase gene of the fetus result in reduced birth weight. *Nature Genet* 1998; **19**: 268–70.

91 Slingerland AS, Hattersley AT. Activating mutations in the gene encoding Kir6.2 alter fetal and postnatal growth and also cause neonatal diabetes. *J Clin Endocrinol Metab* 2006; **91**: 2782–8.

92 Meyre D, Boutin P, Tounian A, Deweirder M, Aout M, Jouret B, Heude B, Weill J, Tauber M, Tounian P, Froguel P. Is glutamate decarboxylase 2 (GAD2) a genetic link between low birth weight and subsequent development of obesity in children? *J Clin Endocrinol Metab* 2005; **90**: 2384–90.

93 Freathy RM, Weedon MN, Bennett A, nen E, Relton CL, Knight B, Shields B, Parnell KS, Groves CJ, Ring SM, Pembrey ME, Ben-Shlomo Y, Strachan DP, Power C, Jarvelin MR, McCarthy MI, vey Smith G, Hattersley AT, Frayling TM. Type 2 diabetes TCF7L2 risk genotypes alter birth weight: a study of 24,053 individuals. *Am J Hum Genet* 2007; **80**:, 1150–61.

94 Loos RJF, Beunen G, Fagard R, Derom C, Vlietinck R. Birth weight and body composition in young adult men—a prospective twin study. *International Journal of Obesity* 2001; **25**: 1537–45.

95 IJzerman RG, Stehouwer CDA, van Weissenbruch MM, de Geus EJ, Boomsma DI. Intra-uterine and genetic influences on the relationship between size at birth and height in later life: analysis in twins. *Twin Res* 2001; **4**: 337–43.

96 Loos RJ, Beunen G, Fagard R, Derom C, Vlietinck R. Birth weight and body composition in young women: a prospective twin study. *Am J Clin Nutr* 2002; **75**: 676–82.

97 Poulsen P, Vaag AA, Kyvik KO, Moller Jensen D, Beck-Nielsen H. Low birth weight is associated with NIDDM in discordant monozygotic and dizygotic twin pairs. *Diabetologia* 1997; **40**: 439–46.

98 Bo S, Cavallo-Perin P, Scaglione L, Ciccone G, Pagano G. Low birthweight and metabolic abnormalities in twins with increased susceptibility to Type 2 diabetes. *Diabet Med* 2000; **17**: 365–70.

99 Baird J, Osmond C, MacGregor A, Snieder H, Hales CN, Phillips DIW. Testing the fetal origins hypothesis in twins: the Birmingham twin study. *Diabetologia* 2001; **44**: 33–9.

100 Loos RJF, Phillips DIW, Fagard R, Beunen G, Derom C, Mathieu C, Verhaeghe J, Vlietinck R. The influence of maternal BMI and age in twin pregnancies on insulin resistance in the offspring. *Diabetes Care* 2002; **25**: 2191–6.

101 Dwyer T, Blizzard L, Morley R, Ponsonby A-L. Within pair association between birth weight and blood pressure at age 8 in twins from a cohort study. *BMJ* 1999; **319**: 1325–9.

102 Poulter NR, Chang CL, MacGregor AJ, Snieder H, Spector TD. Association between birth weight and adult blood pressure in twins: historical cohort study. *BMJ* 1999; **319**: 1330–3.

103 Ijzerman RG, Stehouwer CDA, Boomsma DI. Evidence for genetic factors explaining the birth weight—blood pressure relation: Analysis in twins. *Hypertension* 2000; **36**: 1008–12.

104 Christensen K, Stovring H, McGue M. Do genetic factors contribute to the association between birth weight and blood pressure? *J Epidemiol Community Health* 2001; **55**: 583–7.

105 Loos RJF, Fagard R, Beunen G, Derom C, Vlietinck R. Birth weight and blood pressure in young adults: a prospective twin study. *Circulation* 2001; **104**: 1633–8.

106 IJzerman RG, Stehouwer CDA, de Geus EJ, van Weissenbruch MM, Delemarre-van de Waal H, Boomsma DI. Low birth weight Is associated with increased sympathetic activity: dependence on genetic factors. *Circulation* 2003; **108**: 566–71.

107 Hübinette A, Cnattingius A, Ekbom A, De Faire U, Kramer M, Lichtenstein P. Birthweight, early environment, and genetics: a study of twins discordant for acute myocarial infarction. *Lancet* 2001; **357**: 1997–2001.

108 Poulsen P, Wojtaszewski JFP, Richter EA, Beck-Nielsen H, Vaag A. Low birth weight and zygosity status is associated with defective muscle glycogen and glycogen synthase regulation in elderly twins. Diabetes 2007; db07–0155.

109 Os Jv, Wichers M, Danckaerts M, Van Gestel S, Derom C, Vlietinck R. A prospective twin study of birth weight discordance and child problem behavior. *Biological Psychiatry* 2001; **50**: 593–9.

110 Carlin JB, Gurrin LC, Sterne JA, Morley R, Dwyer T. Regression models for twin studies: a critical review. *Int J Epidemiol* 2005; **34**: 1089–99.

111 Johansson-Kark M, Rasmussen F, Stavola BD, Leon DA. Fetal growth and systolic blood pressure in young adulthood: the Swedish Young Male Twins Study. *Paediatr Perinat Epidemiol* 2002; **16**: 200–9.

112 Johansson M, Rasmussen F. Birthweight and body mass index in young adulthood: the Swedish young male twins study. *Twin Res* 2001; **4**: 400–5.

113 Iliadou A, Cnattingius S, Lichtenstein P. Low birthweight and Type 2 diabetes: A study on 11 162 Swedish twins. *Int J Epidemiol* 2004; **33**: 948–53.

114 Loos RJF, Beunen G, Fagard R, Derom C, Vlietinck R. The influence of zygosity and chorion type on fat distribution in young adult twins—consequences for twin studies. *Twin Res* 2001; **4**: 356–64.

115 Fagard RH, Loos RJF, Beunen G, Derom C, Vlietinck R. Influence of chorionicity on the heritability estimates of blood pressure: a study in twins. *J Hypertens* 2003; **21**: 1313–8.

116 Melnick M, Myrianthopoulos NC, Christian JC. The effects of chorion type on variation in IQ in the NCPP twin population. *Am J Hum Genet* 1978; **30**: 425–33.

117 Kyvik KO, Christensen K, Skytthe A, Harvald B, Holm NV. The Danish Twin Register. *Dan Med Bull* 1996; **43**: 467–70.

118 Kyvik KO, Green A, Beck-Nielsen H. Concordance rates of insulin dependent diabetes mellitus: a population based study of young Danish twins. *BMJ* 1995; **311**: 913–7.

119 Vågerö D, Leon D. Ischeamic heart disease and low birth weight: a test of the fetal-origins hypothesis from the Swedish Twin Registry. *Lancet* 1994; **343**: 260–3.

120 Phillips DIW. Can twin studies assess the genetic component in type 2 (non-insulin-dependent) diabetes mellitus? *Diabetologia* 1992; **36**: 471–2.

121 Reed T, Christian JC, Wood PD, Schaefer EJ. Influence of placentation on high density lipoproteins in adult males: the NHLBI twin study. *Acta Genet Med Gemellol (Roma)* 1991; **40**: 353–9.

122 Loos RJF, Beunen G, Fagard R, Derom C, Vlietinck R, Phillips DIW. Twin studies and estimates of heritability. *Lancet* 2001; **357**: 1445.

123 McNeill G, Tuya C, Smith WCS. The role of genetic and environmental factors in the association between birthweight and blood pressure: evidence from meta-analysis of twin studies. *Int J Epidemiol* 2004; **33**: 995–1001.

124 Bergvall N, Iliadou A, Johansson S, de Faire U, Kramer MS, Pawitan Y, Pedersen NL, Lichtenstein P, Cnattingius S. Genetic and shared environmental factors do not confound the association between birth weight and hypertension: a study among Swedish twins. *Circulation* 2007; **115**: 2931–8.

125 Spector TD, Williams FM. The UK Adult Twin Registry (TwinsUK). *Twin Research and Human Genetics* 2006; **9**: 899–906.

126 Doyle P, Leon D, Maconochie N, Morton S, de Stavlova B. Twins and the fetal origins hypothesis. Patterns of growth retardation differ in twins and singletons. *BMJ* **319**: 517.

127 Phillips DIW, Davies MJ, Robinson JS. Fetal growth and the fetal origins hypothesis in twins—problems and perspectives. *Twin Res* 2001; **4**: 327–31.

128 Phillips DIW, Osmond C. Twins and the fetal origins hypothesis. Many variables differ between twins and singleton infants. *BMJ* 1999; **319**: 517.

129 Stein AD, Zybert PA, van der Pal-de Bruin K, Lumey L. Exposure to famine during gestation, size at birth, and blood pressure at age 59-áy: evidence from the dutch famine. *Eur J Epidemiol* 2006; **21**: 759–65.

130 Seckl JR, Holmes MC. Mechanisms of Disease: glucocorticoids, their placental metabolism and fetal 'programming' of adult pathophysiology. *Nature Clinical Practice Endocrinology & Metabolism* 2007; **3**: 479–88.

131 Bleker OP, Kloosterman GJ, Huidkoper BL, Breur W. Intrauterine growth of twins as estimated from birthweight and fetal biparietal diameter. *Eur J Obst Gynecol Reprod Biol* 1977; **7**: 85–90.

132 Keirse MJNC. Epidemiology and aetiology of the growth retarded baby. *Clin Obstet Gynecol*, 1984; **11**: 415–35.

133 Nyirenda MJ, Lindsay RS, Kenyon CJ, Seckl JR. Glucocorticoid exposure in late gestation permanently programs rat hepatic phosphoenolpyruvate carboxykinase and glucocorticoid receptor expression and causes glucose intolerance in adult offspring. *J Clin Invest* 1998; **101**: 2174–81.

134 Gatford KL, Wintour EM, De Blasio MJ, Owens JA, Dodic M. Differential timing for programming of glucose homeostasis, sensitivity to insulin and blood pressure by in utero exposure to dexamethasone in sheep. *Clin Sci* 2000; **98**: 560.

135 Lopuhaä CE, Roseboom TJ, Osmond C, Barker DJP, Ravelli ACJ, Bleker OP, van de Zee JS, van der Meulen JHP. Atopy, lung function, and obstructive airways disease after prenatal exposure to famine. *Thorax* 2000; **55**: 555–61.

136 Roseboom TJ, van der Meulen JHP, van Montfrans GA, Ravelli A, Osmond C, Barker DJP, Bleker OP. Maternal nutrition during gestation and blood pressure in later life. *J Hypertens* 2001; **19**: 29–34.

137 McKeown T, Record RG. The influence of placental size on foetal growth in man, with special reference to multiple pregnancy. *J Endocrinol* 1953; **9**: 418–26.

138 Klebanoff MA, Graubard B, Kessel SS, Berendes HW. Low birth weight across generations. *JAMA* 1984; **1984**: 2423–7.

139 Carr-Hill R, Campbell DM, Hall MH, Meredith A. Is birth weight determined genetically? *BMJ* 1987; **295**: 687–9.

140 Emanuel I, Filakti H, Alberman E, Evans SJW. Intergenertional studies of human birthweight from the 1985 birth cohort. Do parents who were twins have babies as heavy as those born to singletons? *Br J Obstet Gynaecol* 1992; **99**: 836–40.

141 Godfrey KM, Barker DJP, Robinson S, Osmond C. Maternal birthweight and diet in pregnancy in relation to the infant's thisness at birth. *Br J Obstet Gynaecol* 1997; **104**: 663–7.

142 Ounsted M, Scott A, Ounsted C. Transmission through the female line of a mechanism constraining human fetal growth. *Ann Hum Biol* 1986; **13**: 143–51.

143 Glinianaia SV, Magnus P, Skjaerven R, Bakketeig LS. The relationship between maternal birthweight and gestational age in twins and singletons and those of their offspring in Norway. *Paediatr Perinat Epidemiol* 1997; **11**: 26–36.

144 Kiely JL. The epidemiology of perinatal mortality in multiple births. *Bull N Y Acad Med* 1990; **66**: 618–37.

145 Buekens P, Wilcox A. Why do small twins have a lower mortality rate than small singletons? *Am J Obstet Gynecol* 1993; **168**: 937–41.

146 Eriksson JG, Forsén T, Tuomilehto J, Winter PD, Osmond C, Barker DJP. Catch-up growth in childhood and death from coronary heart disease: longitudinal study. *BMJ* 1999; **318**: 427–31.

147 Gluckman PD, Hanson MA, Beedle AS. Early life events and their consequences for later disease: a life history and evolutionary perspective. *Am J Hum Biol* 2007; **19**: 1–19.

148 Ong KK, Preece MA, Emmett PM, Ahmed ML, Dunger DB, ALSPAC Study Team. Size at birth and early childhood growth in relation to maternal smoking, parity and infant breast-feeding: longitudinal birth cohort study and analysis. *Pediatr Res* 2002; **52**: 863–7.

149 Wilson RS. Twin growth: initial deficit, recovery, and trend in concordance from birth to nine years. *Ann Hum Biol* 1979; **6**: 205–20.

150 Buckler JM, Green M. A comparison of the early growth of twins and singletons. *Ann Hum Biol* 2004; **31**: 311–2.

151 **Andrew T, Hart DJ, Snieder H, de Lange M, Spector TD, MacGregor AJ.** Are twins and singletons comparable? A study of disease-related and lifestyle characteristics in adult women. *Twin Res* 2001; **4**: 464–77.

152 **Ong KK, Loos RJF.** Rapid infancy weight gain and subsequent obesity: Systematic review and hopeful suggestions. *Acta Paediatr* 2006; **95**: 904–8.

Chapter 5

Discussant chapter—summary of the theoretical approaches to family-based studies in life course epidemiology

Hazel M Inskip

Abstract

Many approaches have been used to disentangle familial influences on health and disease within a life course epidemiological approach. Chapters 2 to 4 describe three specific approaches to family studies, namely, intergenerational, sibling, and twin studies. All can be used to assist in distinguishing between genetic and environmental influences mainly within the classical nature-nurture paradigm. This chapter summarizes the three approaches, describes links across the methods, and draws on other examples to highlight some of the areas discussed and to explore other issues, such as birth order effects. All three chapters use the example of influences on birth weight to exemplify the use of their specific study types, intergenerational, sibling or twin, but they also consider outcomes occurring later in the life course. As in all branches of epidemiology a variety of methods in different contexts is required for us to see consistent patterns emerge. Conflicting evidence points to our lack of understanding and for alternative hypotheses to be explored.

5.1 Introduction

The family– that dear octopus from whose tentacles we never quite escape nor, in our inmost hearts, ever quite wish to.

Dodie Smith[1]

The tentacles of the family have a long reach. Throughout the life course our families contribute factors that influence many of our attributes and our physical and mental health. Thus, almost by definition, life course epidemiology requires an understanding of familial influences. A simple schema of the classical distinction between genetic (nature) and environmental (nurture) influences operating within families is given in Figure 5.1.

Genes are transferred from parent to child at conception, though their impact is lifelong. Nurture operates from even before conception (the health and lifestyle of the mother before pregnancy influencing both conception itself and later fetal development) then the mother nurtures the fetus *in utero*, and parents (often with grandparental support) nurture the child to adulthood

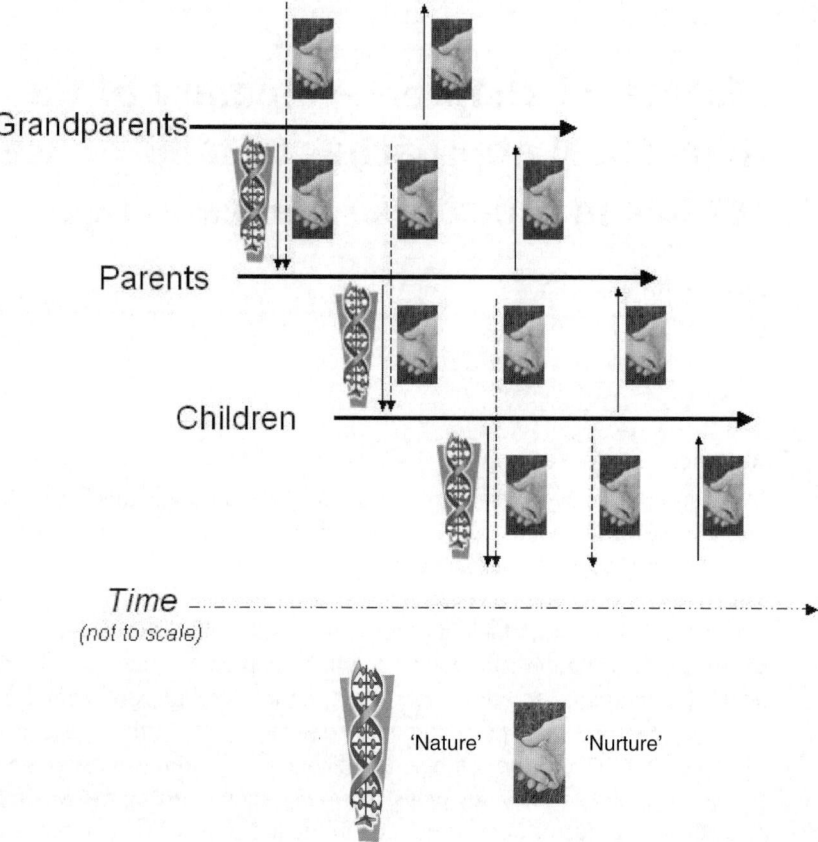

Fig. 5.1 Schematic representation of the classical understanding of 'nature' (genetic influences) and 'nurture' (environmental influences) operating within families.

and beyond. Roles can reverse in older age with children caring for their parents, and, indeed, the health and well-being of parents can be influenced by their children at many stages of life.[2] Even people separated from their family at birth retain the genetic, pre-conceptional and intrauterine influences on their health, and at a later stage their health may be affected by their own offspring. A further layer of influences comes from those exerted by siblings (and twins) on each other. The nature-nurture distinctions have, however, become blurred in recent years, as we increasingly understand gene-environment interactions[3–5] and explore epigenetic mechanisms.[6–8] Thus genetic expression may be modified by environmental influences altering the pathways to disease, and those environmental influences may themselves be derived from within the family. An individual's health trajectory is bound up inextricably with family influences in a variety of ways.

Assessing these influences in life course epidemiology requires a multi-faceted approach. No single study can reasonably include all the 'tentacles' of family life; collecting data on the wide range of cultural and physical exposures and genetic profiles of multiple generations is a daunting task (discussed in more detail in Chapter 6). Thus we end up approaching it in a variety of ways, but by doing so endeavour to build up the jigsaw, looking for links and consistency between the pieces.

5.2 Intergenerational studies

In Chapter 2, the intergenerational transfer of characteristics was described. The primary example used to illustrate such mechanisms was birth weight. Great imagination has been used in designing studies to explore these relationships and a range of methods is described in that chapter.

5.2.1 Studies of parental influences

Probably the simplest form of intergenerational study is the examination of how parental factors affect outcomes in their offspring. These can be extended down the generations to examine grandparental (and great-grandparental, etc.) effects.

Simple correlation of phenotypic characteristics across generations is informative but it can be hard to tease out how these characteristics are transmitted. In relation to birth outcomes, such as birth weight, different correlations between birth weights down the maternal and paternal lines indicate the strength of intrauterine influences.

Examining effects occurring later in the offspring's lives means that the influences operating post-natally and through childhood and beyond need to be considered too. Analyses of the Southampton Women's Survey showed that the extent to which a woman complied with dietary recommendations prior to pregnancy is a key influence on the way in which she follows the infant feeding guidelines when her child is 6 and 12 months of age.[9] In a traditional family where most childcare is performed by the mother, feeding and nurture may be more strongly associated with the way the maternal grandmother nurtured the mother than the paternal grandmother nurtured the father. Correlations therefore may be stronger along the maternal than paternal line due to a multiplicity of influences, and not simply those operating *in utero*.

5.2.2 Other intergenerational study designs

Teasing out the relative contributions of genetic and environmental influences, and determining the actual genetic mechanisms and the specific environmental factors involved is complex, and studies involving the direct parental lines do not address all the issues. Thus more ingenious study designs incorporating maternal twins, maternal cousins, sibships, adopted offspring, egg donation, and surrogate mothers have been employed to enable partitioning of the genetic and environmental influences. Recent exploration of Mendelian randomization[10] has provided a complementary approach to more classical epidemiology but the drawback to this method is the general requirement for particularly large sample sizes.

Examining maternal cousins who share maternal grandparents allow comparisons to be made between pairs of mothers who share some genetic and environmental factors but have differences in some of their intrauterine experiences, as well as those occurring throughout their lives. In Chapter 2, the influence of grandparental smoking *in utero* for the one sister but not for the other was explored in relation to the birth weights in the subsequent generation. Such studies assume that the sisters share the same parental socio-economic background and childhood home environment, but this is a strong assumption. For instance, birth order can have profound effects; in the Southampton Women's Survey,[9] there was a strong effect of birth order on the compliance with infant feeding recommendations, with earlier born siblings eating diets that followed the recommendations more closely than for those born later. Thus although there will be similarity between the childhood environment shared by sisters, their experiences are not identical.

5.2.3 Studies of obesity and outcomes later in life

While studies of birth weight focus on disentangling the genetic, and pre-conceptional and intrauterine environmental influences, they are less complicated than studies of effects later in life.

For some outcomes, the timing of the measurement is also important. For example, those obese at one age are not necessarily obese at other times in their lives, so obesity is not always a lifetime experience. While obesity does track to some extent other influences, such as parental obesity, and racial differences can affect the degree of tracking.[11, 12] The lifetime experience accumulates and contributes to later outcomes, and there will be a greater number of influences that contribute to outcomes occurring at older ages. Genetic and intrauterine exposures may be important influences on outcomes in early life, but these generally become diluted by influences at later ages on outcomes occurring later in life. A notable exception though, as discussed in Chapter 3, is that, contrary to expectation, heritable influences for psychological and behavioural outcomes appear to strengthen as age increases.[13]

5.2.3.1 Maternal smoking *in utero* in relation to obesity

In Chapter 2, examples of effects of maternal and paternal smoking on childhood body mass index (BMI) and other childhood outcomes are described. Maternal, but not paternal, smoking when the offspring is *in utero* leads to lower birth weight. Maternal smoking during pregnancy is also associated with later obesity in the offspring.[14] However, countering this, higher (rather than lower) birth weight is also associated with later obesity.[15] Thus it appears that the mechanism relating maternal smoking and obesity does not operate through the smoking effect on birth weight. As noted in Chapter 2 however, an analysis of the Avon Longitudinal Study of Parents and Children (ALSPAC)[16] indicated that maternal smoking may not have a direct intrauterine effect in relation to later obesity, as the effects of paternal and maternal smoking were similar. Somewhat conversely, Al Mamun *et al.*[17] have shown that levels of obesity in adolescents whose mothers stopped smoking in pregnancy were similar to those of mothers who had never smoked; this indicates a specific intrauterine effect of maternal smoking. Replication of the maternal-paternal smoking difference and further studies of women who gave up smoking in pregnancy are needed to untangle these effects. Large studies will be required, however, as maternal and paternal smoking are highly correlated,[18] and only a proportion of women who smoke manage to give up the habit during pregnancy.

5.2.3.2 Obesity and diabetes

Obesity is a complex phenomenon. The standard measure of obesity uses body mass index defined as weight/height^2, but this does not distinguish between lean and fat mass, or between central and peripheral adiposity. A similar conundrum to that operating for maternal smoking, birth weight and obesity, exists in understanding the relationships between birth weight, obesity and Type 2 diabetes. Higher birth weight babies are at lower risk of diabetes in later life,[19, 20] yet larger babies are more likely to become obese,[15] and obesity is a major risk factor for diabetes.[21] However, the birth weight association with diabetes may be due to low birth weight being associated with a reduction in lean rather than fat mass,[22, 23] or the differential fat distribution about the body[24, 25] in conjunction with the pattern of growth after birth.[19, 20] Teasing out the genetic and intrauterine influences on birth weight and obesity as well as understanding the pathways through infancy, childhood, and adulthood to obesity and diabetes requires varied epidemiological approaches among which intergenerational studies make an important contribution.

5.2.4 Parenting

The quality of parenting is a profound influence exerted by parents on their children. In epidemiology the word 'nurture' covers all the environmental influences that are not genetic in origin. In lay language, the nurturing of a child is more-or-less synonymous with parenting (see Figure 5.1). Parenting and the quality of child-parent relationships have long been recognized as influencing health in the offspring. Various aspects have been studied such as physical abuse, warmth of the relationship, discipline and control, and parental divorce. Such influences not only affect mental and physical health[26] of the offspring, but also affect subsequent relationships with the next generation.[27] Parenting thus has consequences across more than one generation, and typifies an intergenerational contribution to life course epidemiology.

The effects may operate in the reverse direction too; as noted in Chapter 2 depression in the parents is associated with behavioural difficulties in the offspring but it is hard to be clear which is the cause and the effect. In other words, does the parental depression (or precursors of it) cause the offspring's behavioural problems or is it the other way round?[28, 29] Reverse causality is not the only problem though, as reporting bias compounds the issue. Within the ALSPAC cohort,[30] maternal and parental anxiety assessed during the child's first year of life was associated with recurrent abdominal pain in the children aged 6¾ years. However, despite the longitudinal nature of the study, reporting bias could not be ruled out as anxious mothers may over-report recurrent abdominal pain in their children. Disentangling the nature of such relationships is not straight-forward, even in longitudinal analyses.

5.2.5 Summary of intergenerational studies

The effects on a subsequent generation operate through genetic mechanisms and environmental exposures that operate pre-conceptionally, *in utero*, and during the offspring's life course. Intergenerational studies allow the teasing out of aspects of the mechanisms but as they can operate at so many different levels, large studies are required to pin-point particular effects.

5.3 Sibling studies

Sibling studies are a powerful tool because of their similar, but not identical, family environments. In Chapter 3, the theoretical methods underpinning such studies have been clearly laid out. Three particular strategies are described, namely the sibling fixed effects models, behavioural genetic, and genetic linkage studies.

5.3.1 Fixed effects models

The fixed effects approach allows much, though not all, of the familial environmental influences to be taken out of the equation and thus allows the exploration of effects specific to the individual that do not operate across the whole family. Much unexplored confounding can be removed from the analysis, thus strengthening our belief that the results are not simply due to the confounding influences common to both siblings. As noted though, such models only adjust out confounding factors that remain stable within sibling pairs. It is not straightforward to identify the factors that do and do not vary between siblings. The example quoted in Chapter 3 in relation to family income makes the point. Income does vary over time within families but the variation is usually only slight; exploring the effects within families of fluctuations in income, which are generally small, may mean that the influence of income *per se* is missed.

5.3.1.1 Birth order and family size

An effect that differs between non-twin sibling pairs as a *sine qua non* is birth order. Associations have been reported between birth order (and/or family size) and a number of conditions developing later in life, for example, schizophrenia,[31] atopy,[32] obesity,[33–35] and various cancers, such as lymphoma, leukaemia, breast cancer and melanoma,[36–37] but the relationships are not always consistent. Some of the associations are specifically with first born or only children, which may point to a maternal factor relating to primiparity rather than an effect of sibling relationships.

However, the 'hygiene hypothesis' suggests that first (and higher order) born and only children are at increased risk of atopy due to poorer development of their immune system as they are not subjected to infections brought into the house by older siblings.[32, 38–39] While there is some evidence for this, there are enough inconsistencies in the findings from studies that questions remain.[40] There have been various studies that have challenged the hypothesis; in relation to asthma *per se*, a study of more than half a million military conscripts in Israel found that asthma prevalence was strongly related to family size but not to birth order.[41] Studies of this size allow exploration of both family size and birth order, which is not often possible in smaller studies.

5.3.1.2 Random effect models

An additional approach to sibling studies has been to use random as well as fixed effect models (discussed in more detail in Chapter 11). For example, Mann *et al.*[42] used random effects cross-sectional time-series linear regression analysis to estimate the within- and between-families effects simultaneously. Using data on 600 sibling pairs they showed that the between- and within-family effects of birth weight on systolic blood pressure in children were of similar size. The analyses included adjustment for a variety of confounding factors, adding to the robustness of the analysis. Further studies using a similar approach to explore possible mechanisms underlying the association of birth weight with blood pressure and other cardiovascular outcomes are described in Chapter 13.

5.3.2 Behavioural genetics

The behavioural genetics approach to sibling studies allows for exploration of the amount of the the variation between siblings that is made by genetic and environmental factors. The method aims to partition the phenotypic variation into three components: genetic factors, environmental factors shared by the siblings due to their shared family, and environmental factors specific to each individual sibling. Estimates of heritability can be obtained, and by subtraction the components of variation due to the environmental influences can be derived. Different types of siblings are needed, in which the genetic and environmental contributions will vary. Thus half-siblings, adopted siblings, and siblings raised apart bring different genetic and environmental contributions to the analyses.

These methods allow a disentangling of the genetic and environmental components of a particular characteristic, usually at a fixed age. However, examining the way in which the components vary through the life course, by conducting analyses at different ages, informs our understanding about when particular influences are strongest. Trends in the components over time can also be informative as they can reveal cohort effects or point to underlying environmental influences that have affected one generation more than another.

Behavioural genetics methods do allow some estimation of within and between family effects. In other words, an attempt can be made to pinpoint where the environmental influences operate most strongly. Family-level influences are not as strong as many researchers would expect and perhaps the family environment itself creates differences between siblings, though these differences appear in models as within-sibling effects. These add another layer of complexity to the simplistic nature-nurture diagram given in Figure 5.1. For example, as described above, birth order is a strong effect in many analyses. It is undeniably an effect operating within a family context but in behavioural genetics analyses it operates as a within-sibling effect.

5.3.3 Genetic linkage studies

The final methodological approach to sibling studies relates to genetic linkage studies. Such studies focus on families in which more than one member of the family is affected by the disease of interest.

However, as noted in chapter 2, they are hard to conduct as their statistical power tends to be low and it is difficult to infer genetic susceptibility when the disease can be due to different sets of predisposing genes. Few diseases can be attributed to a single allele but, for such diseases, linkage studies are particularly valuable in dissecting out the influences in relation to timing of onset and progression of the disease.

5.3.4 Summary of sibling studies

Sibling studies provide an important contribution to the nature-nurture debate. Full siblings can be used in fixed effect models but different types of siblings can inform our understanding using a behavioural genetics approach. However, discerning the similarities in and differences between environmental influences operating between and within siblings is a challenge.

5.4 Twin studies

Classically, twin studies have been seen as a gold standard for assessing heritability. The standard approach is to compare the similarity of monozygotic twins with the similarity of dizygotic twins. If monozygotic twins are more similar to each other than are dizygotic twins then the genetic heritability is considered to be high. Calculating the correlation coefficient for the factor of interest among dizygous twins and comparing this with the correlation among monozygous twins allows an estimate of the percentage of the factor that is due to heritable influences. However, as we know, the disaggregation of genetic and environmental factors is not simple, and interactions between them muddy the waters in such analyses. Genetic modelling does, however, allow a more sophisticated approach to identifying genetic and various environmental influences and their interactions.

There is much similarity between twin and sibling studies and they can complement each other. However, the assumption that dizygotic twins are as similar in their environmental influences as are monozygotic twins is a strong one, and within families and in society, dizygotic twins may be treated differently to monozygotic twins. Even the prenatal environment may differ between the two types of twins, and different-sex twins may be more different to each other than like-sex twins in other ways than just their sex.

5.4.1 Different types of twins

Classical twin studies have focused on the differences between monozygous and dizygous twins, but this approach ignores important differences between types of monozygous twins. Their fetal life can differ markedly due to variations in placentation, leading to three different processes by which monozygous twins can be nurtured in fetal life (see Chapter 4 for more detailed explanation). Such differences can inform our understanding of fetal growth and development and the influence of materno-fetal nutrient supply through the placenta. However, it is important to remember that a woman carrying two or more fetuses at the same time provides a different pre-natal environment than in a singleton pregnancy. Twins are far more likely to be premature than singletons, and maternal nutrition to the two fetuses is more likely to be compromised than for a woman supplying a single fetus. Zygosity has an impact on birth weight and so do chorionicity and site of umbilical cord insertion. Thus care is needed when we extrapolate from twin studies to influences on singletons.[43]

Birth order was discussed above in relation to differences between siblings. While twins share the same number of younger and older siblings as each other (not counting the other twin), birth order effects within twin pairs cannot be ignored. For example, second-born twins are at a higher risk of perinatal death and cerebral palsy than their co-twins,[44, 45] whereas first-born twins are more likely to be left-handed.[46]

5.4.2 The contribution of twin studies to life course epidemiology

Life course epidemiology requires an understanding from before conception to death. A crucial time window of development is the pre-natal period. Early studies that led to the 'fetal origins' hypothesis[47] showed that birth weight was strongly and inversely correlated with many later chronic diseases. The hypothesis has widened to include pathways of growth and development in childhood and as such forms a component of life course epidemiology. Many early criticisms of the hypothesis were that the associations were entirely due to genetic factors. The classical twin study approach was therefore used to tease out the genetic and environmental contributions to the associations between birth weight and later outcomes (see Chapter 4 and Chapter 13 for specific examples of this approach with respect to the birth weight-cardiovascular disease association). Standard analyses used the fixed effects approach, in a similar way to that described in Chapter 3 for the analysis of sibling studies. Contrasting the findings for monozygous and dizygous twins allows the genetic and environmental effects to be dissected. But, as we have seen, monozygous twins are not identical in the prenatal environment and so the classical distinction between environment and genes is far from clear-cut.

Taking the comparison of twins further, differences and similarities within twin pairs can be exploited to examine the relationships between factors such as birth weight and later disease. Chapter 4 contains a description of the use of analyses of twins who were concordant for low or for high birth weight to explore relationships between birth weight and adult blood pressure[48] (additional examples are provided in Chapter 13). Differences in birth weight within twin pairs were not associated with differences in adult blood pressure and so the exploration of concordant pairs was of interest. However, differences in birth weights within pairs of twins are not usually large and so teasing out the effects of differences and concordance in birth weights is not straightforward; it mirrors the difficulties, described in Chapter 3 and noted above in Section 5.3.1, in exploring the effect of differences in family income by analysing siblings.

5.4.3 Summary of twin studies

Analyses of twin studies require care. The classical twin study approach provides an important contribution to the nature-nurture debate, but it does have its limitations. We are increasingly able to use more sophisticated models for identifying the components due to differences between pairs and within pairs.[49] The challenges, though, include gaining data on sufficient numbers of twins so that analyses have high statistical power, the degree to which results from twin studies can be extrapolated to singletons, and the influences of chorionicity and site of cord insertion.

5.5 Types of family studies

Three main types of family studies are described in Chapters 2 to 4, namely intergenerational, sibling, and twin studies. A concept that underlies all three types is that of testing differences between individuals. This is particularly true of sibling and twin studies whose strength derives from examining the differences between siblings within families, or between twins within twin pairs. However, it is also true of much of the intergenerational work; while some studies focus on the influence of maternal factors on the offspring, there are intergenerational analyses that examine the difference between paternal and maternal influences, or differences between the maternal influences operating on maternal cousins. This is unlike much classical epidemiology, which tends to relate risk factors operating on the individual to later development of disease within the same individual.

All the types of study give insights into the genetic and environmental components that influence particular characteristics or disease outcomes. A particular focus of such studies is on the pre- and post-natal influences. The genetic influences come from both parents; the intrauterine experience is undeniably influenced by the mother, and is shared by twins and to some extent by siblings; and the early childhood experience is influenced both by parents and siblings and, for twins, by the co-twin. These effects have a long reach and determine not only physical characteristics such as adult height and weight, but also physical and mental health. The tentacles of family life are indeed inescapable, and understanding the strength of each particular familial influence is part of the challenge of life course epidemiology.

References

1 Smith DG. *Dear Octopus—A comedy*. Act III, Scene 2. Samuel French, London, 1938.
2 Gould E. Decomposing the effects of children's health on mother's labor supply: is it time or money? *Health Economics* 2004; **13**: 525–41.
3 Ottman R. Gene-environment interaction and public health. *American Journal of Human Genetics* 1995; **56**: 821–3.
4 Khoury MJ, Wagener DK. Epidemiological evaluation of the use of genetics to improve the predictive value of disease risk factors. *American Journal of Human Genetics* 1995; **56**: 835–44.
5 Boks MP, Schipper M, Schubart CD, Sommer IE, Kahn RS, Ophoff RA. Investigating gene environment interaction in complex diseases: increasing power by selective sampling for environmental exposure. *International Journal of Epidemiology* 2007; **36**: 1363–9.
6 Holliday R. Epigenetics: a historical overview. *Epigenetics* 2006; **1**: 76–80.
7 Godfrey KM, Lillycrop KA, Burdge GC, Gluckman PD, Hanson MA. Epigenetic mechanisms and the mismatch concept of the developmental origins of health and disease. *Pediatric Research* 2007; **61**: 5R–10R.
8 Gluckman PD, Hanson MA, Beedle AS. Non-genomic transgenerational inheritance of disease risk. *Bioessays* 2007; **29**: 145–54.
9 Robinson S, Marriott L, Poole J, Crozier S, Borland S, Lawrence W, *et al.* Dietary patterns in infancy: the importance of maternal and family influences on feeding practice. *British Journal of Nutrition* 2007; **98**: 1029–37.
10 Davey Smith G, Ebrahim S. 'Mendelian randomization': can genetic epidemiology contribute to understanding environmental determinants of disease? *International Journal of Epidemiology* 2003; **32**: 1–22.
11 Kvaavik E, Tell GS, Klepp KI. Predictors and tracking of body mass index from adolescence into adulthood: follow-up of 18 to 20 years in the Oslo Youth Study. *Archives of Pediatric Adolescent Medicine* 2003; **157**: 1212–8.
12 Freedman DS, Khan LK, Serdula MK, Dietz WH, Srinivasan SR, Berenson GS. Racial differences in the tracking of childhood BMI to adulthood. *Obesity Research* 2005; **13**: 928–35.
13 McGue M, Bouchard TJ. Genetic and environmental influences on human behavioral differences. *Annual Review of Neuroscience* 1998; **21**: 1–24.
14 Huang JS, Lee TA, Lu MC. Prenatal programming of childhood overweight and obesity. *Maternal and Child Health Journal* 2007; **11**: 461–73.
15 Baird J, Fisher D, Lucas P, Kleijnen J, Roberts H, Law C. Being big or growing fast: systematic review of size and growth in infancy and later obesity. *BMJ* 2005; **331**: 929–31.
16 Leary SD, Davey Smith GD, Rogers IS, Reilly JJ, Wells JC, Ness AR. Smoking during pregnancy and offspring fat and lean mass in childhood. *Obesity* 2006; **14**: 2284–93.
17 Al Mamun A, Lawlor DA, Alati R, O'Callaghan MJ, Williams GM, Najman JM. Does maternal smoking during pregnancy have a direct effect on future offspring obesity? Evidence from a prospective birth cohort study. *American Journal of Epidemiology* 2006; **164**: 317–25.
18 Clark AE, Etilé F. Don't give up on me baby: spousal correlation in smoking behaviour. *Journal of Health Economics* 2006; **25**: 958–78.

19 Fall CHD. Developmental origins of cardiovascular disease, type 2 diabetes and obesity in humans. In: Wintour M, Owens J, editors. *Early life origins of health and disease.* Springer Science and Business Media, London. pp. 8–27, 2006.

20 Eriksson JG. Epidemiology, genes and the environment: lessons learned from the Helsinki Birth Cohort Study. *Journal of Internal Medicine* 2007; **261**: 418–25.

21 Haffner SM. Relationship of metabolic risk factors and development of cardiovascular disease and diabetes. *Obesity* 2006; **14**: 121S–127S.

22 Hediger ML, Overpeck MD, Kuczmarski RJ, McGlynn A, Maurer KR, Davis WW. Muscularity and fatness of infants and young children born small- or large-for-gestational-age. *Pediatrics* 1998; **102**: E60.

23 Gale CR, Martyn CN, Kellingray S, Eastell R, Cooper C. Intrauterine programming of adult body composition. *Journal of Clinical Endocrinology and Metabolism* 2001; **86**: 267–72.

24 Law CM, Barker DJ, Osmond C, Fall CH, Simmonds SJ. Early growth and abdominal fatness in adult life. *Journal of Epidemiology and Community Health* 1992; **46**: 184–6.

25 Kuh D, Hardy R, Chaturvedi N, Wadsworth ME. Birth weight, childhood growth and abdominal obesity in adult life. *International Journal of Obesity and Related Metabolic Disorders* 2002; **26**: 40–7.

26 Stewart-Brown SL, Fletcher L, Wadsworth ME. Parent–child relationships and health problems in adulthood in three UK national birth cohort studies. *European Journal of Public Health* 2005; 15: 640–6.

27 Roberts R, O'Connor T, Dunn J, Golding J, The ALSPAC Study Team. The effects of child sexual abuse in later family life; mental health, parenting and adjustment of offspring. *Child Abuse and Neglect* 2004; **28**: 525–45.

28 Elgar FJ, McGrath PJ, Waschbusch DA, Stewart SH, Curtis LJ. Mutual influences on maternal depression and child adjustment problems. *Clinical Psychology Review* 2004; **24**: 441–59.

29 Ramchandani P, Stein A, Evans J, O'Connor TG, ALSPAC study team. Paternal depression in the postnatal period and child development: a prospective population study. *Lancet* 2005; **365**: 2201–5.

30 Ramchandani PG, Stein A, Hotopf M, Wiles NJ, ALSPAC Study Team. Early parental and child predictors of recurrent abdominal pain at school age: results of a large population-based study. *Journal of the American Academy of Child and Adolescent Psychiatry* 2006; **45**: 729–36.

31 Gaughran F, Blizard R, Mohan R, Zammit S, Owen M. Birth order and the severity of illness in schizophrenia. *Psychiatry Research* 2007; **150**: 205–10.

32 Strachan DP. Family size, infection and atopy: the first decade of the 'hygiene hypothesis'. *Thorax* 2000; **55**: S2–S10.

33 Wang H, Sekine M, Chen X, Kanayama H, Yamagami T, Kagamimori S. Sib-size, birth order and risk of overweight in junior high school students in Japan: results of the Toyama Birth Cohort Study. *Preventive Medicine* 2007; **44**: 45–51.

34 Stettler N, Tershakovec AM, Zemel BS, Leonard MB, Boston RC, Katz SH, *et al.* Risk factors for increased adiposity: a cohort study of African American subjects followed from birth to young adulthood. *American Journal Clinical Nutrition* 2000; **72**: 378–83.

35 Ravelli GP, Belmont L. Obesity in nineteen-year-old men: family size and birth order associations. *American Journal of Epidemiology* 1979; **109**: 66–70.

36 Altieri A, Castro F, Bermejo JL, Hemminki K. Number of siblings and the risk of lymphoma, leukemia, and myeloma by histopathology. *Cancer Epidemiology, Biomarkers and Prevention* 2006; **15**: 1281–6.

37 Hemminki K, Mutanen P. Birth order, family size, and the risk of cancer in young and middle-aged adults. *British Journal of Cancer* 2001; **84**: 1466–71.

38 Strachan DP. Hay fever, hygiene, and household size. *BMJ* 1989; **299**: 1259–60.

39 Johnston SL, Openshaw PJ. The protective effect of childhood infections. *BMJ* 2001; **322**: 376–7.

40 von Mutius E. Allergies, infections and the hygiene hypothesis—the epidemiological evidence. *Immunobiology* 2007; **212**: 433–9.

41 Goldberg S, Israeli E, Schwartz S, Shochat T, Izbicki G, Toker-Maimon O, *et al.* Asthma prevalence, family size, and birth order. *Chest* 2007; **131**: 1747–52.

42 Mann V, De Stavola BL, Leon DA. Separating within and between effects in family studies: an application to the study of blood pressure in children. *Statistics in Medicine* 2004; **23**: 2745–56.

43 Morley R, Dwyer T, Carlin J. Studies of twins: what can they tell us about the developmental origins of adult health and disease? In: Wintour M, Owens J, editors. *Early Life Origins of Health and Disease*. Springer Science and Business Media, London. pp. 29–41, 2006.

44 Smith GC, Fleming KM, White IR. Birth order of twins and risk of perinatal death related to delivery in England, Northern Ireland, and Wales, 1994-2003: retrospective cohort study. *BMJ* 2007; **334**: 576–78.

45 Topp M, Huusom LD, Langhoff-Roos J, Delhumeau C, Hutton JL, Dolk H, SCPE Collaborative Group. Multiple birth and cerebral palsy in Europe: a multicenter study. *Acta Obstetricia et Gynecologica Scandinavica* 2004; **83**: 548–53.

46 James WH, Orlebeke JF. Determinants of handedness in twins. *Laterality* 2002; **7**: 301–7.

47 Barker DJP. *Mothers, babies and health in later life*. Churchill Livingstone, Edinburgh, 1998.

48 Loos RJ, Fagard R, Beunen G, Derom C, Vlietinck R. Birth weight and blood pressure in young adults: a prospective twin study. *Circulation* 2001; **104**: 1633–8.

49 Carlin JB, Gurrin LC, Sterne JA, Morley R, Dwyer T. Regression models for twin studies: a critical review. *International Journal of Epidemiology* 2005; **34**: 1089–99.

Part II

The practicalities of undertaking family-based studies

Chapter 6

Birth cohorts: a resource for life course studies

Anne-Marie Nybo Andersen, Mia Madsen and Debbie A Lawlor

> Life is to be understood backwards, but it is lived forwards.
> [Livet skal forstaaes baglaens, men leves forlaens]
>
> Søren Kierkegaard, Danish Philosopher, 1813–1855

Abstract

In this chapter we discuss issues concerned with the design and practicalities of setting up birth cohorts for life course studies. The demand for a blueprint of the ideal birth cohort study is perhaps intuitive but, using examples from older birth cohorts, we question the extent to which standardization of data collection and study protocols across contemporary and planned birth cohorts is desirable or feasible.

We discuss different approaches, difficulties and strengths of these different approaches, the determination of scientific priorities, definition of the birth cohort (including which family members are key participants), data collection and samples size, as well as the ethical considerations specific to the establishment of a birth cohort.

The advantages of a scientific focus on specific exposures in each birth cohort study, of documentation of birth cohort data, and of collaborative studies using data from several birth cohorts are emphasized.

6.1 A blueprint for the ideal birth cohort study: is it possible and desirable to develop?

In the two decades around the turn of the millennium a significant number of birth cohorts have been initiated and more are in the phase of planning.[1-6] This trend reflects a renewed interest in how the earliest phases of life affect adult health. In particular, there has been increasing interest in the roles of growth patterns in the intrauterine period and the first years of life on later life health and disease, following the seminal work published by Barker and colleagues during the 1980s and 1990s.[7]

While the inverse association between birth weight and a number of chronic diseases in adult life, particularly cardiovascular diseases, seemed to be indisputable, many researchers questioned the causality in the associations found[8–10] (see Chapter 13 for a detailed discussion of the scientific debates around this association and how family-based studies have contributed to some aspects of this debate). A number of the issues raised about whether these associations were causal, and if so, their importance with respect to disease prevention, might be possible to answer with studies that are better able to control for potential confounding factors and that have more detailed information on intrauterine, perinatal, infant and childhood exposures and conditions, compared to the earlier cohorts examining the developmental origins of adult disease. Thus, an obvious answer to this scientific debate was to create new studies, designed to address research questions around determinants of fetal and infant growth and their association with long-term health, with prospectively collected data on putative or alleged confounding factors, as well as what might be the key causal risk factors during the developmental period. This reasoning became an important justification for launching many new birth cohorts around the turn of the millennium, notwithstanding the fact that these new cohorts would not be able to provide data to address research questions concerned with developmental origins of adult disease, such as cardiovascular disease, until around year 2060.

In the meantime, creative epidemiologists began to 'dig up' old cohorts with information, not only on birth weight, but also on some of the suspected factors that could explain the association, whether it was the possible key causative risk factors or confounders of this association. In the search for these older existing cohorts, it became apparent that a wave of birth cohorts was established around the 1950s to 1960s. Examples include the Aberdeen Children of the 1950s cohort,[11] the Danish Metropolit Cohort[12] and its Swedish counterpart from Stockholm,[13] the British 1958 birth cohort,[14] the Perinatal Collaborative Study from US,[15, 16] and the Copenhagen Perinatal Cohort.[17, 18] Some of the cohorts were medically oriented and intended to focus on perinatal health, whereas others were established within the field of sociology and psychology with scientific foci on mental health and learning disabilities.

While some of these cohorts had carried out data collection sweeps regularly all through the period from their initiation to the present date and had expanded their research focus far beyond the initial aims of determining factors associated with perinatal outcomes,[14] other birth cohorts that were established around the middle of the last century remained dormant after addressing their original (short-term) aims and have been recently revitalized in order to address the questions relating to the current interest in developmental origins of later health and disease.[11, 12]

Many of these newly established birth cohorts and revitalized older cohorts focused primarily on extending Barker and colleagues' work in relation to cardiovascular risk factors and outcomes, however, there was also emerging interest in the developmental origins of a much wider range of health outcomes. For example the Prenatal Determinants of Schizophrenia (PDS) study is a rejuvenation of an existing birth cohort—the Child Health and Development Study (CHDS). The CHDS was initiated in 1959 with the original purpose of investigating prenatal and perinatal determinants of child health and development, and data collection included biological samples from both child and parents. Apart from a few small sub-samples, follow-up beyond childhood was never carried out. Using information from the Kaiser Foundation Health Plan, which provided health care to a large proportion of the cohort, the tracing of cohort members and identification of cases of schizophrenia was initiated in the late 1990s[19] and the established PDS has now contributed important findings regarding a number of prenatal determinants of schizophrenia.[20]

With respect to considering what should be included in a blueprint for the ideal birth cohort study at least two points can be made from the above discussion of how current birth cohorts have arisen:

- Birth cohorts are not necessarily scientifically exploited to their full potential, which, with respect to both time and research topics, goes beyond the original a priori research questions that resulted in these cohorts being established.

- We cannot imagine what interesting scientific questions will evolve two or ten decades from now and, therefore, how today's birth cohorts could contribute informative data to key research questions in the future. Consequently, we have no way of being able to ensure that they do indeed include relevant data for future priority research questions.

To further elaborate on these points let us imagine that we are in the year 2080. Let us further imagine that there is a strong intergenerational transfer of intellect and imagination in the family of epidemiologists, and therefore that epidemiologists seven decades from now are as adept at finding old birth cohorts and exploiting them to address key research questions as the current family of epidemiologists. Our hypothetical 2080 epidemiologist might tell the following story:

> In the two decades around the turn of the millennium a significant number of prenatal birth cohorts with collection of biological material, including DNA, were initiated. These included the Avon Longitudinal Study of Parents and Children (ALSPAC),[1] the Danish National Birth Cohort,[2] the Norwegian MoBa study (Norwegian National Birth Cohort),[3] Generation R from Rotterdam,[5] and the National Children's Study from the US.[6] The establishment of these new cohorts reflected an understanding that the development of disease should be understood using a life course perspective, which emphasized effects on health related outcomes of biological (including genetic), environmental and social exposures during gestation, infancy, childhood, adolescence, adulthood and across generations.[21] Furthermore, the developments within molecular genetics and computing power had led to an increased focus on how genes and environment interact and contribute to individuals' risk of disease.
>
> In addition to the interests in developmental origins of health and disease and life course epidemiology, the aim to study gene-environment interactions in a prospective setting became a further justification for initiating many of these new birth cohorts. This was despite the fact that the public health importance of gene-environmental interactions had been questioned and that power calculations suggested that most of the birth cohorts with sample sizes around 5,000–10,000 were too small to address specific gene-environment interactions.[22] Nowadays, we would also question whether these studies had adequate power to determine main effects for some key rare exposures and outcomes.
>
> Some epidemiologists around the turn of the Millennium came up with what they thought was an obvious solution to the problem of insufficient power, which was to call for standardization and close co-ordination of the data collection in the different birth cohorts, thus making data suitable for pooled analyses.[23] This was—fortunately—only partly done.
>
> I have seen the results from the great pooled analyses of these Millennium birth cohorts, including the remarkable contribution they made to understanding the developmental and life course origins of cardiovascular disease in the 2050s and 2060s. However, once I started to use the data from these studies for my own research I also discovered problems. Standardization of data collection was not actually exact across all studies for all variables, even when it was intended to be so from the study initiation. For some variables this was unsurprising and necessary, for others it was a not understandable—to me at least. I learnt at first hand how these differences can make pooling of data and cross-cohort comparisons scientifically dubious.
>
> On the other hand, in a few areas, e.g. dietary habits, standardized and validated instruments for exposure data collection were used in a majority of the cohorts. The associations found between these exposures and some specific outcomes in separate cohorts were approximately the same, however, the exposure measurements were—from what we know now—measured with considerable error and therefore all of the cohorts with these identical measures are subject to a number of—identical—biases. This is such a shame because it means we really have no historical cohorts with accurate measures of these exposures.

Though not very well justified at the time a few single cohorts had—fortunately—included some pieces of information, which have now proved very valuable: one of the cohorts broke rank and collected information on organic food intake (in addition to the standard cohort collaboration diet questions) and the famous research group on organic food and dementia from Uganda have found the information in that cohort very valuable. Another of the cohorts had information on hours spent in an aircraft (by then at an altitude of approx. 30,000 feet) during intrauterine life and infancy and we are very excited about examining the effect of this exposure on future health (it's a shame the information is only available in one of the cohorts).

Some areas that got attention in all cohorts were tobacco smoking (both parents and offspring) and animals in the household during childhood. These exposures have no real relevance today, when tobacco growth and consumption no longer exists anywhere and no one keeps animals in the house, but were obviously important at the time when tobacco smoking was common and animals were frequently kept as pets.

Can you believe that none of these cohorts had information on maternal use of cosmetics containing endocrine disruptors despite evidence that some scientists had begun to suspect its detrimental effects, and whilst there was much chatter in the media at the turn of the Millennium about the changing formation of the family, the only information on parental relations in the majority of these cohorts was whether the 'parents' were married to each other or not and whether the participants were brought up in single parent families or not.

This story of the future epidemiologist might seem fanciful but experience from existing older cohorts demonstrates that it probably isn't far from reality. Documents from the 1950s and 1960s prove that the Aberdeen Children of the 1950s cohort and the Metropolit cohort from Copenhagen were planned and designed in close collaboration between the leading sociologists in Aberdeen and Copenhagen: R Illsley and K Svalastoga.* However, a recent attempt to undertake some pooled analyses using just a small fraction of these almost 50 year old data by one of the authors (A-MNA) and Professor David Leon from the London School of Hygiene and Tropical Medicine, highlighted insurmountable problems relating to lack of data consistency. What initially seemed to be minor differences in the data, e.g. the categorization of birth weight and father's social position, both measures, wisely, customized to their respective contexts, turned out to create impenetrable problems. Thus, separate analyses of the relation between paternal social position at birth and the mortality of cohort members displayed entirely different associations, and it was not possible to determine whether these differences were real or an artefact resulting from the classification of the social position of the fathers. Furthermore, in a number of the published associations from these two studies[24–30] it would have been ideal to have been able to adjust for maternal smoking during pregnancy. Contemporary epidemiologists would also be interested in using these cohort studies to examine the effect of modifiable maternal behaviours during pregnancy (including smoking, alcohol consumption, diet and physical activity) on later outcomes in the offspring, but these data were not recorded in either study. Given present day knowledge of the impact of smoking during pregnancy, and at other stages of the life course, on health outcomes, it is inconceivable that smoking data would not be collected today in any cohort study. However, in the 1950s smoking was only just emerging as a major health risk factor.

---

* The documentation was found in copies the correspondence about establishment of the Metropolit cohort, which in year 2000 was handed over from the founders of the cohort to M Osler and B Holstein at Department of Social Medicine, University of Copenhagen.

With the purpose of making a blueprint for the ideal birth cohort study at least two points could be made from our futuristic story:

- If data from birth cohorts are to be pooled, very strict protocols for the data collection might be necessary, but this might not be possible. Even small differences in the data collection method may hamper comparability and cast doubt on whether differences in associations are real or due to differences in data collection.

- Given that birth cohorts might appropriately be considered a research resource for now and many decades in the future, and that we cannot second guess what research priorities will be in future decades, if birth cohorts all stick rigidly to collecting the same data its possible that none will be suitable for future research questions.

So, is it sensible to develop a blueprint for the ideal birth cohort study? A conclusion based on the points in the discussion above is not obvious. Very strict standardization across all birth cohorts might not be feasible and variety in cohort data may very well be desirable in the long term as this will increase the chance of being able to find data to address future research questions not yet conceived. Also measurement standardization might result in error standardization across all cohorts. On the other hand, very large numbers and comparable data will allow us to address prevailing and future research questions with greater precision and to use cross-cohort comparisons to help causal understanding.

6.1.1 Current and future research priorities: lessons from forestry

The above stories highlight what for us should be one guiding principal in establishing and running birth cohorts: *Birth cohorts should be seen as research resources for now and for many future decades.*

The longitudinal nature of birth cohorts requiring decades of follow-up before results relating even to current research priorities (e.g. the developmental origins of cardiovascular disease), made the Norwegian epidemiologist, Leiv Bakketeig, use the metaphor of 'forest planting' in his description of birth cohorts at the first meeting in Norwegian Epidemiological Association in 1990 (personal communication). Applying this metaphor, a lesson from history can illustrate the risk associated with thinking of birth cohorts only in terms of their initial research aims: Around the turn of the 18th century when the British, with Lord Nelson at their helm, eradicated the Danish Navy, the King ordered forests to be planted in Denmark so a new navy could be built. These trees are only just now ready for harvest, but are not of great value for military purposes (certainly not against the original intended target, who are now more friendly and collaborative with the Danes).

6.1.2 Combining standardisation with diversity: a possible solution

If we agree that birth cohorts should be considered as important research resources for today's and the future's epidemiologists then it becomes intuitive that we should strive for some standardization but not at the extent of removing all diversity. Within the restrictions of research resources, ethical considerations and considerations of maintaining high levels of participation one solution might be to agree on standard protocols for data collection of a restricted list of variables related to contemporary research questions and where we have a very high level of confidence that our measurements tools are accurate (so we do not replicate measurement error across all cohorts). Investigators of each individual study could then add any other variables that will differ between studies and that would reflect differing local contexts and research priorities and also the thoughts of individual study investigators regarding what future researchers might be interested in. Of course there will still be the potential for problems with such an approach.

Individual study investigators would have to decide whether the 'common standard list of data collection' should take priority over their local research interests. But we feel there is benefit in greater communication across investigators of contemporary birth cohorts to try and standardise some measurements where this is feasible and advantageous for today's priorities without trying to make all of these cohorts fit a single blueprint.

There are, indeed, some good examples of such an approach. The International Childhood Cancer Cohort Consortium (I4C) is an international collaboration initiative that brings together ongoing and new birth cohorts with the aim of improving understanding of the origin of childhood cancers. Since childhood cancers are rare, but important diseases, collaboration is necessary to obtain precise estimates of the effect of key exposures. The idea of the consortium is to standardize selected protocol elements of all studies that belong to it (e.g. timing and measurement of key exposures, type and handling of bio-specimens, etc.), whilst still allowing the respective birth cohorts to be unique in other respects.[31]

Similarly, the website http://www.birthcohorts.net, which will be developed further in the years to come, is an attempt to build an infrastructure, gathering information on existing data in the various birth cohorts that exist across the world. A key aim of the website is to facilitate collaborations particularly amongst researchers interested in examining gene-environment interaction effects on disease outcomes, since such studies necessarily require large sample sizes and independent replication. This aim is achieved by making detailed information about design and data in the existing cohorts easily accessible. The existing birth cohorts are heterogeneous in design and focus, but for specific purposes pooling of data from multiple cohorts may be feasible where the website information demonstrates sufficient consistency for the key variables of interest to the specific research question. A prerequisite for such a strategy is, however, that the cohorts are well documented and that the website is regularly updated.

6.1.3 Birth cohort documentation

Once we acknowledge that the research outcomes of many of the primary hypotheses of birth cohorts will not emerge until six to seven decades after the cohort's initiation, and that birth cohorts should be thought of as resources for developing hypotheses over many future decades, the need for very clear documentation about all data collected is obvious. Such documentation does, however, require considerable resource, which funders and investigators must be aware of.

6.1.4 Summary

This introduction has highlighted the arguments in favour and against developing a formal 'blueprint' for the birth cohort. We would argue that some standardization is valuable but we would also argue against a single blueprint and we have tried to demonstrate the importance of diversity across birth cohorts. A further metaphor from forestry is perhaps useful here. The photographs in Figure 6.1 show a plantation (Figure 6.1a) and a rainforest (Figure 6.1b). Both of these have their uses, but whereas the plantation produces one outcome the rainforest (with some standardization, but much diversity) supports a wide range of ecosystems. In particular we emphasize the importance of thinking of birth cohorts as a resource for now and for many decades in the future. This clearly has important consequences for funders and researchers. What follows in the rest of this chapter are some reflections on practicalities to consider when setting up birth cohort studies. For the purposes of these reflections, we define birth cohorts as a population, defined at birth, *in utero* or even before conception, on which systematic and prospective collection of data has taken place or is intended.

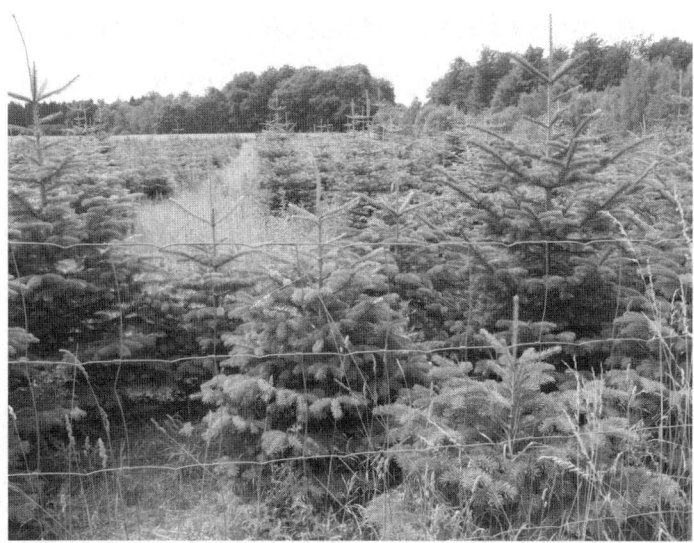

Fig. 6.1a Plantation.

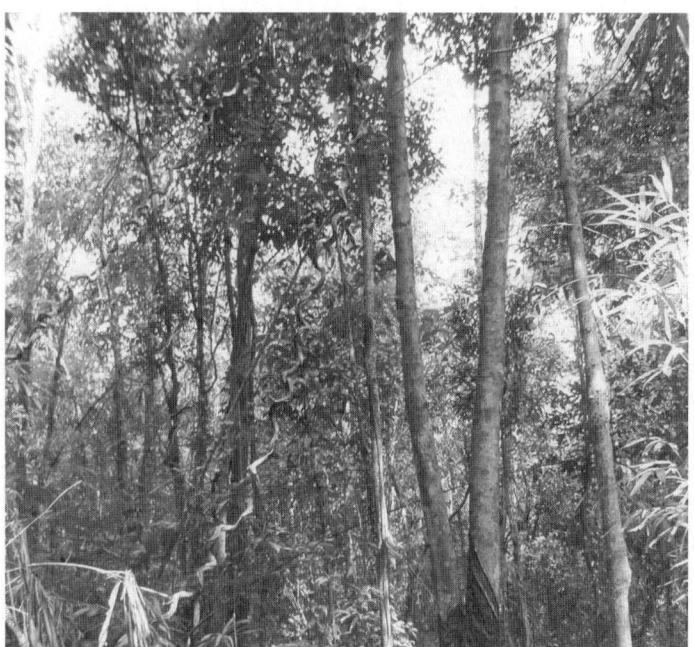

Fig. 6.1b Rain forest.

Both photos by Nybo & Nissen.

6.2 The practicalities of establishing birth cohort studies

6.2.1 A narrow scientific focus or infrastructure for future research?

Establishment of a birth cohort of a significant size represents a huge investment for a society, for the researchers involved, and for the funding bodies. Despite our strong comments above regarding the importance of birth cohorts as a resource for many decades, only very rarely would it be the case that the partners are willing to commit themselves to investment in the project on a very long-term basis. Even when very extensive resources are available consideration needs to be given to the balance between contemporary scientific focus and building a research infrastructure. Some of the issues in addressing this balance are illustrated by two examples of birth cohorts that have been planned in the last decade.

The National Children's Study, a US birth cohort that is currently being formed, serves as an example of a cohort with extensive financial resources and that involved very elaborate planning (the planning process has been documented in various reports[6]). This cohort is planned to include 100,000 children, some of them recruited before conception, others during intrauterine life or at birth. Currently, follow-up is planned (and budgeted) to continue until the key participants are aged 21 years. By means of a wide range of 'state of the art' meetings and literature reviews a list of scientific priorities, with justifications, has been made. Despite this extensive and evidence based development process for the study (something many would consider essential for such an investment), decision making has been difficult and controversial, with a piece in *Science*, ironically stating: 'Researchers are planning a major study of mothers and children: after two years they've narrowed the possible objectives of the study down to 70'.[32]

Compared to the National Children's Study, The Danish National Birth Cohort had a tiny fraction of the resources for planning, design, and implementation. Because of this, and the particularly favourable opportunities in Denmark for obtaining data from administrative and health registers, the principal investigators quite quickly agreed that initial resources should be used to collect data on exposures during pregnancy, infancy and early childhood that could not be obtained from the existing registers. The population administrative and health registers in Denmark provide individual level data on prescribed medication, a variety of measures of socioeconomic position, environmental exposures for the home address, type of day-care facility, hospitalizations (with dates, key diagnoses, and procedures) and mortality data. Much of this data is available from 1977 and citizen unique IDs allow study participants to be linked accurately to these register based data. Of importance for family-based life course studies it is possible to link families (intergenerationally and by siblings) using these registers. Thus, for example, the key participants (the offspring) of the Danish National Birth Cohort can be linked to data on several aspects of their parent's and in some cases grandparent's medical history. The additional data that were collected in the birth cohort (i.e. that those planning the study knew could not be obtained from population registers) included individual life style habits (e.g. use of alcohol, tobacco, and other recreational drugs), use of over-the-counter medication, specific occupational exposures in certain jobs, nutrition, and 'soft' outcomes such as developmental milestones and diseases and ailments not leading to secondary health care.

The scope of exposures during pregnancy/intrauterine life on which data were collected was broad, but for a number of selected exposures, the data collected were particularly detailed. This was the case for, e.g., infections and fever during pregnancy and maternal binge drinking, as a number of selected present-day scientific questions were planned that related to these exposures. Principal investigators of the cohort were interested in the role of infections and fever during pregnancy for fetal survival and for the risk of schizophrenia in the offspring and in how episodes of maternal binge drinking affected the fetus and future health of the child. Detailed data on infections and fever has allowed a study of how intensity, number and timing of fever episodes affect fetal survival to be completed,[33] while the question of schizophrenia has to wait for the cohort to reach young adult age. Likewise, detailed information on the number and timing of episodes of maternal binge drinking (high blood-alcohol levels) in susceptible time windows of fetal development have made it possible to examine the effects of these on fetal survival.[34]

The broad approach towards much of the data collection in the Danish National Birth Cohort has advantages in enabling the birth cohort to address scientific questions that emerge. For example, in 2004 the Danish National Board of Health published guidelines regarding physical exercise during pregnancy.[35] Almost concurrently, similar guidelines were disseminated in the UK, Norway and the US.[36-38] While the general health effects of physical exercise are well-documented, sparse literature is available about the impact on fetal health.[39] The new guidelines encouraged pregnant women to participate in regular moderate activity during their pregnancy, but pregnant women wanted to know whether this was harmful to the developing fetus. Using the data on maternal physical activity in the cohort, a series of studies were initiated two of which have been published.[40,41] One study that was very widely reported in the media suggested that higher levels of physical activity in early pregnancy were associated with greater risk of miscarriage.[40] However, these studies are somewhat limited by the fact that the information collected on maternal physical activity was designed without a specific research project in mind, and is thus less detailed than one might have wished. Nonetheless, the findings with respect to miscarriage are useful in addressing an important question that emerged and suggest that some caution may be warranted with respect to encouraging women to increase their levels of physical activity during pregnancy until future research has clarified whether this is indeed safe for the developing fetus.

Our experience, both in the development of a new birth cohort (the Danish National Birth Cohort) and in working on revitalized birth cohorts set up some decades ago such as the Aberdeen Children of the 1950s cohort[11] and the Danish Metropolit cohort,[12] has made us realize that both in the short-term and the long-term very few research projects that use data from multidisciplinary birth cohorts will be able to genuinely state that the data were designed for that specific project. Perhaps paradoxically, we believe that this fact is a further argument against a standard blue-print for a cohort study and in favour of different birth cohorts undertaking very detailed measurements of some characteristics that reflect specific local scientific interests at the planning stage of data collection. Such an approach with the prioritization of a few selected characteristics to be measured in great detail in order to answer very specific research questions, might, at first glance, seem to limit the potential of birth cohort data for future research, on closer inspection we feel is actually a sensible strategy in the multi-cohort scientific society that we live in today, where different birth cohorts can complement each other. No single cohort is likely to be able to collect very detailed data on all possible exposures, outcomes and confounders that are relevant to today's and the future research communities needs. However, if we produce a family of cohorts across the world that include some standardized measurements and a variety of different characteristics that are measured in greater detail in some cohorts but in less detail in other studies we increase the possibility that across all cohorts more research questions will be answerable. For many questions it would then be possible to examine 'accurate' associations with little measurement error in one or two cohorts and 'precise' associations with more measurement error in other cohorts. The value of the very detailed exposure data measures (that would inevitably be at the expense of sample size) would be balanced by larger cohort studies with less detailed exposure data.

6.2.2 What drives the research agendas: the available data fallacy

While the specific focus on perinatal and infant health often serves to secure the funding of the birth cohorts, it has shortcomings. The available data tend to set an agenda for the research questions: The large number of studies[42–46] using birth weight as a predictor of later health was possible because birth weight has been registered in birth certificates in many populations for a long time and therefore serves as a proxy measure of intrauterine nutrition (discussed in more detail in Chapter 13). There is, however, some evidence that shorter gestational length is the important determinant for the associations found between birth weight and later disease outcomes[47, 48] and researchers increasingly suggest that birth weight per se is not the risk factor of interest, rather it is a proxy for the main risk factor, which could be one or more of genetic variation, epigenetic effects, maternal nutrition or intrauterine nutrition. However, since these data are often unavailable or obtained with greater measurement error, birth weight continues to be the exposure of choice in many studies, with these studies then generating an industry of questions about what the associations actually mean (see Chapter 13).

Similarly, the recent interest in the association of childhood intelligence has, at least in part, resulted from the availability of childhood IQ measurements in many studies conducted in the 1960s. An important scientific concern in the 1960s was whether improvements in obstetric and perinatal care, which were increasing the chance of preterm infants surviving, might result in later problems (particularly problems with cognition and development) in these surviving infants. This concern resulted in IQ scores being measured in children in many cohort studies in the 1960s.[12, 13, 49] Thus, this is another measure that is available in many populations and easily accessible for quantitative analyses. Consequently, the number of studies relating IQ around age 7–11 (when a number of school test are routinely performed) or IQ around age 18 (when conscription tests take place, often restricting these studies to male populations) to different health outcomes is high and increasing as the children and young adults in these cohorts reach adulthood.[50–52]

These comments should not be seen as critical of the researchers involved in this work, indeed two of the authors of this chapter (AMNA and DAL) have contributed several papers to the literature on the associations of both birth weight and childhood/early life IQ with later health outcomes. Nor do these comments detract from our earlier assertions that we believe birth cohorts should be seen as research resources for current and future generations of researchers. Rather we feel it is important to emphasize that once data are collected for one reason, they tend to be used for many other reasons, and that the possibility of over emphasizing the importance of specific exposures (simply because they are there) should be considered by researchers.

A slightly different issue concerns the tendency to link early life exposures with later health outcomes without fully considering the possibility that the early life exposure is merely a marker for later life exposures that are the real causal risk factors. For example, maternal alcohol drinking during pregnancy is associated with cognitive function in the offspring and a number of investigators have suggested that lower cognitive function is a long-term consequence of exposure to alcohol during intrauterine life.[53] It is, however, likely that a child exposed to alcohol during fetal life is also exposed to parental alcohol abuse in childhood, which may well explain any behavioural and cognitive dysfunction associated with maternal alcohol during pregnancy. In terms of health promotion/disease prevention one could argue that interventions aimed at reducing maternal alcohol consumption during pregnancy would (if effective) have will have beneficial effects for the offspring whether it was maternal alcohol consumption during pregnancy or the postnatal period that mattered most. However, we would argue that if the postnatal exposure is mainly (or also) important then interventions would need to be targeted both during the pregnancy and postnatal periods and would need to include both parents. Another example of this potential problem with causal inference related to exposures at particular times in the life course could be maternal nutrition, shown to be associated with both short- and long-term health of the offspring.[54, 55] However, maternal nutrition during pregnancy and nutrition during childhood are most likely correlated to some extent.

If the birth cohorts aim to serve the purpose of being an infrastructure for life course research and avoid being a source for self-perpetuating research on fetal exposures, just as much effort should be put into the collection of exposure data throughout infancy, childhood, and adolescence as during pregnancy. Such a life course approach, with repeated measurements throughout the life course, does not only involve a great commitment from the participants, but also obliges the principal investigators of the birth cohorts and the funding bodies to a long term obligation.

6.2.3 When to start?

Most of the older birth cohorts, those enrolling participants up to the 1970s, enrolled participants at birth, whereas more recent cohorts have generally recruited participants antenatally (using the potential of antenatal clinic visits). These latter studies have the advantage of being able to prospectively collected data for ante- and peri-natal exposures and outcomes. However, antenatal recruitment also has a number of disadvantages.

First, these studies are rarely able to collect complete prospective data on the most frequent adverse pregnancy outcome—miscarriage—because the period from the enrolment of a pregnant woman to the potential occurrence of a miscarriage is very short and because in many countries the first antenatal clinic visit (often between 12–16 weeks gestation) is at or after the most common period for miscarriage.

Second, to exploit the full potential of a birth cohort to determine life course influences on future health and well-being it would be optimal to start before conception and ideally recruit both prospective mothers and fathers.[56] This relates to the very definition of life course epidemiology, which is to examine exposures from conception to adulthood (and across generations) on health outcomes. It also relates to the fact that in both mothers and fathers preconceptual exposures and exposures around the time of conception could plausibly affect offspring outcomes. Environmental factors have a direct influence on the fertilising sperm cell up to three months before conception. Maternal exposures around the time of conception (e.g. supplementation, physical strain) have been shown to affect offspring health.[57, 58] The fact that both mothers and fathers are affected also highlights the importance of recruiting both parents into a birth cohort.

It is, however, a great challenge to get a cohort of a certain size established before conception, primarily due to the fact that any couples who are planning to get pregnant and who are also known to clinicians/researchers (and therefore 'easy' to recruit) tend to have fertility problems. To obtain a suitably large birth cohort pre-conceptually from a general population sample would be a huge undertaking. For example, in a Danish study that sought to study the effects of time to pregnancy on different outcomes, the researchers had to approach 52,552 members of trade unions in order to obtain a final sample of 430 couples who had no known reproductive problems, wanted to have a child within the next year, and succeeded in conceiving during the study period.[59] Another somewhat different approach was employed in the Southampton Women's Survey,[60] in which women of reproductive age were included irrespective of their plans of pregnancy. Those of the included women who did become pregnant after the initial data collection were invited to take part in the pregnancy phase of the study. Obviously this is a big effort and requires a large sample to start with in order to get a sufficient number of births, but it is good example of a truly general population pre-conception cohort.

In addition to the Southampton Women's Survey, at least two of the next large-scale birth cohort initiatives are planning to enrol all or a part of their study population prior to conception. The National Children's Study in the United States expects to include about 25% of their study participants before pregnancy, a group constituted by women considered to be at high probability of becoming pregnant within the near future.[61] Even more ambitious are the intentions of the

Chinese Children and Families Cohort Study, who are aiming at enrolling a total of 300,000 newly married couples.[62] These pre-pregnancy cohorts are likely to yield some important gains in our knowledge of the effects of periconceptional exposures on later health and disease.

Before considering who are participants of a birth cohort it is useful to consider how timing of recruitment to a birth cohort might influence selection bias in some contexts. As discussed below birth cohorts can be used to examine the life course epidemiology of outcomes in parents as well as children. For example, a new clinical examination will take place in the ALSPAC cohort mothers between 2008–2010 (on average 16 years since their index pregnancy). The initial planned aims of this clinic follow-up are to determine the obstetric, genetic and lifestyle characteristics that influence metabolic and vascular traits in women in their mid-40s (a group in whom rates of CHD have recently been shown to be increasing in the UK). By definition to be in this cohort women must have had at least one pregnancy and therefore one could argue that for genetic and lifestyle exposures findings will not necessarily be generalizable to the general population of women. That said, the women who we will include will have a median age of 44 and interquartile range of 41–49 years at the time of examination. Current Office of National Statistics show that for UK women in that age range 85-88% will have at least one child (http://www.statistics.gov.uk/statbase/Product.asp?vlnk=5768). These statistics also show fertility rates increasing in recent years in the UK. Therefore findings should be relevant to the large majority of UK women. A further potential advantage of pre-conceptual cohorts is that they are less select than birth or antenatal cohorts in respect of the parents. However, it should be acknowledged that those being planned are restricted either to married couples and/or women or couples who declare an intention to get pregnant in the near future.

6.2.4 Who is the participant in the birth cohort?

Traditionally, data collection in epidemiological studies on adults is restricted to the single individual under study. This is not the case in birth cohort studies. Even in the situation where the child (or child-to-be) is be considered to be the key (or only) participant of the birth cohort, the distinction between fetus and the mother is subtle, and even in the first decade of extra-uterine life it is difficult to make a distinction between the life (and exposures) of the child and its family. Furthermore, it is an assumption within life course epidemiology that adverse effects of the environment on health, not only accumulate over the lifespan of the individual, but also across generations.[21] Thus, the family of the child becomes relevant both in terms of an intergenerational perspective and because it constitutes an important aspect of the child's environment. In addition, the potential of sibling studies to understand life course mechanisms (see Chapters 2, 3 and 13), and of sibling relationships as important exposures for health and well-being of the 'key' individual (see Chapters 14 and 16) raises the possibility of collecting data on siblings as well as the index child. For studies that recruit participants antentally or preconceptually over an extended period siblings will naturally occur, and even for cohorts that recruit at birth there will be twins and higher order births. Increasingly, birth cohorts are exploited for the potential not only to examine the index child but also their parents for future health outcomes (see discussion above regarding ALSPAC mothers). For all of these reasons the participants of a birth cohort can be difficult to define.

The main participants in a birth cohort are to some extent determined by the time at which the cohort begins. Thus, for pre-conceptional cohorts women of reproductive age and/or their male partners are recruited and form the initial cohort. These men and women remain in the cohort irrespective of whether they go on to have a child, but for those that do have a child that child becomes a cohort participant. In prenatal cohorts pregnant women are recruited and therefore these are the primary cohort members but once their offspring are born these too become cohort participants, and frequently researchers attempt to enrol fathers in the cohort too. By contrast birth cohorts such as the UK 46, 58 etc., have recruited only the individual born at a particular time, though in the case of the 1958 birth cohort routinely available data on participants parents and offspring has been recently obtained and linked to the cohort,[63, 64] and in the 1946 birth cohort data on first pregnancies to the female participants has been routinely collected. Thus, previous and subsequent generations can become cohort participants some time after the initial cohort initiation.

Inevitably, when dealing with the practical work of data collection in birth cohorts, the question about how to define the family of the child is brought to attention. Is a family defined by genes or by the persons around you in your home? And how relevant are distant relatives? Even the question about how to define the 'home' of the child may constitute a problem, at least in a Danish context, where a substantial share of biological parents (more than 20%) live apart by the time the child is 11 years old[65] and often choose to let the child move between two homes on a regular basis.

These issues need to be addressed when deciding who to recruit (in the context of limited research resources) and how to identify family relationships within the cohort dataset. Bearing in mind the use of birth cohorts by many researchers now and in the future decisions about who is recruited and how families are linked in the dataset must be well documented.

6.2.4.1 Mothers

As the birth cohorts most often begin at birth or during pregnancy, definition of the mother is, with the exception of a small number of cases of pregnancies established through oocyte donation, straightforward. Mothers/pregnant women are relatively easily approached in connection with antenatal care visits or on the delivery wards, which is a great advantage when making the initial contact to potential study participants. The fact that most children of divorced parents maintain contact with their mothers, and a majority live with their mothers,[65] makes it practical to address the mothers when collecting information about the infant and child.

6.2.4.2 Fathers

Inclusion of the father in the data collection is, from a scientific point of view, desirable for obvious reasons. Not only does the biological father deliver half of the genetic material, he also influences the surroundings in which a child grows up. Non-biological fathers will similarly have important influences on the environment of a growing child. The reason why fathers are not always included in birth cohorts is pragmatic rather than scientific and reflects the fact that most birth cohorts are established through antenatal care or delivery wards, where the person in focus is the pregnant woman/mother. This is further compounded by the fact that in general women respond more often to research studies than do men. The practical problem of trying to obtain informed consent from two adults (rather than one), to establish a birth cohort, may be an additional reason why fathers are not involved in some birth cohorts, as was the case in the Danish National Birth Cohort. Finally, although the figures often mentioned about unexpected paternal identity are probably exaggerated,[66] another issue that might be a disincentive for some fathers is the possibility that in birth cohorts that want to collect DNA, there may be a fear that this will be used to test for paternity.

Both biological and social (non-biological) fathers (and mothers) are of interest in birth cohort studies since some research questions will be best (or only) answered with one type of parent and others will require information on both type of parent. Ideally we would want to collect information on both biological and non-biological mothers and fathers. It is, however, important that we can distinguish the two, and sensitive questions that serve this purpose for each particular birth cohort are important. Statistical sensitivity methods for dealing with possible non-paternity in statistical associations are discussed in Chapter 10.

Despite these difficulties, fathers have been successfully recruited in several birth cohorts. In ALSPAC a pragmatic decision was taken to recruit fathers via the mother who was asked to deliver study documents and questionnaires to her partner at the time of the study recruitment and in subsequent follow-up assessments. This approach has resulted in valuable data on fathers (partner of the mother at recruitment and each follow-up questionnaire), but with fewer questionnaire responses at each time point than mother questionnaire responses for each family unit. The lower response from father will result from a combination of factors—mothers may not have a partner or may not forward the questionnaire to them and in general men are less likely to respond to questionnaire surveys than are women. It is interesting to note that for these questionnaire data the difference in response between mothers and partners has remained constant across the 16 year duration of the study and the pattern of attrition of both is, to date, identical. To date follow-up clinic examinations have been conducted on children only (though as noted above a clinical examination of mothers is funded and will take place 2008–2010). DNA was extracted, where possible, from maternal obstetric samples for mothers, and supplemented where necessary by opportunistic samples when mothers attend clinic with their child. Initially, it was only planned to obtain DNA samples from ALSPAC fathers of the 10% children in focus subsample and therefore to date DNA is only available on ~1000 fathers, compared with over 10,000 mothers and offspring. Core funding is now available to obtain DNA from all remaining fathers (partners) and a variety of measures, including the use of saliva samples, will be used to boost the father's DNA bank. Genetically true biological trios can be determined for analysis in ALSPAC, but strict anonymity would always be maintained for such analytical datasets.

By contrast, a number of different methods are being used to encourage direct participation by fathers in the Born in Bradford study (http://www.borninbradford.nhs.uk/), which is a new bi-ethnic birth cohort that aims to recruit 10,000 families of European and Pakistani origin, via the antenatal clinic. These methods include involvement of community men's health workers and men's health clinics, as well as, having the local football and rugby teams as sponsors of the study and using the local media and work places in order to promote the study and explain why the involvement of fathers is important. In this study it was decided that questions about biological paternity were insensitive and might risk reducing recruitment rates and therefore this has not been asked in the recruitment interviews. As with ALSPAC it is hoped to collect samples for DNA extractions from both parents and the index child; reassurances that these would not be used for paternity testing will be given.

6.2.4.3 Siblings

A birth cohort recruited over a longer time span has the possibility to include more children from the same family. Both siblings and twin pairs constitute a valuable resource in birth cohorts (see Chapters 3, 4, and 11), as the often shared environment, intrauterine life and the genetic con- and discordance may elucidate genetic and environmental contributions to health related phenomena[67–69] (the use of such studies in relation to cardiovascular disease is discussed in Chapter 13). However, considerable numbers of sibling/twin pairs/groups are required for adequate statistical power to distinguish between and within group effects with precision and therefore large birth cohorts (or record linkages) are necessary to exploit these methods.

In the Danish National birth cohort, the number of women who participated with more than one pregnancy was 9,380, resulting in more than 9,000 sibling pairs. In addition, more than 4,000 twins resulted from the enrolled pregnancies. Thus, this very large cohort has by virtue of its size incredible potential for answering key life course epidemiology mechanistic questions in the future. However, one important issue when dealing with siblings is the increasing prevalence of reconstituted families, which can make it difficult to get a clear picture of the family constellation, including 'half-paternal siblings', 'half-maternal siblings', 'step siblings', co-habiting, and non-co-habiting siblings. This information is important when making assumptions about shared environment and shared genes, as one does in between and within sibling/twin studies (see Chapters 3, 4, and 11) and collecting this information in detail requires resources, sensitivity and careful documentation.

As well as sibling/twin groups being recruited as part of the cohort, many birth cohorts will collect information (usually from the mother) about existing children and/or previous pregnancies at the time of recruitment of the index pregnancy/birth and will continue to collect information on new pregnancies/births that occur after the index birth. Such information is valuable for understanding the impact of birth order, home environment, and family relationships and size on the index participant.

6.2.4.4 Offspring of index child

There has been a recent increase in research interest in examining inter-generational exposure-disease associations, and several studies have now shown that both maternal and paternal cardiovascular mortality are associated with offspring birth weight.[70, 71] In addition, maternal anthropometric factors such as her intrauterine growth, height, and leg length have been found to have enduring intergenerational effects on offspring growth, which cannot be fully explained by later biological or socioeconomic characteristics of the mother[72–74] (see also Chapters 2, 10, and 15). Such associations are complex and may reflect a dynamic interplay between many factors, including the effect of *in utero* influences, genomic, and epigenetic processes. In addition, parents and offspring are likely to share socio-economic environments as well as a tendency to certain behavioural patterns. These complexities are discussed in more detail in Chapters 2, 10, 13, and 15.

As discussed in previous chapters it is rare for studies to have prospectively collected data on health and development across the life course on multiple generations. In recent years, a few studies have, however, collected data suitable for this purpose, e.g. the 1958 birth cohort, where information on the offspring of cohort members have been collected in addition to data on the parents of the cohort members,[75] and in the 1946 birth cohort prospective information on the first born offspring of female participants has been collected. The Aberdeen children of the 1950s cohort[76] and the Metropolit cohort[77] also now have data on three generations. Though it should be noted that for the Aberdeen Children of the 1950s it was only possible to link offspring to female members of the original cohort and that the Metropolit cohort only ever included males. As the younger birth cohorts grow older, the options for obtaining intergenerational data will increase and if we indeed wish to collect prospective data on the next generation we need to consider systems to collect these data. The challenge of this task depends on how early we want to identify the offspring of a cohort member, as prenatal identification poses a significantly greater challenge than establishing contact after the birth of the offspring. It also depends on our desire to have complete prospectively collected perinatal and later life course data on all offspring of the index cohort. Within a 'Developmental Origins of Health and Disease (DOHaD)' framework prenatal identification must be considered to be ideal. In contemporary Western populations first births occur to women between the full age range of under 16 to over 40 years, with a peak occurring around mid-20s-early-30s. Few funding bodies are likely to be prepared to fund data collection on the relatively small numbers of new 'participants' when index participants are under 18 years of age or older than 40, but even restricting the data collection period to a

10 year span (say between mean age 20–30 of index participants) is daunting. Furthermore, data collection from the male index participants requires by definition recruiting their partners (the mother of their offspring) as well as their offspring. It would also be useful to recruit fathers of the offspring of the female index participants. Thus, the original cohort potentially increased both in width and length over a very extended time-period. A pragmatic approach would be to use several mechanisms to try and obtain data on this next generation:

(i) Obtain consent to link to and abstract information from routine data sources and medical records, including abstraction of obstetric data. This consent could be collected when the cohort members reach 17–18 years of age and have to reconfirm the consent to participate in the study that was originally provided by their mothers/parents.

(ii) Include questions about pregnancies and new babies in data collection sweeps, particularly during the periods when numbers will be relatively small (i.e. when mothers are very young and when older). In cases where male index participants are becoming a parent or have become a parent ask them to pass on a questionnaire to their partner (the mother of the baby) so that she and her baby can be enrolled & asked for consent to link the mother (and her child) to medical, including obstetric, and other data collection procedures. Consider also asking female index participants who are pregnant or have become a parent to pass on a questionnaire to the father of their child.

(iii) Set up specific research clinic tests in antenatal clinics to 'capture' any female participants and the female partners of male participants when they become pregnant, but running these clinics over a limited (e.g. 5 or 10 year period) to coincide with the time of maximum fertility of the index 'children' i.e. when they are aged 20–25 or 25–30. This approach may be more feasible in cohorts restricted to geographically well-defined areas and with a relatively short recruitment period for the original index cohort.

(iv) Use existing cohort clinic facilities (those used to complete follow-up examinations of index cohort participants) to examine both index participants and their offspring (at whatever age they might be) on a regular (e.g. 5 or 10 year) basis. For example, the geographically restricted ALSPAC study has a dedicated study clinic with staff who have completed regular examinations of the participants from age 7. Whilst, participants are likely to move away from home in young adulthood, they are also likely to maintain contact with home and may be willing to come back to regular clinics with their children. The 1946 UK birth cohort, which is geographically representative of mainland Britain, is currently completing a 60–62 year follow-up examination of participants by using dedicated (MRC and Wellcome Trust funded) research clinic facilities that exist across major centres in the UK. These clinics could (with funding) also be used to examine cohort offspring.

6.2.5 Size matters

The Danish National Birth Cohort[78] and the Norwegian MoBa cohort[79] were the first to set the magical goal of recruiting 100,000 pregnant women to the cohort. This was done based on power calculations showing that this sample size would allow precise estimation of the association of risk factors for rare, but serious diseases, such as acute leukaemia, and some congenital malformations, and this sample size would also provide sufficient statistical power to examine gene-environment interaction on relatively frequent or continuous outcomes in a prospective setting. The US National Children's Study has now set the same goal.[80]

These large sample sizes do provide greater statistical power than smaller studies and enable some hypotheses to be tested that could not be appropriately done with smaller studies. However, there are some limitations of such large studies that also need to be acknowledged. There are finite resources for scientific research and in general larger studies tend to be conducted at the expense of: (i) the quality in measurement of exposures and potential confounding factors (for example questionnaires rather than clinical examination might be the most frequently used method for obtaining data on the whole cohort), (ii) the frequency of repeat measurements across the life course of these exposures, and (iii) the total number of exposures/confounders that are measured. Furthermore, in very large cohort studies that do not have the opportunity of population wide register data on outcomes, the proportion of attrition might be greater with larger numbers. The strategies often used to minimize attrition in a cohort, such as continuous contact with the cohort members and incentives such as birthday cards and book tokens, is simply not realistic in very large cohorts.

For example, the costs of sending just one post card to all children in the Danish National Birth Cohort would be more than £100,000 (equivalent to €150,000 and US$200,000 at 2008 exchange rates). Likewise, rigorous clinical examinations of the total cohort are not very realistic. In contrast to that the Danish National Birth cohort, the ALSPAC cohort, which is a tremendous endeavour, has managed to do regular follow-ups on more than 10,000 children and has rich data on almost every aspect of life of these children and their mothers. Interestingly, whilst the sample size of ALSPAC seems modest in contemporary times, when we are planning birth cohorts of 100,000, at the time it was being planned (in the late 1980s) it seemed very large and when the offspring were in early infancy intensive examination follow-up was restricted to a 10% sub-sample of the cohort, the so-called Children in Focus. This approach was subsequently stopped and by the time the children were aged 7 the whole cohort was regularly (initially every year and then every second year) invited to detailed clinic follow-up examinations each lasting 3–4 hours.

For the follow-up of the Danish National Birth Cohort at age 11, which is currently being planned, internet based multimedia questionnaires are being considered. Using this data collection method it is possible to reach a large proportion of the cohort at relatively low cost and it has additional advantages: interactive and instructive computer programs with the use of pictures and speech reduce the requirement for literacy, which normally applies when using written questionnaires. This may reduce a differential selection favouring the academically strongest respondents. Validity is further enhanced by the fact that filters and validations can be integrated in the questionnaire. For the 11-years follow-up (and hopefully future follow-up sweeps), the Danish National Birth Cohort are further planning to take an approach similar to the ALSPAC Children in Focus sample. Random and strategic sampled sub cohorts will be approached for clinical examinations, assuming that necessary funds can be secured. MoBa (the Norwegian National Birth cohort) is still in the process of recruiting the last participants for the study and as of February 2008, 98,531 pregnancies had been recruited. Currently, the earliest recruited children have reached 7 years and a questionnaire based data collection has been launched. In conjunction with this, an ambitious collection of milk teeth among all participants is being carried out.

One of the reasons why it has been possible in Denmark and Norway to establish cohorts of 100,000 magnitude is the existence of up-to-date and well-functioning population and health registers and unique person identification numbers that make it practical and economically feasible to trace all cohort members and to do register-based follow-up on a regular basis. In addition, other external sources can be exploited such as Geographical Information Systems (GIS), where centrally registered environmental data like water quality or air pollution can be linked to address of residence.

6.2.6 **Attrition matters**

6.2.6.1 A birth cohort is for life—making participants 'partners' in the study at recruitment

It is almost inevitable that over the life course of a birth cohort participants will drop out or be lost to follow-up. This attrition matters for two reasons. First, we have discussed earlier how very large birth cohorts are now regarded as important for providing precise estimates of the effects of risk factors for rare diseases and for examining main genetic effects and gene-environment interactions of even quite common outcomes. If there is considerable attrition in the cohort over time even the very large birth cohorts may end up with insufficient statistical power to be able to address important questions about aetiology. Second, if attrition is differential (that is if amongst those who are lost to follow-up there are important differences in the magnitude or direction of the associations of interest) not only will effect estimates be imprecisely estimated they may also be biased. Broadly speaking, there are two ways in which the effects of attrition can be minimised. One is design methods that can be used to minimize voluntary drop-out and loss to follow-up. The second is analytical methods that can be employed to try and assess the extent of any likely bias and/or to impute missing values due to attrition. Methods to prevent attrition in the first place are better than trying to deal with any effects through statistical methods, which often have un-testable assumptions. However, in reality both approaches often need to be done in many uses of birth cohorts.

Chapter 10 describes some statistical methods that can be employed to assess and deal with missing data. We also refer readers to http://www.missingdata.org.uk, and would suggest that they continue to look at this site into the future as more and more work is done in this area. In this section we will focus on methods that can be used to minimize attrition in the first place. One way of keeping attrition to a minimum level is to create a feeling of attachment to the cohort. This is might be easier in a cohort of a limited size than in a large cohort. As well as the potential threat to precision and the validity resulting from loss to follow-up, in birth cohorts that has had extensive data collection during the early phases of life every withdrawal later-on from the cohort represents a loss of substantial investment. It may therefore be sensible to ensure that those who enrol in the birth cohort (most often the mother or a parent) have a full understanding of the long-term commitment that is being requested. This approach could mean that those who are then enrolled in the cohort are not fully representative of the source population (assuming that parents who are prepared to volunteer to the long-term commitment of a birth cohort for themselves and the children differ from those not prepared to make this commitment). However, as long as some variation and exposure contrast, for key exposures, is maintained in the recruited cohort, having a cohort that are more likely to remain may be more important than one that is truly representative of the source population.

There are also methods that can be employed to try both to gain commitment and maintain a high level of representativeness of the source population. For example, in Bradford in the North of England, a new bi-ethnic birth cohort is currently being established—the Born in Bradford cohort (http://www.borninbradford.nhs.uk/). Bradford is one of the poorest cities in England and approximately 50% of births each year are to parents of South Asian origin (including first, second and third generation migrants). In order to gain long-term commitment and a highly representative cohort a very large amount of work was done prior to starting recruitment that aimed to encourage the community of Bradford to feel they were partners in the study. This included meetings with community leaders, engaging local football and rugby teams to support the study, persuading the Lord Mayor of the City to make it his 'Appeal of the Year', extensive coverage in local media, providing means for the community to say what key areas should be researched in the study and working with health care and social care providers across the city. The study is still in the recruitment phase and at this stage it is impossible to judge how successful this approach will be both in terms of maintaining high levels of participation and of the participants (and wider community) truly feeling that they have a say in areas of research that are undertaken. This study, somewhat like the Scandinavian countries with population registers, hopes to maintain high levels of participant data by obtaining consent to link health service and child development data into the main study data bank, and has also worked closely with workers who collect these data to ensure high standards of measurement and data entry. The aim is to encourage these staff, as well as the participants, to feel partners in the development and use of the birth cohort, as well as to promote translation of research findings into clinical practice.

6.2.6.2 Methods to keep participants engaged after recruitment

Making commitments for the unknown future is of course difficult. Some parents who initially feel a high level of commitment at the time of recruitment may feel less so as time goes on. Furthermore, once the offspring reaches an age where they can decide for themselves whether or not they want to attend a clinical follow-up examination or complete a questionnaire, they may have very different views to the parents about involvement in the study. Consequently methods to maintain high levels of participants following recruitment continue for the whole life of the birth cohort. Methods that have been employed to maintain high levels of participation include:

- Sending birthday and Christmas cards each year to remind participants of the study, make them feel part of it and to keep current contact details up to date.
- Sending regular newsletters about research that has been published from the study and planned future follow-up to participants on a regular basis.
- Involving participants in the organisation of the study. For example, in the ALSPAC study parents are represented on the 'ALSPAC Law and Ethics Committee' and a 'Teenage Advisory Panel', which consists of the offspring participants in the study and liaises with the study youth workers, provides a forum for the participants to comment on how the study is run, pilot new data collection tools with their peers in the study and suggest new research areas. As noted above in the Born in Bradford Study major attempts have been made from its initiation to allow the community of Bradford to inform research priorities now and into the future.
- Working with schools when the offspring participants are in school so that the follow-up clinics can be educational and so that the children are not penalized for missing school to attend the clinic.
- Offering remuneration of travel expenses to clinic visits. For local travel this is relatively inexpensive but at the time that cohort participants become very geographically mobile (in young adulthood) this could be extremely expensive, and therefore important to offer. Some birth cohorts have used extraordinary measures to keep attrition at a low level. For example, the Dunedin cohort has traced its members throughout the world and offered air tickets to secure that cohort members took part in follow-up examinations. For the participants this has clear advantages since it provides a 'free' trip 'home' to see family and friends. On this level it might be seen as inappropriate inducement (see below).
- Offering incentives/gifts to attend follow-up clinic. On the one hand it does not seem unreasonable to offer a small gift to study participants who often give up considerable lengths of time to complete questionnaires and attend clinic follow-up visits. On the other hand, this is contentious since it might be seen as inducing participants to undergo tests that they would not otherwise have volunteered for. Incentives such as book tokens or record tokens might be

seen as less problematic than financial gifts, though from the participants' point of view this might be seen as insulting, as it implies they are not able to make responsible decisions about how to spend money. Ethical guidance from appropriate study review bodies should be used to determine the appropriateness of gifts.
- Targeted personal initiatives. In order to limit a differential drop-out of less resourceful participants the ALSPAC study, for instance, has created a special team that deals specifically with this group through a more personalized and intensive contact.

To our knowledge, there is very little research in general concerning the effectiveness and cost-effectiveness of different methods for maintaining participants in research, and none that has specifically looked at this in birth cohorts. Of course lack of research evidence does not imply that these methods are not effective, and for some of the initiatives listed above, in particular providing participants with feedback on how their data has contributed to research, should be considered good practice irrespective of their effect on attrition.

6.2.6.3 Maintaining participation during adolescence and early adulthood

A specific issue in birth cohorts is the fact that the basic population, the offspring, has to give consent to their participation in the cohort when they reach a certain age. The age of consent varies between countries but is around the time of life (16–20 years) when individuals often rebel against authority and when they become much more geographically mobile. The very time when one has to gain personal consent for participants to stay in the study, and to be able to obtain information on their contact detail, coincides with an age when many might be expected to ignore or refuse such requests.

In order to avoid a large proportion of the cohort withdrawing at that stage, frequent interaction with the participants during the years of early adolescence and feed-back about issues of relevance to them may be of value. An alternative approach might be to avoid contact with the cohort in the years around puberty and in young adulthood and plan to re-engage the cohort at an older age. However, since this period is an essential one in the life course (because of the major changes in social, geographical, behavioural, and biological characteristics at this time) this strategy would be a major loss to a life course study. As noted above we are not aware of any evaluations of different methods to avoid attrition in birth cohorts in general and so are not aware of any studies that have evaluated the effectiveness of different methods to maintain participation during adolescence/early adulthood.

6.2.6.4 Offering different levels of participation

In many birth cohorts (and other prospective cohorts) participation at different levels has been used to maintain overall high levels of participation. For example, in the Danish National Birth Cohort withdrawal has—until now—been kept to a minimum of less than 1% by making it possible to withdraw from single elements of the data collection. Also, it is possible to withdraw from the project at three levels: not to participate in a certain data collection sweep, not to be contacted from the project anymore, and finally a complete withdrawal with data that has already been collected being destroyed and therefore no longer available for use in future studies. Of course, the absence of data from some aspects of the study can also cause lack of statistical power and bias in some areas of research. However, the presence of other data in the study in these circumstances can allow one to examine statistically the likely extent of any bias.

6.2.6.5 Use of record linkage to medical and other databases avoid attrition

As noted previously in the Danish National Birth Cohort, and in some other birth cohorts (e.g. MoBa and the Aberdeen Children of the 1950s cohort) the ability to link all study participants to hospital admission, prescribing, birth, census, and other databases, means that for many outcomes almost complete 'participation' is possible with no effort to complete questionnaires or attend clinic on the part of the participants. This ability emphasizes the importance of trying to avoid participants making a complete withdrawal from the study, with withdrawal of consent to use previously collected data and link these to available routine databases (see above). The value of this record linkage is appreciated across the world and efforts to widen such linkage in countries where this is currently limited (for example the UK) are currently underway.

6.2.7 Ethics matter

A fierce debate about protection of confidentiality, individual's rights, and research ethics has preceded the initiation of several of the new birth cohorts.

The area of reproduction has always been one for considerable ethical discussion, with issues about assisted reproduction, prenatal diagnosis and treatment of disease, antenatal screening, and abortion occupying much of the activity of official bodies for ethics, such as the Danish Council of Ethics Council, which is a governmental organization serving to promote and qualify the ethical debate in the field of biomedicine.[81] In some cases, birth cohorts are examined in this context with their initiation raising concerns about the medicalization of pregnancy and childbirth and about risk factor epidemiology potentially increasing the anxiety of pregnant women.

The prospective and far-reaching perspective for a birth cohort, as well as the collection of bio-specimens serving a not yet specified purpose, entail the collection of a generic informed consent from the participants. Naturally, this may add to a feeling of insecurity about what the data could be used for both among study participants and, in the case of the Danish National Birth Cohort, among the GPs who had to hand out the invitations to participate to pregnant women. Finally, the dream birth cohort of the epidemiologists,[82] covering information on all aspects of life, with the overconfident ambition to both integrate and disentangle how social, psychological, biological, and genetic factors act together in the creation of people's lives may evoke associations of the 'Big Brother is watching you'.

While it is important to recognize these concerns when planning a birth cohort, the experience from the Danish National Birth Cohort was that the discussion ended when the cohort was a reality. No need to say, that this does not imply that the responsibility for keeping these concerns in mind and taking them seriously should be disregarded. The birth cohorts represent a huge financial and human investment, and their prospective nature make them entirely dependent of goodwill from the cohort members, the funding bodies as well as from the public in general. Furthermore, past examples demonstrate that sometimes medical research has been unethical and it is without question that all birth cohorts at the time of establishment and throughout their life should have procedures to secure public scrutiny and approval of what the data is used for, such as Research Ethics Committee (REC), Institutional Review Board (IRB) or external review boards.

Some of the early ethical concerns when a new birth cohort is first being developed may change as the study progresses. For example, a particular concern in the Danish debate was that results from the cohort would increase anxiety during pregnancy both among the participating women as well as among future pregnant women by linking this or that exposure to adverse pregnancy outcome. However, well-designed and sufficiently powered studies are just as likely to refute existing concerns in the lay population. Thus, a number of the first papers published from the Danish National Birth Cohort demonstrated that previously suspected hazardous exposures (for example, fever and infection during pregnancy and caffeine consumption during pregnancy) had no elevated risk for specific adverse outcomes.[33, 83–85, 41] Such results could reassure and relieve anxiety.

6.2.7.1 Disclosure of results to study participants

One area of particular ethical concern in any observational epidemiological study is the individual's right to access to their own data or be informed of results of tests completed in the study. Interestingly in some countries (for example in France) this right of access is indisputable, whereas in others (for example the UK) there is no clear guidance and considerable debate, with some researchers and ethicists feeling strongly that it is unethical to reveal results collected for research purposes to 'healthy' study volunteers. The argument here is that the clinical meaning/utility of any results outside of the clinical context may be disputed—some participants who are ill could be falsely reassured by a clinic visit, whereas others who are told that a study test result is 'abnormal' may be made incredibly anxious, when in fact further medical assessment demonstrate no problem. Furthermore, even if there is clear evidence of an 'abnormality' there may be no known effective treatment and it is questionable that such results should be given to 'healthy' research volunteers. In these debates others argue that it is unethical not to disclose results that have clinical meaning and an established effective treatment.

Even in areas where there is a strong principle of individual's right to access information collected in research studies, for birth cohorts there are still ethical issues that require consideration. There is the question of who the data belong to—the mother, the father, the child, all of them? Genetic data may be of particular relevance here since providing one member of a family with such data might *de facto* provide information on other family members who may not want to know this information. There is the responsibility of the study team not to cause harm and disclosure of results without providing sufficient personal information on their meaning could cause harm. Yet decisions to disclose or not disclose information from clinical examinations in observational studies could in some contexts lead to harm (either by potentially delaying beneficial treatment or prevention in the case of non-disclosure or by potentially providing false reassurance or increased anxiety over a false 'abnormal' result in the case of disclosure).

From our experience of working on different cohort studies, in different countries and discussing these issues with other researchers from a number of different areas it seems that there is no agreed way to deal with the question of disclosure. We believe good principles in this area include: (i) making sure that participants understand that the measurements are being taken for research purposes and should not be considered to be health screening or to replace any usual medical care; (ii) if a decision has been made to disclose some results, informed consent to do so should be obtained from relevant participants prior to the test being undertaken (those who agree to the test but not to being informed of their results should not have these disclosed); (iii) if results are to be disclosed making sure that adequate information is provided to participants about their meaning at the time of disclosure and what further action they should take (this would include informing them which results would be disclosed. For example, some ethics committees/IRBs may support only disclosing results of a particular test when it has reached a given threshold for which there is an evidence base to suggest it has clinical meaning and an established treatment). Finally, as with all ethical decisions, issues about disclosure of results should be reviewed by and agreed with relevant ethics committees/IRBs.

6.2.7.2 Sharing data

One of the themes of this chapter has been the importance of viewing birth cohorts as a resource for a wide-range of researchers now and into the future. This ideal is encouraged by governments in many countries and by other research funders who are increasingly encouraging or insisting that anonymized datasets from cohort studies are made 'publicly' available to all researchers. The logic of this—in terms of the largest and best return for public money spent on collecting the data—is compelling. However, it also raises ethical issues. How widely available should the data be made? Should politicians, insurance companies, and industry, for example, be able to access these data without express permission from the study participants? Currently, in most studies consent is given for the data to be used for (health) research and participants might not be happy for groups beyond this to be able to access the study data.

There is also an important issue of whether such datasets can be made truly anonymous, given the extensive and often repeatedly collected data in birth cohort/life course studies. This will be an issue particularly for studies in relatively small confined geographical areas. Here combining even a relatively small number of data items (all of which would be relevant to many researchers)—gender, month of birth, height, area of residence, name of school—might make it possible to identify individuals. Furthermore, making 'genome wide' data on individuals widely available could compromise anonymity. To our knowledge there are no examples of researchers trying to find out which individuals in a cohort particular data belong to and then using this connection in an inappropriate way. Nonetheless, there is an important issue of honesty with participants and this includes informing them of who has access to their data and the nature of this access.

The issues of broad access to data from birth cohorts is one that is currently being widely debated in many countries and clearer guidance may become available in the future.

6.3 Conclusions: diversity is desirable

The message of this chapter is that birth cohorts are long-term investments in necessary infrastructure for the epidemiological research that take a life course perspective on development of health and disease. Birth cohorts should, like forests, display diversity. The long-term benefits of such diversity has potentially important advantages over the short-term profit of very large data sets, constructed by pooling identical data from different birth cohorts. Though, if resources are available a combination of standardized data collection in some areas, together with diversity and flexibility, could support both aims.

Since financial and human resources are not unlimited and because exhaustion of participants should be avoided as the maintenance of a birth cohort ultimately depends on good will from participants, the best data collection strategy of birth cohorts might be a hypothesis-driven approach with a focus on a restricted number of well-defined exposures, for which associated health outcomes could be investigated. The data collected on these exposures should be as detailed and specific as possible; ideally they should be collected before birth, in infancy, during childhood, adolescents and during adulthood. In addition detailed measurement of potential confounders for these exposures should be given priority. A variety of additional exposures measured in less detail, if funding allows, should also be included.

A substantial part of this chapter has been concerned with the practical issues (perhaps more correctly termed difficulties) of establishing and maintaining birth cohorts, together with a description of some of the ways that these have been (or might be addressed) in different cohorts. However, our main conclusion would be to highlight three characteristics that we believe are essential to achieving the ideals of a birth cohort: **dedication**, **documentation**, and **data sharing**.

Dedication: dedication is required by the funders, researchers, and participants. As this chapter outlines, birth cohorts require an incredible amount of commitment and work by all three, particularly in the early stages of planning, developing, recruitment, and data collection. The major outcomes from this effort will be in the future, and often achieved by the next generation of researchers with impacts on population health in future generations. Thus a high level of altruism is required by everyone involved in initiating a birth cohort. Not only do funders, researchers, and participants need to be aware of the commitment involved, they have to have the necessary dedication to 'the cause' of the birth cohort. If there are doubts about this dedication then it may be best not to think about starting or being involved with a birth cohort.

Documentation: the second characteristic of an ideal birth cohort would be good documentation of the population from which the cohort arises, the context and research ideas in which the cohort was planned and how these change over the life of the cohort, of the data collection procedures used (including decisions about which data not to collect), the connection between different participants, and of the data storage and analysis. This is in accordance with the understanding that birth cohort provides an infrastructure for epidemiological research that is designed to be utilized over a long period of time and by a large number of researchers. At the initiation and at each data collection the cohort leads should ask themselves 'if I were given this dataset, and all its documentation, without having been involved in its collection would it all make sense to me?' This leads to the third characteristic of the ideal birth cohort,

Data sharing: ideally, data from all birth cohorts should be accessible to researchers with good research ideas. This requires appropriate data protection in order to secure confidentiality, but also procedures that fulfil these requirements and also facilitate easy access by researchers. Easy access to all documentation concerning the data is clearly part of this process. These and other measures to facilitate analyses of pooled data from different birth cohorts should balance the advantages of diversity with the need for cohort data with very large sample sizes.

Regarding the actual scientific relevance of the data we collect now to research questions in sixty years time, no guarantee can be given. We can only hope that diversity will increase the likelihood for an existence of relevant data somewhere out there, that proper documentation will make the data useable, and that the data are maintained in a way that keeps them accessible for future researchers with a good idea.

The question whether the experiences of the birth cohorts that grow up now will apply to the future generations is difficult to answer. To that end we would like to give the very last words to Søren Kierkegaard:

> Philosophy is perfectly right in saying that life must be understood backwards. But then one forgets the other clause—that it must be lived forwards. The more one thinks through this clause, the more one concludes, that life in temporality never becomes properly understandable, simply because never at any time does one get perfect repose to take a stance: backwards.
>
> (Søren Kierkegaards Skrifter [Søren Kierkegaards Writings] Vol 18, p 306)

Acknowledgements

AMNA would like to acknowledge the co-PIs in the Danish National Birth Cohort: Peter Aaby, Mads Melbye, Sjurdur Olsen, Thorkild IA Sørensen, and particularly the principal PI Jørn Olsen as well as the principal PI for the Metropolit study Merete Osler for scientific inspiration and discussions about birth cohorts over the last decade.

DAL is extremely grateful to Jean Golding, University of Bristol, whose dedication, documentation, and data sharing has allowed her and many others to exploit the value of the ALSPAC cohort. She is also grateful to Professor John Wright, Professor Neil Small, Pauline Rayner, and Jane West, Bradford Royal Infirmary and University of Bradford, and others from the Born in Bradford Study, who invited her to be part of the Research Collaborators group and who have been unstinting in their dedication and documentation over the last 12 months as this cohort begins.

Thanks also to Professor David Leon, London School of Hygiene and Tropical Medicine, for valuable discussions with both AMNA and DAL, and for making the comparison of Aberdeen and Metropolit data possible during a research stay of AMNA in London.

Thanks to the Søren Kierkegaard Research Center, University of Copenhagen, for helping with an authorized translation of the quote that ends the chapter.

The comments and views expressed in this chapter are, however, the authors'.

References

1 Golding, J, Pembrey, M, Jones, R. ALSPAC—the Avon Longitudinal Study of Parents and Children. I. Study methodology. *Paediatr Perinat Epidemiol* 2001; **15**: 74–87.

2 Olsen, J, Melbye, M, Olsen, SF, Sorensen, TI, Aaby, P, Andersen, AM, Taxbol, D, Hansen, KD, Juhl, M, Schow, TB, Sorensen, HT, Andresen, J, Mortensen, EL, Olesen, AW, Sondergaard, C. The Danish National Birth Cohort—its background, structure and aim. *Scand J Public Health* 2001; **29**: 300–7.

3 Magnus, P, Irgens, LM, Haug, K, Nystad, W, Skjaerven, R, Stoltenberg, C. Cohort profile: the Norwegian Mother and Child Cohort Study (MoBa). *Int J Epidemiol* 2006; **35**: 1146–50.

4 Najman, JM, Bor, W, O'Callaghan, M, Williams, GM, Aird, R, Shuttlewood, G. Cohort Profile: The Mater-University of Queensland Study of Pregnancy (MUSP). *Int J Epidemio* 2005;. **34**: 992–7.

5 Hofman, A, Jaddoe, VW, Mackenbach, JP, Moll, HA, Snijders, RF, Steegers, EA, Verhulst, FC, Witteman, JC, Buller, HA. Growth, development and health from early fetal life until young adulthood: the Generation R Study. *Paediatr Perinat Epidemiol* 2004; **18**: 61–72.

6 http://www.nationalchildrensstudy.gov/. http://www.nationalchildrensstudy.gov/. (2007).

7 Barker DJP. *Mothers, Babies, and Disease in Later Life*. BMJ Publishing Group, London, 1994.

8 Lucas, A, Fewtrell, MS, Cole, TJ. Fetal origins of adult disease-the hypothesis revisited. *BMJ* 1999; **319**: 245–9.

9 Huxley, R, Neil, A, Collins, R. Unravelling the fetal origins hypothesis: is there really an inverse association between birthweight and subsequent blood pressure? *Lancet* 2002; **360**: 659–65.

10 Tu, YK, West, R, Ellison, GT, Gilthorpe, MS. Why evidence for the fetal origins of adult disease might be a statistical artifact: the 'reversal paradox' for the relation between birth weight and blood pressure in later life. *Am J Epidemiol* 2005; **161**: 27–32.

11 Batty, GD, Morton, SM, Campbell, D, Clark, H, Smith, GD, Hall, M, Macintyre, S, Leon, DA. The Aberdeen Children of the 1950s cohort study: background, methods and follow-up information on a new resource for the study of life course and intergenerational influences on health. *Paediatr Perinat Epidemiol* 2004; **18**: 221–39.

12 Osler, M, Lund, R, Kriegbaum, M, Christensen, U, Andersen, AM. Cohort profile: the Metropolit 1953 Danish male birth cohort. *Int J Epidemiol* 2006; **35**: 541–5.

13 Stenberg, SA, Vagero, D. Cohort profile: the Stockholm birth cohort of 1953. *Int J Epidemiol* 2006; **35**: 546–8.

14 Power, C, Elliott, J. Cohort profile: 1958 British birth cohort (National Child Development Study). *Int J Epidemiol* 2006; **35**: 34–41.

15 **The Collaborative Perinatal Study of the National Institute of Neurological and Communicative Disorders and Stroke.** *The First Year of Life*. Johns Hopkins University Press, Baltimore, 1979.

16 **The Collaborative Perinatal Study of the National Institute of Neurological Diseases and Stroke.** *The Women and theirPregnancies*. W.B. Saunders Company, Philadelphia, 1972.

17 Zachau-Christiansen B. *The Influence of Prental and Perinatal Factors on Development during the First Year of Life*. Poul A. Andersens Forlag, Helsingør, 1972.

18 Villumsen AAL. *Environmental Factors in Congenital Malformations*. University of Copenhagen, 1970.

19 Susser, ES, Schaefer, CA, Brown, AS, Begg, MD, Wyatt, RJ. The design of the prenatal determinants of schizophrenia study. *Schizophr Bull* 2000; **26**: 257–73.

20 Bresnahan, MA, Brown, AS, Schaefer, CA, Begg, MD, Wyatt, RJ, Susser, ES. Incidence and cumulative risk of treated schizophrenia in the prenatal determinants of schizophrenia study. *Schizophr Bull* 2000; **26**: 297–308.

21 Ben-Shlomo, Y, Kuh, D. A life course approach to chronic disease epidemiology: conceptual models, empirical challenges and interdisciplinary perspectives. *Int J Epidemiol* 2002; **31**: 285–93.

22 Clayton, D, McKeigue, PM. Epidemiological methods for studying genes and environmental factors in complex diseases. *Lancet* 2001; **358**: 1356–60.

23 Kogevinas, M, Andersen, AM, Olsen, J. Collaboration is needed to co-ordinate European birth cohort studies. *Int J Epidemiol* 2004; **33**: 1172–3.

24 Osler, M, Andersen, AM, Due, P, Lund, R, Damsgaard, MT, Holstein, BE. Socioeconomic position in early life, birth weight, childhood cognitive function, and adult mortality. A longitudinal study of Danish men born in 1953. *J Epidemiol Community Health* 2003; **57**: 681–6.

25 Andersen, AM, Osler, M. Birth dimensions, parental mortality, and mortality in early adult age: a cohort study of Danish men born in 1953. *Int J Epidemiol* 2004; **33**: 92–9.

26 Osler, M, Nordentoft, M, Andersen, AM. Birth dimensions and risk of depression in adulthood: cohort study of Danish men born in 1953. *Br J Psychiatry* 2005; **186**: 400–3.

27 Lawlor, DA, Davey Smith, G, Clark, H, Leon, DA. The associations of birthweight, gestational age and childhood BMI with type 2 diabetes: findings from the Aberdeen Children of the 1950s cohort. *Diabetologia* 2006; **49**: 2614–17.

28 Lawlor, DA, Clark, H, Davey Smith, GD Leon, DA. Intrauterine growth and intelligence within sibling pairs: findings from the Aberdeen children of the 1950s cohort. *Pediatrics* 2006; **117**: e894–e902.

29 Lawlor, DA, Ronalds, G, Clark, H, Davey Smith, G, Leon, DA. Birth weight is inversely associated with incident coronary heart disease and stroke among individuals born in the 1950s: findings from the Aberdeen Children of the 1950s prospective cohort study. *Circulation* 2005; **112**: 1414–18.

30 Wiles, NJ, Peters, TJ, Leon, DA, Lewis, G. Birth weight and psychological distress at age 45–51 years: results from the Aberdeen Children of the 1950s cohort study. *Br J Psychiatry* 2005; **187**: 21–8.

31 Brown, RC, Dwyer, T, Kasten, C, Krotoski, D, Li, Z, Linet, MS, Olsen, J, Scheidt, P, Winn, DM. Cohort Profile: The International Childhood Cancer Cohort Consortium (I4C). *Int J Epidemiol* 2007; **36**: 724–30.

32 Kaiser, J. Everything You Wanted to Know About Children, for $2.7 Billion. *Science* 2003; **301**: 162–3.

33 Nybo Andersen, AM, Vastrup, P, Wohlfahrt, J, Andersen, PK, Olsen, J, Melbye, M. Fever in pregnancy and risk of fetal death: a cohort study. *Lancet* 2002; **360**: 1552–6.

34 Strandberg-Larsen, K, Nielsen, NR, Gronbaek, M, Andersen, PK, Olsen, J, Andersen, AM. Binge drinking in pregnancy and risk of fetal death. *Obstet Gynecol* 2008; **111**: 602–9.

35 National Board of Health. *Physical Activity—a handbook on prevention and treatment*. National Board of Health, Copenhagen, Denmark, 2004.

36 RCOG. *Antenatal care: routine care for the healthy pregnant woman, Clinical Guideline*. London, UK, 2006.

37 The Directorate for Health and Social Affairs. *Guidelines for Antenatal Care*. The Directorate for Health and Social Affairs, Oslo, Norway, 2005.

38 ACOG committee opinion. Exercise during pregnancy and the postpartum period. Number 267, January 2002. American College of Obstetricians and Gynecologists. *Int J Gynaecol Obstet* 2002; **77**: 79–81.

39 Kramer, MS, McDonald, SW. Aerobic exercise for women during pregnancy. *Cochrane Database Syst Rev* 2006; **3**: CD000180.

40 Madsen, M, Jorgensen, T, Jensen, ML, Juhl, M, Olsen, J, Andersen, PK, Nybo Andersen, AM. Leisure time physical exercise during pregnancy and the risk of miscarriage: a study within the Danish National Birth Cohort. *BJOG* 2007; **114**: 1419–26.

41 Juhl, M, Andersen, PK, Olsen, J, Madsen, M, Jorgensen, T, Nohr, EA, Andersen, AM. Physical exercise during pregnancy and the risk of preterm birth: a study within the Danish National Birth Cohort. *Am J Epidemiol* 2008; **167**: 859–66.

42 Lawlor, DA, Ronalds, G, Clark, H, Davey Smith, G, Leon, DA. Birth weight is inversely associated with incident coronary heart disease and stroke among individuals born in the 1950s: findings from the Aberdeen Children of the 1950s prospective cohort study. *Circulation* 2005; **112**: 1414–18.

43 Gale, CR, Martyn, CN. Birth weight and later risk of depression in a national birth cohort. *Br J Psychiatry* 2004; **184**: 28–33.

44 Hemachandra, AH, Howards, PP, Furth, SL, Klebanoff, MA. Birth weight, postnatal growth, and risk for high blood pressure at 7 years of age: results from the Collaborative Perinatal Project. *Pediatrics* 2007; **119**: e1264–e1270.

45 Hardy, R, Kuh, D, Langenberg, C, Wadsworth, ME. Birthweight, childhood social class, and change in adult blood pressure in the 1946 British birth cohort. *Lancet*, 2003; **362**: 1178–83.

46 Stavola, BL, Hardy, R, Kuh, D, Silva, IS, Wadsworth, M, Swerdlow, AJ. Birthweight, childhood growth and risk of breast cancer in a British cohort. *Br J Cancer* 2000; **83**: 964–8.

47 Nybo Andersen, AM, Osler, M. Birth dimensions, parental longevity and early adult mortality in a cohort of Danish men born in 1953. *Int J Epidemiol* 2004; **33**: 92–99.

48 Dalziel, SR, Parag, V, Rodgers, A, Harding, JE. Cardiovascular risk factors at age 30 following pre-term birth. *Int J Epidemiol* 2007; **36**: 907–15.

49 Leon, DA, Lawlor, DA, Clark, H, Macintyre, S. Cohort profile: the Aberdeen children of the 1950s study. *Int J Epidemiol* 2006; **35**: 549–52.

50 Batty, GD, Deary, IJ, Schoon, I, Gale, CR. Mental ability across childhood in relation to risk factors for premature mortality in adult life: the 1970 British Cohort Study. *J Epidemiol Community Health* 2007; **61**: 997–1003.

51 Hart, CL, Taylor, MD, Davey Smith, G, Whalley, LJ, Starr, JM, Hole, DJ, Wilson, V, Deary, IJ. Childhood IQ and all-cause mortality before and after age 65: prospective observational study linking the Scottish Mental Survey 1932 and the Midspan studies. *Br J Health Psychol* 2005; **10**: 153–65.

52 Kuh, D, Richards, M, Hardy, R, Butterworth, S, Wadsworth, ME. Childhood cognitive ability and deaths up until middle age: a post-war birth cohort study. *Int J Epidemiol* 2004; **33**: 408–13.

53 Spohr H-L, Steinhausen H-C. *Alcohol, Pregnancy and the Developing Child.* Cambridge University Press, Cambridge, 1996.

54 Harding, JE. The nutritional basis of the fetal origins of adult disease. *Int J Epidemiol* 2001; **30**: 15–23.

55 Demmelmair, H, von Rosen, J, Koletzko, B. Long-term consequences of early nutrition. *Early Hum Dev* 2006; **82**: 567–74.

56 Susser, E, Terry, MB. A conception-to-death cohort. *Lancet* 2003; **361**: 797–8.

57 Lumley, J, Watson, L, Watson, M, Bower, C. Periconceptional supplementation with folate and/or multivitamins for preventing neural tube defects. *Cochrane Database Syst Rev* 2001; CD001056.

58 Hjøllund, NH, Jensen, TB, Bonde, JPE, Henriksen, TB, Andersson, AM, Kolstad, HA, Ernst, E, Giwercman, A, Skakkebæk, NE, Olsen, J. Spontaneous abortion and physical strain around implantation: a follow-up study of first—pregnancy planners. *Epidemiology* 1999; **11**: 18–23.

59 Bonde, JP, Hjollund, NH, Jensen, TK, Ernst, E, Kolstad, H, Henriksen, TB, Giwercman, A, Skakkebaek, NE, Andersson, AM, Olsen, J. A follow-up study of environmental and biologic determinants of fertility among 430 Danish first-pregnancy planners: design and methods. *Reprod Toxicol* 1998; **12**: 19–27.

60 Inskip, HM, Godfrey, KM, Robinson, SM, Law, CM, Barker, DJ, Cooper, C. Cohort profile: the Southampton Women's Survey. *Int J Epidemiol* 2006; **35**: 42–8.

61 National Children's Study Reseach Plan. Volume 1. http://www.nationalchildrensstudy.gov/research/research_plan/upload/Research_Plan_Volume_1.pdf., 2008.

62 **International Childhood Cancer Cohort Consortium Workshop.** http://www.nationalchildrensstudy.gov/research/workshops/upload/Meeting-Report-International-Childhood-Cancer-Cohort-Consortium-Workshop.pdf., 2008.

63 **Hypponen, E, Smith Davey, G, Shepherd, P, Power, C.** An intergenerational and lifecourse study of health and mortality risk in parents of the 1958 birth cohort: (II) mortality rates and study representativeness. *Public Health* 2005; **119**: 608–15.

64 **Hypponen, E, Smith Davey, G, Shepherd, P, Power, C.** An intergenerational and lifecourse study of health and mortality risk in parents of the 1958 birth cohort: (I) methods and tracing. *Public Health* 2005; **119**: 599–607.

65 **Petersen AN, Jensen MS.** Temaartikel. Børn og deres familier de seneste 20 år. [Children and their families in 20 years]. In: Statistics Denmark. *Statistisk 10-aars oversigt.* Statistics Denmark, Copenhagen, 2000.

66 **Macintyre, S, Sooman, A.** Non-paternity and prenatal genetic screening. *Lancet*, 1991; **338**: 869–71.

67 **Basso, O, Nohr, EA, Olsen, J, Christensen, K.** Relationship of maternal body mass index and height to twinning. *Obstet Gynecol* 2005; **106**: 411.

68 **Williams, S, Poulton, R.** Twins and maternal smoking: ordeals for the fetal origins hypothesis? A cohort study. *BMJ* 1999; **318**: 897–900.

69 **Lawlor, DA, Clark, H, Davey Smith, G, Leon, DA.** Intrauterine growth and intelligence within sibling pairs: findings from the Aberdeen children of the 1950s cohort. *Pediatrics* 2006; **117**: e894–e902.

70 **Davey Smith, G, Harding, S, Rosato, M.** Relation between infants' birth weight and mothers' mortality: prospective observational study. *BMJ* 2000; **320**: 839–40.

71 **Davey Smith, G, Hart, C, Ferrell, C, Upton, M, Hole, D, Hawthorne, V, Watt, G.** Birth weight of offspring and mortality in the Renfrew and Paisley study: prospective observational study. *BMJ* 1997; **315**: 1189–93.

72 **Lawlor, DA, Davey Smith, G, Ebrahim, S.** Association between leg length and offspring birthweight: partial explanation for the trans-generational association between birthweight and cardiovascular disease: findings from the British Women's Heart and Health Study. *Paediatr Perinat Epidemiol* 2003; **17**: 148–55.

73 **Emanuel, I, Kimpo, C, Moceri, V.** The association of maternal growth and socio-economic measures with infant birthweight in four ethnic groups. *Int J Epidemiol* 2004; **33**: 1236–42.

74 **Emanuel, I, Kimpo, C, Moceri, V.** The association of grandmaternal and maternal factors with maternal adult stature. *Int J Epidemiol* 2004; **33**: 1243–8.

75 **Hypponen, E, Davey Smith, G, Shepherd, P, Power, C.** An intergenerational and lifecourse study of health and mortality risk in parents of the 1958 birth cohort: (I) methods and tracing. *Public Health* 2005; **119**: 599–607.

76 **Batty, GD, Morton, SM, Campbell, D, Clark, H, Davey Smith, G, Hall, M, Macintyre, S, Leon, DA.** The Aberdeen Children of the 1950s cohort study: background, methods and follow-up information on a new resource for the study of life course and intergenerational influences on health. *Paediatr Perinat Epidemiol* 2004; **18**: 221–39.

77 **Osler, M, Lund, R, Kriegbaum, M, Christensen, U, Andersen, AM.** Cohort profile: the Metropolit 1953 Danish male birth cohort. *Int J Epidemiol* 2006; **35**: 541–5.

78 **Olsen, J, Melbye, M, Olsen, SF, Sorensen, TI, Aaby, P, Andersen, AM, Taxbol, D, Hansen, KD, Juhl, M, Schow, TB, Sorensen, HT, Andresen, J, Mortensen, EL, Olesen, AW, Sondergaard, C.** The Danish National Birth Cohort—its background, structure and aim. *Scand J Public Health* 2001; **29**: 300–7.

79 **Magnus, P, Irgens, LM, Haug, K, Nystad, W, Skjaerven, R, Stoltenberg, C.** Cohort profile: the Norwegian Mother and Child Cohort Study (MoBa). *Int J Epidemiol* 2007; **35**: 1146–50.

80 **Landrigan, PJ, Trasande, L, Thorpe, LE, Gwynn, C, Lioy, PJ, D'Alton, ME, Lipkind, HS, Swanson, J, Wadhwa, PD, Clark, EB, Rauh, VA, Perera, FP, Susser, E.** The National Children's Study: a 21-year prospective study of 100,000 American children. *Pediatrics* 2006; **118**: 2173–86.

81 Homepage in English: http://www.etiskraad.dk/sw293.asp. http://www.etiskraad.dk/sw293.asp., 2007.
82 **Davey Smith, G.** Lifecourse epidemiology of disease: a tractable problem? *Int J Epidemiol* 2007; **36**: 479–80.
83 **Albertsen, K, Andersen, AM, Olsen, J, Gronbaek, M.** Alcohol consumption during pregnancy and the risk of preterm delivery. *Am J Epidemiol* 2004; **159**: 155–61.
84 **Benn, CS, Melbye, M, Wohlfahrt, J, Bjorksten, B, Aaby, P.** Cohort study of sibling effect, infectious diseases, and risk of atopic dermatitis during first 18 months of life. *BMJ* 2004; **328**: 1223.
85 **Bech, BH, Obel, C, Henriksen, TB, Olsen, J.** Effect of reducing caffeine intake on birth weight and length of gestation: randomised controlled trial. *BMJ* 2007; **334**: 409.

Chapter 7

Family-based life course studies in low- and middle-income countries

G David Batty, Cesar G Victora and Debbie A Lawlor

Abstract

We briefly describe the growing impact of non-communicable disease in low- and middle-income countries (LMIC) which, together with existing infectious illnesses and a rising incidence of violence, represents a triple health burden. Birth cohort studies, and in particular those with family-based elements, clearly have a role in identifying risk factors for chronic disease. Existing studies from LMIC are described. We identified sixteen birth cohort studies, all but one of which had a known intergenerational element—that is, data on the parents, usually the mother, of the cohort members—although the depth of information was typically modest. With the exception of one large-scale twin registry, we were unable to find examples of twin or sibling studies from LMIC offering sufficient size and breadth of data to facilitate explorations of multiple influences on chronic disease and risk factors. We advance a number of reasons for adding to the very sparse research base outside of industrialized nations, and attempt to provide solutions for some of the methodological complications that might accompany such endeavors. Finally, we suggest that, on the basis of what we regard as a clear need for a greater geographical representation of family-based life course studies, the involvement of a central overseeing body—such as the World Health Organization—that has the respect of all countries and the capacity to develop strategic plans for 'global' life course and transgenerational epidemiology, would be beneficial.

7.1 Introduction

Rates of non-communicable diseases such as cardiovascular disease (CVD) and many malignancies are declining in most industrialized countries, however, they remain the leading causes of death.[1] Whilst inadequate infrastructure in some countries make routine collection of health data difficult, there is growing evidence that non-communicable disease rates are increasing in low- and middle-income countries (LMIC).[2] The predictions are that such disorders will become the predominant cause of mortality by 2020, representing 70% of all deaths.[3,4] As has been highlighted,[5,6] what is often ignored in considering such statistics—whether they be from developed or developing countries—is the impact of less lethal, but equally debilitating diseases such as psychiatric illness: for instance by the same year it is estimated that clinical depression, will become the major cause of disability adjusted life years in developing societies.[3] Furthermore, recent evidence suggests that depression has a greater impact on overall health than cardiovascular disease in all regions of the world.[7] The added presence of communicable diseases—HIV/AIDS, malaria, tuberculosis, acute respiratory infections, diarrhoeal disease, and other, vaccine-preventable illnesses—and, in women, serious obstetric complications, has raised well-documented concerns of a dual burden of disease amongst the world's poor.[5, 8] Indeed, the rising epidemic of violence in many LMIC has led some commentators to draw attention to a triple-health burden.[9]

A large number of studies using observational designs (chiefly, cohort and case-control), representing a research tradition beginning in the 1930s[10] and 1940s,[11] have been conducted in middle- and older-aged persons in high income countries. These have offered crucial insights into understanding the aetiology of non-communicable diseases. Notable examples include work pioneered in Germany[10] and subsequently extended by Doll and Bradford Hill that identified the link between cigarette smoking and lung cancer, heart disease, and other adverse health outcomes,[12–15] and, more recently, studies establishing the causal associations of both high blood pressure[16] and dyslipidaemia[17] with cardiovascular disease. These findings have been instrumental in the development of interventions (lifestyle and pharmacological) that have resulted in population-level declines in these risk factors, treatment of those at highest risk, and ultimately decreases in cardiovascular disease and smoking-related cancer morbidity and mortality rates.

Despite these successes there are debates about the extent to which these now established, major adult risk factors, when measured solely in mid-life, fully explain the variation in important chronic diseases.[18–20] Some investigators have argued that these risk factors explain most of the geographical and secular variations in non-communicable diseases, such as CVD, and that there is no need to search further.[21, 22] However, this focus on adult risk factors, which is consistent with a degenerative model of non-communicable disease epidemiology, pays scant attention to processes—within *and* between generations—that lead up to the peak or optimal phenotypic state that are usually a feature of adolescence or early adulthood, and that are increasingly recognized as relevant to non-communicable disease risk in adulthood. These optimal phenotypic states include peak bone mass (usually attained post-puberty), peak respiratory function (usually attained in early 20s), and peak arterial function (usually attained by age 15–20 years).[23] Life course epidemiology- an approach to understanding disease processes that originated in the field of psychiatry and was applied to somatic chronic disease in the late 1980s-explicitly recognizes the *development* of anatomical and physiological systems, in addition to how rapidly one degenerates from this optimum, as having important relevance to the likelihood of developing non-communicable diseases.

7.2 The rise of life course chronic disease epidemiology and the family-based approach in high income countries

Support for the importance of developmental processes in the aetiology of adult non-communicable diseases—in this illustration, CVD—can be found in studies employing diverse research designs. First, pathological investigations have revealed evidence of atherosclerosis—the precursor to coronary heart disease—in males as young as 15 years of age.[24, 25] Second, levels of established mid-life risk factors for CVD and selected cancers (physical inactivity, smoking, obesity), seem to 'track' between childhood and adulthood, such that children at high risk tend become adults at high risk.[26–29] Third, for adult-targeted lifestyle modification designed to reduce coronary heart disease rates, results are typically modest,[30] suggesting that earlier intervention may have some benefit. Finally, in a small but growing literature, several of the classic markers of disease risk identified in adult populations—smoking, raised blood pressure, obesity—also seem to be predictive of later CVD and cancer risk when measured in younger populations who are followed into middle- and older-age.[31]

7.2.1 Birth and family-based cohort studies

A birth cohort study, on which much of the understanding of life course influences on health is based, can be defined as the collection of data at follow-up survey, through passive (e.g., hospital admissions, death registration, or educational records) and/or active (e.g., medical examination, psychiactric interview) means over a given period (often decades), of a group of individuals born around the same time (this may stretch to a few days, or, in some studies, years). In Latin, *cohors* refers to a group of warriors within a roman legion.[32] Alternative terms for cohort study include longitudinal or panel study. The growing use of this research design has, however, led to the 'life course study' being incorrectly name-checked as a study design in its own right[33–36] when it is simply a cohort study.

Birth cohort studies have also been referred to as pregnancy cohorts or family-based cohorts, recognizing that for some (e.g., Avon Longitudinal Study of Parents and Children[37, 38] and Mater-University of Queensland Study of Pregnancy[39]) recruitment was of mothers in early pregnancy—sometimes by identifying those who were seeking to become pregnant. Using this approach, information on parents and children is gathered during the follow-up period so facilitating analyses of intergenerational influences on health. Such studies differ from many birth cohorts (e.g., from a high income country, the UK 1946,[40] 1958[41]) that recruited infants at birth in that they are better able, through prospective data gathering as opposed to distant recall, to evaluate the impact, if any, of pre-natal (and even pre-conception) exposures—maternal alcohol consumption, smoking, dietary intake, physical activity patterns, illicit drug use, weight change— on the future health of the index child (so called trans-generational or intergenerational influences) and also the mother. A third category of investigations includes panel or cross-sectional studies of infants/children (e.g., from a LMIC, the Young Lives study[42]), that are then followed up prospectively; the above mentioned issue of recall bias is even more acute in this type of study.

7.2.2 Life course approach to chronic disease epidemiology

Prompted by this body of work pointing to the importance of both developmental and degenerative processes in the aetiology of adult disease, a 'life course' paradigm has been proposed which offers a framework for identifying the long term effect on adult disease of social, physiological, behavioural, and psychological processes operating during gestation, childhood, adolescence, adulthood, and between generations.[23] This approach therefore emphasizes a combination of measures of developmental and degenerative processes from across the life span and, ideally, between generations. The last two decades have witnessed a marked rise in research output in this area as evidenced by the increasing number of publications worldwide over the last 20 years citing the use of birth cohort studies (Figure 1a). There has also been a comparable increase in family based studies judging by the growing literature in the fields of twin (Figure 7.1b), intergenerational (Figure 7.1c) and sibling research (Figure 7.1d).

7.3 Existing birth cohorts in LMIC: an overview with a focus on family-based studies

In Table 7.1 we describe a series of birth cohort studies from LMIC which have already contributed towards the understanding of chronic disease aetiology, or have the potential to do so. For the purposes of comparison, we also describe some birth cohort studies from industrialized societies.

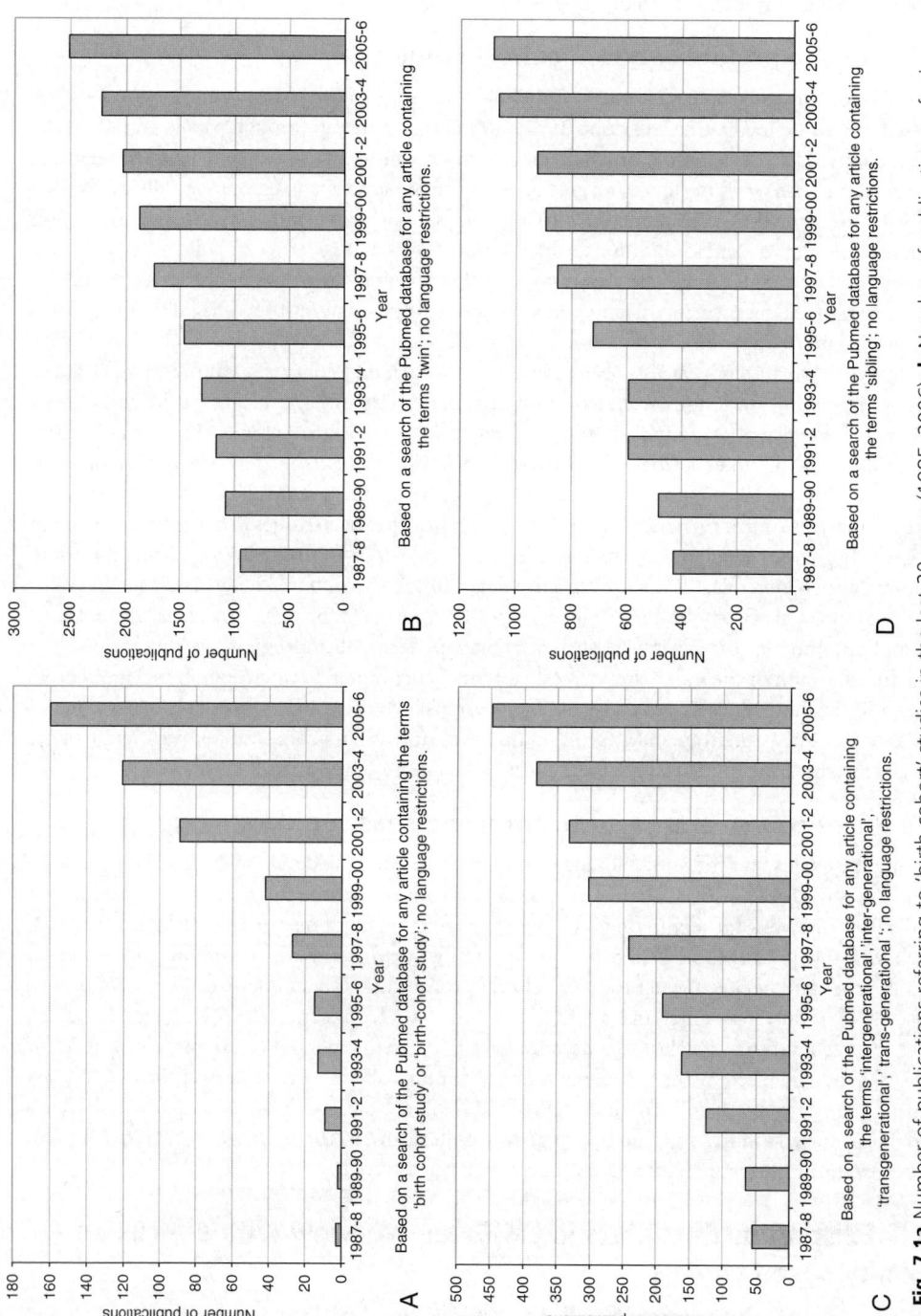

Fig. 7.1a Number of publications referring to 'birth cohort' studies in the last 20 years (1985–2006); **b** Number of publications referring to 'twin' studies in the last 20 years (1985–2006); **c** Number of publications referring to 'inter-generational' studies in the last 20 years (1985–2006); **d** Number of publications referring to 'sibling' studies in the last 20 years (1985–2006).

Our criteria for including studies were that they should have recruited at least 1000 participants and that, to our knowledge, they remain research active (i.e., still collecting follow-up data on participants). The list of birth cohorts from LMIC is—we hope—exhaustive, while several cohorts from high-income nations could not be included owing to page constraints (thus these examples are illustrative rather than exhaustive). Unsurprisingly, for reasons already stated, in comparison to cohorts from high-income societies, in addition to being fewer in number, they are also generally smaller in size, and less mature; however, in general, they offer similarly detailed and valuable data.

An additional important feature of Table 7.1 is that it highlights the regions of the world with few or no birth cohorts; unrepresented are north Africa, and the Middle East. To our knowledge there is also only one birth cohort in south Asia[43] where there are likely to be marked differences in exposures and developmental processes across different countries in this region. Similarly, we are aware of only one east Asian cohort, the Taiwan Birth Cohort Study,[44] which currently falls within the jurisdiction of the Republic of China. There is a solitary birth cohort from sub-Saharan Africa[45–47] and one from the former Soviet Union[48,49] where the considerable social upheaval and major substance abuse problems amongst adults[50–53] is likely to have significant impact upon the development of future generations. This sole offering from the former Soviet Union is the Republic of Belarus-based Promotion Of Breastfeeding Intervention Trial (PROBIT),[48] a very large scale randomised controlled trial (N = 17,046 mother-infant pairs) of a breast feeding promotion intervention with detailed data collection on both parents and offspring at the time of birth of the infant. The long-term follow-up of this trial means that is can be utilized as an intergenerational study. Using its randomized controlled trial design, it has already shown itself to be extremely useful in exploring the health consequences of breast feeding in the offspring,[54] while analysing the data as a prospective cohort design has added to the growing literature on the role of other perinatal and early life characteristics in the development of asthma and other atopic disease.[55] The use of large scale intervention studies of adults in this manner is not uncommon.[56] The closest match to this is the much smaller Human Capital Study,[57] that started as a nutritional intervention trial in four rural villages in 1960s Guatemala. In general, the afore-described cohort studies feature representative, rather then convenience, samples.

7.3.1 Intergenerational studies

Of these sixteen studies from LMIC (Table 7.1), all but one (South Delhi Cohort[43]) were found to have family-based characteristics and these are described in more detail in Table 7.2 (intergenerational only). These are the Taiwan Birth Cohort Study,[44] the Human Capital Study,[57] the 1982, 1993, and 2004 Pelotas Birth Cohort Study,[58,59] the 1978/9 Ribeirão Preto Birth Cohort Study,[60] 1994 Ribeirão Preto Birth Cohort Study,[60] 1997/8 São Luis Birth Cohort Study,[60] the Cebu cohort,[61,62] Birth to Twenty Cohort,[45–47] Young Lives studies (Ethiopia, India, Peru, and Vietnam),[42] and the PROBIT.[48] Most of the data collected on the parents of study participants, which enables an assessment of the intergenerational transmission of risk factors for chronic diseases (see Chapter 2), is modest in depth and scope. For instance, the only parental data in the Ribeirão Preto and São Luis studies is maternal smoking, and the Human Capital Study only has data on maternal stature. By contrast, in the Pelotas[42,58] studies and the Young Lives cohorts, detailed information on minor psychiatric illness in the mother and social networks (Young Lives only[63,64]) were ascertained. Some other investigations of the health consequences in the offspring of maternal psychiatric illness exist[65–67]—probably the most examined relation in intergenerational cohorts from LMIC—although in samples that were too small in size to meet the entry criteria here. Data on fathers is particularly sparse (a characteristic also of many life

Table 7.1 Birth cohort studies from affluent and LMIC (reproduced with permission based on a modification of a previously published table, Batty GD, Alves JG, Correia J, Lawlor DA. Examining life-course influences on chronic disease: the importance of birth cohort studies from low- and middle-income countries. *Braz J Med Biol Res* 2007; **40**: 1277–86[114])

Name[key citation]	Location	Birth year(s)	Cohort size at induction	Family-based element? (Y/N)
Affluent countries				
British Cohort Studies[41, 115–118]	UK	1946, 1958, 1970, ~2000	5362–20,000	Y (intergenerational)
Avon Longitudinal Study of Parents and Children[37,38]	England	1991/2	13 971	Y (intergenerational, sibling)
Aberdeen Children of the 1950s study[108,109]	Scotland	1950–6	12150	Y (intergenerational, sibling)
Northern Finland Birth Cohort[83]	Finland	1966	12,058	Y (intergenerational, sibling)
Danish National Birth Cohort[119]	Denmark	1997–2003	Births to 100,000 women	Y (intergenerational)
National Collaborative Perinatal Project[120]	US*	1959–66	633	Y (intergenerational, sibling)
Dunedin Multidisciplinary Health & Development Study[121]	New Zealand	1972/3	1037	Y (intergenerational)
Mater-University of Queensland Study of Pregnancy[39]	Australia	1981/4	7223	Y (intergenerational, sibling)
LMIC				
South Delhi Cohort[43]	India	1969–72	8181	N
Human Capital Study[57]	Guatemala	1969–77	1301	Y (intergenerational)
1982 Pelotas Birth Cohort Study[58,59]	Brazil	1982	5914	Y (intergenerational)
1993 Pelotas Birth Cohort Study[59]	Brazil	1993	5249	Y (intergenerational)
2004 Pelotas Birth Cohort Study[59]	Brazil	2004	2403	Y (intergenerational)
1978/9 Ribeirão Preto Birth Cohort Study[60]	Brazil	1978/9	6748	Y (intergenerational)
1994 Ribeirão Preto Birth Cohort Study[60]	Brazil	1994	2846	Y (intergenerational)
1997/8 São Luis Birth Cohort Study[60]	Brazil	1997/8	2542	Y (intergenerational)
Cebu cohort[61,62]	Philippines	1983/4	2080	Y (intergenerational)

Birth to Twenty Cohort ('Mandela's children')[45-47]	South Africa	1990	3273	Y (intergenerational)
Young Lives[42]	Ethiopia	~2001	1999	Y (intergenerational)
Young Lives[42]	India	~2001	2011	Y (intergenerational)
Young Lives[42]	Peru	~2001	2052	Y (intergenerational)
Young Lives[42]	Vietnam	~2001	1999	Y (intergenerational)
Promotion Of Breastfeeding Intervention Trial[48]	Belarus	1996–1997	17,046	Y (intergenerational)
Taiwan Birth Cohort Study[44]	Taiwan (Rep. China)	2003	2048	Y (intergenerational)

Only cohorts with over 1000 study participants at induction and for which investigators continue to be research active were included in this table. The cited cohorts from high income countries is illustrative of those available but not exhaustive, while the cited cohorts from low and middle income countries is intended to be fully comprehensive. *only selected sites active.

Table 7.2 Examples of data collected in birth cohort studies from LMIC with an intergenerational element

Name[key citation]	Examples of data collected on parents	Examples of data collected on offspring (core cohort)	Published parental-offspring association[citation]
Human Capital Study[57]	Maternal stature	Height and weight throughout childhood	Maternal stature as a determinant of offspring stunting[122]
1982 Pelotas Birth Cohort Study[58,59]	Maternal minor psychiatric disorder and other morbidities (inc. during pregnancy), age, reproductive history, height pre-pregnancy weight, smoking, alcohol consumption, skin color. Paternal education, smoking and alcohol consumption	Weight, standing and sitting height, body composition, blood pressure, oral health, drug use, body image, age at first intercourse, smoking, alcohol intake, exercise, diet, mortality, etc.	Maternal smoking as a determinant of offspring intrauterine growth retardation and prematurity[123]
1993 Pelotas Birth Cohort Study[59]	Maternal and paternal education, smoking, paternity status, parental beatings. Maternal exercise, alcohol consumption, pre-pregnancy weight	Exercise, television viewing, use of video games, length, head and abdominal circumferences, mortality	Maternal pre-pregnancy weight and offspring physical activity[124]
2004 Pelotas Birth Cohort Study[59]	Maternal height and weight, smoking and alcohol intake. Paternal education	Mortality, weight, length, head, chest and abdominal circumferences	None identified as yet
1978/9 Ribeirão Preto Birth Cohort Study[60]	Maternal smoking only	Birth characteristics, post-natal growth, CVD risk factors	Maternal smoking and offspring overweight/malnutrition[125]
1994 Ribeirão Preto Birth Cohort Study[60]	Maternal smoking only	Birth characteristics, post-natal growth	None identified as yet
1997/8 São Luis Birth Cohort Study[60]	Maternal smoking only	Birth characteristics, post-natal growth	None identified as yet
Cebu cohort[61,62]	Maternal stature, age & education	Height	Maternal growth as a determinant of offspring stunting[126]

Birth to Twenty Cohort[45-47]	Maternal/caregiver stress and health, age	Growth, physical activity, health, cognition, blood pressure, body composition, genetic material	None identified as yet
Young Lives[42]*	Maternal age, education, minor psychiatric illness, social networks, social capital	Birth weight, post-natal growth, infant feeding, and detailed data on illness/injury	Maternal mental health as a determinant of offspring childhood growth[63]
Promotion of Breastfeeding Intervention Trial[48]	Maternal and paternal age, education, occupation, weight, height, smoking	Birth weight, post-natal growth, infant feeding, childhood atopy, wheezing, cognition, metabolic and vascular outcomes, DNA being collected from parents and offspring	Various analyses on-going: parental anthropometry vs. offspring growth and size; parental behaviours vs. health outcomes in offspring
Taiwan Birth Cohort Study[44]	Maternal education, occupation, and income; plus hypertension, diabetes and herbal medicine use during pregnancy	Birthweight, gestational age, infant feeding	None to date were identified

Only cohorts with over 1000 study participants at induction and which continue to be research active were included in this table. The cited cohorts from high income countries is illustrative of those available but not exhaustive, while the cited cohorts from low and middle income countries is intended to be fully comprehensive. *Although the Young Lives study is based on four cohorts drawn from different countries, they have a shared methodology.

course studies in industrialized countries—see Chapter 6), despite increasing interest in both understanding the direct impact of fathers on the health of their offspring, and of comparing the relative magnitude of maternal–offspring associations to paternal–offspring associations (Chapter 2).

The most commonly studied outcome in the intergenerational studies reviewed is offspring size or growth, with findings that maternal smoking during pregnancy is related to lower birth weight and both overweight and malnutrition later in life (Table 7.2). Parental size has also been related to offspring size in these studies in an attempt to distinguish the relative contributions of genetic and environmental factors to stunting (Table 7.2).

7.3.2 Twin studies

We identified few studies of twins from LMIC, and sibling studies were seemingly more scarce (Table 7.1).[68] The twin cohorts that exist had, for example, set out to examine gene environment influences on blood pressure variation in twins from Barbados[69] and Madras (India),[70] and the prevalence of epilepsy in proband and non-proband twins.[71] While most of these studies are, again, small in scale and ambition, being designed to test a single hypothesis or research question, they nonetheless point to the feasibility of establishing such a study in countries with, at best, a modest research culture and infrastructure. Exceptional in this regard is the Sri Lankan Twin Registry[72, 73] which probably represents the first such large-scale registry in the developing world. An island with wide genetic diversity, Sri Lanka's five main populations exhibit both European and Asian origins. A cohort of 4,600 twin pairs was initially established through a media-advertised competition, and this has been supplemented by birth registration-based cohorts through hospitals. There is also a nationwide population-based younger twin cohort (1992–1997) traced through the Department of Birth and Death Registration.[72, 73] The Sri Lankan twin cohorts are specifically being utilized to identify genetic and life course environmental determinants of common mental disorders, suicidal ideation and alcohol use.[74]

7.4 Establishing and maintaining family-based birth cohort studies in LMIC: a justification

Given some of the methodological difficulties of establishing and maintaining birth cohorts even in affluent nations (see Chapter 6), together with the likelihood that some risk factors may well be equally important in both industrialized countries and LMIC, one could argue that limited research funds should be preferentially directed towards studies that evaluate population-specific interventions aimed at reduction of risk factors for important non-communicable disease in LMIC (e.g. smoking prevention programmes, interventions for improving antenatal care, re-housing studies). While this approach has it obvious merits, we believe that there are several important reasons for supporting birth cohorts in LMIC, particularly those with a family-based element. These include the possibility that the composition of exposures may differ between countries at varying stages of the economic transition; some exposures, particularly occupational, may be unique to LMIC; there may be between-country differences in confounding structure; important exposure-disease association that may realistically be expected to differ from those seen in higher income societies, such as fetal growth and adult CVD, have yet to be well investigated in cohorts drawn from LMIC; economic transition may modify exposure-disease associations; and, finally, replication of very well established exposure-disease from western populations in those relationships apparent in LMIC may have important positive political ramifications.

7.4.1 Composition of exposures

There are fundamental differences in the composition of important exposures across countries. For example, in industrialized societies, most physical activity in children and adults is accumulated in leisure where it is vigorous and time-limited. By contrast, in LMIC, energy expenditure for all age groups is largely occupational in nature or produced whilst undertaking essential activities of daily living (including transportation) where it is typically of longer duration but of lower intensity. These differences may have important implications for findings from life course epidemiology, in that the association of maternal energy balance during pregnancy on offspring health during infancy and later life may differ between industrialized and LMIC countries. Similarly, while tobacco consumption in western populations mainly comprises inhalation from cigarettes, in south Asia over one-third of tobacco intake is smokeless.[75] The consumption of traditional forms such as betel quid, tobacco with lime, and tobacco tooth powder is increasing. Further, when tobacco smoke is inhaled, 'bidis' are more common than cigarettes in selected countries such as India. Although smaller than cigarettes, bidis potentially deliver a higher dose of cancer-causing agents.[76] The effect of maternal tobacco intake during pregnancy on the future health risk of her offspring may therefore differ between countries depending upon the actual mechanism by which tobacco affects a given outcome. In a further example, infants who are not breastfed in high income countries will typically receive formula replacement, whereas the principal substitute in LMIC it is often cow's milk. Of relevance to the developmental origins of disease, there is some evidence that body composition for a given birth size differs between English and Indian infants, with evidence that the so called 'fat-thin insulin resistant' phenotype common in south Asian adults[77–79] may be present at birth.[80] In these various instances, comparison of the exposed and unexposed with respect to a given health endpoint may give rise to different findings in samples drawn from different countries.[58]

7.4.2 Unique exposures

There are some exposures that are relatively unique in LMIC and that might have important influences on developmental and degenerative processes leading to ill-health. For example, cancer-causing occupational exposures, such as benzene,[81] are more common in non-industrialized societies where conditions of occupational hygiene are probably less favourable than in high income countries.[82] The same may be true of wider environmental pollutants, such as pesticides.[83] Contact with such pollutants might have lasting influences across generations via an intrauterine effect if women of reproductive age are exposed. Developing a robust evidence base of the health effects of such exposures is likely to be important in supporting policy aimed at maintaining economic growth that is not at the expense of population health.

7.4.3 Confounding structure

The confounding structure of a given variable may differ across studies drawn from countries at different stages of the economic transition. Taking the example of breast feeding again, while this practice is more common in affluent groups from high income countries, the reverse is the case in developing societies. Given that, in keeping with other behaviours, breast feeding is a highly confounded variable,[84] this is a crucial issue in considering its relation to health outcomes. The occurrence of disparate findings for a given association across studies that have differential confounding structures would raise concerns that confounding is an important alternative explanation. This was the case in a recent detailed comparison of socioeconomic inequalities in mother and offspring characteristics between the Avon Longitudinal Study of Pregnancy (ALSPAC), a UK based pregnancy cohort, and the three Pelotas (Brazil) cohorts (Table 7.1) where notable differences between the UK and Brazil cohorts were indeed evident. Different confounding structures may also explain why breastfeeding does not seem to protect against adolescent overweight/obesity in the 1982[85] and 1993[86] Pelotas birth cohorts, unlike what is found in most studies from developed countries such as the UK.[87]

7.4.4 Relevance of exposure-disease associations

While the relation of fetal and post natal growth with adult disease has, with some exceptions,[43] been examined in most detail in cohorts drawn from affluent societies—in particular the Hertfordshire (UK)[88] and Helsinki (Finland) historical cohorts[89] (Table 7.1)—the findings may in fact have most relevance for LMIC where the higher prevalence of low birth weight, malnutrition, and stunting result in greater population attributable risk. Related examples include the suggestion that childhood diarrhoea and accompanying dehydration may programme salt retention leading to increased blood pressure levels and CVD.[90–92] However, taking the former example, the possible difference in body composition at a given birth weight, and the uncertainty about the biological pathways that link low birth weight and stunted early post natal growth to later disease outcomes, emphasizes the importance of first establishing whether growth parameters during developmental periods relate to adult non-communicable disease outcomes in LMIC in they same way that they do in high-income countries. These findings have major policy implications for low and middle-income countries, where concern about under nutrition leads health workers to promote rapid weight in childhood through the ingestion of high-energy foods.

7.4.5 Effect modification by stage of economic transition

Socioeconomic inequalities in health, such as coronary heart disease, appear to differ by epoch in western societies.[93] Similarly, they are also likely to vary by country at a single point in time. A recent cross-country comparison of socioeconomic variation in insulin resistance in European children[94] serves as a reminder of this. In a more affluent country (Denmark), higher socioeconomic position, as indexed by family income and education, was associated with lower (more favourable) insulin levels, while in countries undergoing marked social, cultural, and economic transition (Portugal and, particularly, Estonia) it was positive.[94] The authors speculated that, in the countries undergoing economic upheaval, life style changes attributable to globalization and urbanization—including a movement from a diet rich in complex carbohydrate and fibre to one in which sugars and fats predominate—may be occurring. That such changes seem to impact most rapidly upon affluent individuals in countries undergoing such transitions, for instance in Latin America and Asia[95] might explain the results.

7.4.6 Politics of study replication

Finally, the replication of established risk factor–disease relationships in LMIC may have important, positive political ramifications. For example, it has been speculated that, outside of the richer nations, the absence of specific data for LMIC has led to the importance of cigarette smoking as a major cause of death being seriously underestimated by the medical profession, the media, and government in those countries.[5] It has been claimed, for example, that smoking, a well established risk factor for CVD in developed nations (see Section 7.1), may be less detrimental to cardiovascular disease outcomes in east Asian countries where cholesterol levels are low.[96] This 'myth' may at least partially explain the very high smoking levels amongst men in particular in these countries.[96] It is hoped that recent analyses of large cohorts drawn from China[97] and Korea,[98] amongst others,[99] that clearly counter this standpoint, together with worrying predictions of future deaths,[2] will bring about a change in political will. Thus, even in the absence of biological plausibly for a different exposure–disease relation, it may be important to replicate in LMIC what most epidemiologists would consider an established association. This also has much relevance to birth cohort studies: smoking is often initiated in adolescence or early adulthood, and a life course approach using birth cohort data should be useful in exploring the country- or population-specific early life predictors of this behaviour (i.e., the determinants of the disease determinants).

7.5 Establishing and maintaining family-based birth cohort studies in LMIC: conceptual and methodological considerations

As outlined, to date, the modest evidence base concerning the inter-generational transmission of adult disease/risk factors has been gleaned from cohort studies based in high income countries (for examples see Table 7.1). This is largely the product of affluence which manifests itself in several ways. First, these societies have the medical research funding to facilitate the initiation and maintenance of cohorts. Second, births typically occur in hospitals, rather than the home, and home visits by a medical practitioner during infancy (often with routine collection of standard data on growth and development) are commonplace, so facilitating systematic documentation of early life characteristics. Third, surveillance of cohort members is less problematic than in LMIC owing to a lower prevalence of internal (predominantly rural to urban) migration and the capacity to trace persons passively through national databases, particularly in the Scandinavian countries where unique person identification numbers have expedited the process (see for example, reports based on Swedish[100–103] and Danish[104, 105] population-based studies). The need for active follow-up of subjects through home visits—which is the norm in cohorts from less developed settings—is one of the explanations for the generally smaller size of many cohorts compared to those from high-income countries.

Despite substantial resources and a supportive infrastructure, maintaining family-based cohorts in high-income countries is still problematic (see also Chapter 6). Some of the most important findings from such cohorts are only likely to emerge seven or more decades after they begin. This is because studies that can really contribute to understanding how risk factors that influence developmental processes combine with those affecting degenerative processes to affect disease risk require cohorts that have collected repeat, detailed information from the parental generation, through gestation, childhood, adolescence, and early adulthood of the offspring to the point at which non-communicable diseases are commonplace. Over this time, loss to follow-up is likely to be considerable. For example, in a 53 year follow-up of the 5,362 infants in the 1946 UK birth cohort, 1,979 (33%) were not approached because they had previously refused to take part, were living abroad, were unable to be traced since the previous follow-up or had died; of the 3,383 approached 3,035 (90%) provided information;[106] this pattern of attrition is in keeping with the response in other birth cohort studies in high income countries.[41] Whilst death is unavoidable and provides an endpoint in a birth cohort, other reasons for attrition, including refusal to take part, moving abroad and loss of contact details could be considered preventable to some degree and have implication for statistical power. As discussed in Chapter 6, birth cohort studies require incredible amounts of dedication from participants, researchers and funding bodies, all of whom need to be willing to not only commit to an investigation for some decades, but also accept delayed gratification that realistically extends into the next generation of scientists and people able to benefit from the research. They also require resources to develop field methods for maximizing participant uptake and for the development of analytical methods for determining the extent to which attrition might bias findings.

Amongst the family-based birth cohorts in LMIC, the three Pelotas (Brazil) studies (established in 1982, 1993, and 2004) have contributed markedly to the knowledge base (for a list of research output see two recent profiles of the studies[58, 107]). Several of the factors cited by the principal investigators on these study as being crucial to the continued successful follow-up of the study participants mirror the characteristics of several studies conducted in high income countries such as ALSPAC[37, 38] and the Mater-University[39] studies: lower than average rates of in- and out-migration; fewer apparent concerns of the inhabitants of Pelotas over personal safety—so common elsewhere in Brazil—resulting in refusal to participate being rare;[58] and the moderate size of the city which makes data collection manageable, whilst maintaining a reasonable level of statistical power.

Here we discuss some issues pertinent to the optimal conduct of family-based studies (these are described in greater detail in Chapter 6). As outlined in chapter 2, it is clear that the ideal intergenerational study will have well measured, detailed characteristics on two or more generations—that is, grandparents, parents, and offspring. In addition, it would also have information on siblings and, by extension since it is intergenerational, cousins. We are not aware of any such resource nor do we see that current pregnancy/birth cohorts are likely to provide this for future researchers. Nonetheless, it is worth giving some consideration to how family-based designs could be strengthened, particularly in LMIC.

7.5.1 Collecting data across two generations

One particularly important issue that warrants mention is the difficulty of obtaining good quality data from fathers as well as mothers. Information on fathers is commonly obtained by using the mother as a proxy, either with the mother reporting, for instance, her partner's smoking, education level, height, weight, and other characteristics (clearly a method prone to inaccuracy), or with the mother passing on questionnaires to her partner (with the result that missing data is more common for fathers than mothers). These issues are further complicated by parental separation during the offspring's life—an increasingly common occurrence—when study administrators need to be able to establish whether information[58] relates to biological (genetic) or 'social' (step) fathers. For example, in the 1982 Pelotas cohort, 8.2% of the mothers were not living with the child's biological father at the time of delivery. When the child had reached four years of age this proportion had increased to 17.2%, and by 15 years to 34.3%. In comparison to fathers, mothers are relatively easy to recruit and survey, including the collection of biological data and accurately measured anthropometric, vascular, respiratory information either during their antenatal clinic visits and/or around the time of birth of their child. The collection of adequate information from fathers could involve the utilization of research clinics on an evening and/or over the weekend to take account of working schedules and possibly the provision of incentives for fathers to attend these clinics (e.g. tickets to sporting events, or even data collection at such fixtures). Clearly, such practices would require additional revenue from funding agencies. Taking the example of the Pelotas study again, recalling parents for follow-up surveys has resulted in approximately 50% attrition. Fathers in particular are the least compliant. As levels of economic migration increase in LMIC—such that younger adults, particularly, relocate to urban environments from rural communities in pursuit of employment and educational opportunities—the previously stable family unit, a potentially great advantage for establishing intergenerational studies in LMIC, will inevitably fracture making research contact with offspring problematic.

7.5.2 Collecting data across three generations

The issue of collection of high quality data over more than two generations is equally difficult in practice. For example, index persons in the original Pelotas birth cohort were born in 1982 and are now aged 25; the second cohort, born in 1993, are now aged 14 years. Whereas the recruitment of parents in these cohorts and the collection of sweeps of clinic data for the offspring has been relatively straightforward since they were all born over a short period of time, the collection of data on the next generation (the offspring of the offspring), whilst potentially an exceptional research resource, is far more complex. In the 1993 cohort, births will occur in small numbers over the coming 4–5 years, the majority over the following 10–15 years and then a reduced number as the current generation age into their 40s. Few funding bodies are likely to provide sustained support over such a protracted period. One solution is to have good routine clinical data sources that can be linked to the study participants and made accessible to researchers. While this approach is being used in the Pelotas cohorts, it relies on near-complete birth registration systems which may not be available in other LMIC. Even then, this would provide information on infants born to mothers but, particularly in their teenage years, it might be unreliable for identifying all offspring of fathers.

In addition to these practical difficulties, the collection of data from one generation to the next will reflect the particular prevailing research interests at that time that may be less relevant subsequently. A good example of this is the Aberdeen *Children of the 1950s* cohort study, which, highly unusually, has information on three generations of women with detailed perinatal and family background information on the index population (12,150 individuals born in Aberdeen, Scotland between 1950–56).[108, 109] In that study there are over 700 variables from the baseline databases that characterize family background, perinatal circumstances, schooling, and the child's cognition and behaviour whilst in school. These include information on the newspapers that the mother and father read, parental hobbies, religious and political affiliations, and their favourite television programmes, but astonishingly—at least to any researcher working in the early 21st century—there is no data on parental smoking pre or post birth of offspring. To researchers in the 1950s and 60s, smoking was not the major health hazard that we now recognize it to be; it was not until 1964 that the first position statement to this effect was released.[110] Likewise, the Pelotas 1982 cohort did not collect any information on exclusive (as opposed to any) breastfeeding, because in the early 1980s the importance of this behaviour had not yet been realized. One wonders what information we are failing to collect in the present generation that future researchers will rue.

Where data are available on multiple generations, care is required that the statistical analyses and interpretation are appropriate (see Chapters 2 and 10). This includes *a priori* specification of sub-group analyses to avoid the temptation to over-emphasize *post-hoc* sub-group analyses (e.g. association of exposure X in fathers with outcome Y in daughters only) when main effects are null; correct understanding of correlation structures across generations; and appropriate methods to deal with repeat measurements and missing data.[111]

7.5.3 Collecting data on siblings and twins

In general, similar issues to those discussed above pertain to the collection of data on siblings in LMIC (and elsewhere). In general, birth/life course cohort studies include siblings when the period of recruitment (of the pregnant mother or birth of the index child) extends over a time period that is sufficiently long enough to allow more that just the index child to be included in the cohort. However, even when this is the case, data are rarely available for every sibling in a family, and, where they do exist they are usually obtained from other family members, most commonly the mother. While there is evidence that use of proxy informants in this way can provide valid information (see Chapter 8), much of this knowledge base comes from high income countries and has largely examined the provision of information by spouses.

It is not inconceivable that methods could be established for the collection of data on siblings in LMIC. For example, the demographic surveillance systems that exist in selected countries in sub-Saharan Africa have increasingly been employed to formulate prospective cohort studies to examine, for example, the emerging HIV epidemic.[112] It should be equally possible to use these systems for family-based life course epidemiology. Utilising a similar approach for genuine twin studies (i.e., those that focus specifically on within and between twin comparisons rather than those that include twins in the context of more general family studies) would necessitate the establishment of twin registers that collect perinatal data on all multiple births and follow-up these individuals over time. This would be particularly problematic in several LMIC where many births occur outside of the hospital; although, as investigators on the Sri Lankan Twin Registry[72,73] have demonstrated, such problems are surmountable.

7.5.4 The concept of family in different countries

In general, the concept of 'family' is similar across most high income countries. However, there are also some important distinctions not only between these societies and LMIC but also between countries within the LMIC classification. For example, in China there is no single word for cousin; instead, several terms are used that distinguish the gender of the individual, whether they are from father's or mother's side of the family, whether they are the offspring of a sister of the father or sister of the mother, and so on. Furthermore, marked differences in household/family structure determined by social factors, such as, as described, the need for some family members to work away from home (either in a different area of their own country or abroad), and the impact of natural and man-made disasters and various disease epidemics (e.g., HIV/AIDS), will have important implications for how life course studies are conducted and their results interpreted. For example, in Chapter 3, the use of within and between sibling comparisons to control for fixed familial characteristics (such as socioeconomic position) is described, but this assumes that siblings are reared in a similar family environment which may not always be the case.

7.6 Conclusions and future directions

We have, we hope, provided some pertinent reasons to correct the evident dearth of existing family-based studies in LMIC, continued support for the few in existence, and the establishment of new ones. The clear need for a broader geographical representation may be addressed by a greater collaboration worldwide in the sharing of ideas, fieldwork experience, cross-country cohort comparisons, and data, in order to carry out the best science in the most efficient manner. This requires the involvement of a central overseeing body—such as the World Health Organization (WHO) which has previously produced reviews of life course chronic disease epidemiology[113]—that has respect of all countries and the capacity to develop strategic plans for 'global' life course epidemiology while addressing such issues as data-sharing. For rapid progress to be made, however, there must be minimal bureaucratic entanglements. An agency such as the WHO should also be mindful of the worrying potential of, and anecdotal evidence for, research 'neo-colonialization'. That is, the practice by some investigators of 'parachuting in' to collect data in LMIC in the absence of full collaboration with existing researchers. Research resources, in their broadest sense, have to be about building local research capacity in LMIC.

Acknowledgements

David Batty is a Wellcome Trust Fellow; part of this manuscript was written while he was a visiting fellow at Instituto Materno Infantil Prof. Fernando Figueira (IMIP), Pernambuco, Brazil. Debbie Lawlor is funded by a Department of Health (UK) Career Scientist Award. The views expressed in this publication are those of the authors and not necessarily those of any funding body.

The authors would welcome any additions to the audit of family-based studies from LMIC (Tables 7.1 and 7.2) if omissions have been made.

References

1 **Anon.** *Mortality statistics: cause, 1995.* The Stationery Office, London, 1997.
2 **Murray CJ, Lopez AD.** Mortality by cause for eight regions of the world: Global Burden of Disease Study. *Lancet* 1997; **349**: 1269–76.
3 **Murray CJL, Lopez AD.** *The global burden of disease.* WHO, Harvard School of Public Health, World Bank, Boston, MA, 1996.
4 **Anon.** *The World Health Report. Making a Difference.* World Health Organization, Geneva, 1999.
5 **Ebrahim S, Smeeth L.** Non-communicable diseases in low and middle-income countries: a priority or a distraction? *Int J Epidemiol* 2005; **34**: 961–6.
6 **Prince M, Patel V, Saxena S, Maj M, Maselko J, Phillips MR, et al.** No health without mental health. *Lancet* 2007; **370**: 859–77.
7 **Moussavi S, Chatterji S, Verdes E, Tandon A, Patel V, Ustun B.** Depression, chronic diseases, and decrements in health: results from the World Health Surveys. *Lancet* 2007; **370**: 851–8.
8 **Yusuf S, Reddy S, Ounpuu S, Anand S.** Global burden of cardiovascular diseases: part I: general considerations, the epidemiologic transition, risk factors, and impact of urbanization. *Circulation* 2001; **104**: 2746–53.
9 **Bradshaw D, Schneider M, Dorrington R, Bourne DE, Laubscher R.** South African cause-of-death profile in transition—1996 and future trends. *S Afr Med J* 2002; **92**: 618–23.
10 **Müller F.** Tabakmissbrauch und lungencarcinoma. *Z Krebsforsch* 1939; **49**: 57–85.
11 **Dawber TR, Meadors GF, Moore FE.** Epidemiological approaches to heart disease: the Framingham study. *Am J Public Health* 1951; **41**: 279–86.
12 **Doll R, Peto R, Boreham J, Sutherland I.** Mortality from cancer in relation to smoking: 50 years observations on British doctors. *Br J Cancer* 2005; **92**: 426–9.
13 **Doll R, Bradford Hill A.** Smoking and carcinoma of the lung; preliminary report. *BMJ* 1950; **2**: 739–48.
14 **Doll R, Bradford Hill A.** The mortality of doctors in relation to their smoking habits; a preliminary report. *BMJ* 1954; **1**: 1451–5.
15 **Doll R, Peto R, Boreham J, Sutherland I.** Mortality in relation to smoking: 50 years' observations on male British doctors. *BMJ* 2004; **328**: 1519–27.
16 **MacMahon S, Peto R, Cutler J, Collins R, Sorlie P, Neaton J, et al.** Blood pressure, stroke, and coronary heart disease. Part 1, Prolonged differences in blood pressure: prospective observational studies corrected for the regression dilution bias. *Lancet* 1990; **335**: 765–74.
17 **Stamler J, Wentworth D, Neaton JD.** Is relationship between serum cholesterol and risk of premature death from coronary heart disease continuous and graded? Findings in 356,222 primary screenees of the Multiple Risk Factor Intervention Trial (MRFIT). *JAMA* 1986; **256**: 2823–8.
18 **Marmot MG, Shipley MJ, Rose G.** Inequalities in death—specific explanations of a general pattern? *Lancet* 1984; **1**: 1003–6.
19 **Yarnell JW.** The PRIME study: classical risk factors do not explain the severalfold differences in risk of coronary heart disease between France and Northern Ireland. Prospective Epidemiological Study of Myocardial Infarction. *QJM* 1998; **91**: 667–76.
20 **Batty GD, Der G, MacIntyre S, Deary IJ.** Does IQ explain socioeconomic inequalities in health? Evidence from a population based cohort study in the west of Scotland. *BMJ* 2006; **332**: 580–4.
21 **Beaglehole R, Magnus P.** The search for new risk factors for coronary heart disease: occupational therapy for epidemiologists? *Int J Epidemiol* 2002; **31**: 1117–22.
22 **Magnus P, Beaglehole R.** The real contribution of the major risk factors to the coronary epidemics: time to end the 'only-50%' myth. *Arch Intern Med* 2001; **161**: 2657–60.

23 Kuh D, Ben Shlomo Y. *A lifecourse approach to chronic disease epidemiology*. Oxford Medical Publications, Oxford, 2004.

24 Enos WF, Holmes RH, Beyer J. Coronary disease among United States soldiers killed in action in Korea; preliminary report. *JAMA* 1953; **152**: 1090–3.

25 Strong JP, Malcom GT, McMahan CA, Tracy RE, Newman WP, III, Herderick EE, *et al*. Prevalence and extent of atherosclerosis in adolescents and young adults: implications for prevention from the Pathobiological Determinants of Atherosclerosis in Youth Study. *JAMA* 1999; **281**: 727–35.

26 Kelder SH, Osganian SK, Feldman HA, Webber LS, Parcel GS, Leupker RV, *et al*. Tracking of physical and physiological risk variables among ethnic subgroups from third to eighth grade: the Child and Adolescent Trial for Cardiovascular Health cohort study. *Prev Med* 2002; **34**: 324–33.

27 Andersen LB. Tracking of risk factors for coronary heart disease from adolescence to young adulthood with special emphasis on physical activity and fitness. *Dan Med Bull* 1996; **43**: 407–18.

28 Webber LS, Srinivasan SR, Wattigney WA, Berenson GS. Tracking of serum lipids and lipoproteins from childhood to adulthood. The Bogalusa Heart Study. *Am J Epidemiol* 1991; **133**: 884–99.

29 Power C, Lake JK, Cole TJ. Body mass index and height from childhood to adulthood in the 1958 British born cohort. *Am J Clin Nutr* 1997; **66**: 1094–1101.

30 Ebrahim S, Davey Smith G. Systematic review of randomised controlled trials of multiple risk factor intervention for preventing coronary heart disease. *BMJ* 1997; **314**: 1666–74.

31 McCarron P, Davey Smith G. Physiological measurements in chidlren and young people, and risk of coronary heart disease in adults. In Dr Alison Gates (ed) *A lifecourse approach to coronary heart disease prevention scientific and policy review*, pp. 49–78. TSO (The Stationery Office), London, 2003.

32 Last J. *A Dictionary of Epidemiology*. Oxford University Press, Oxford, 1995.

33 Lamont D, Parker L, White M. Risk of cardiovascular disease measured by carotid intima-media thickness at age 49–51: lifecourse study. *BMJ* 2000; **320**: 273–8.

34 Brown GW, Craig TK, Harris TO, Handley RV, Harvey AL. Development of a retrospective interview measure of parental maltreatment using the Childhood Experience of Care and Abuse (CECA) instrument—A life-course study of adult chronic depression—1. *J Affect Disord* 2007; **103**: 205–15.

35 Melchior M, Moffitt TE, Milne BJ, Poulton R, Caspi A. Why do children from socioeconomically disadvantaged families suffer from poor health when they reach adulthood? A life-course study. *Am J Epidemiol* 2007; **166**: 966–74.

36 Danese A, Pariante CM, Caspi A, Taylor A, Poulton R. Childhood maltreatment predicts adult inflammation in a life-course study. *Proc Natl Acad Sci USA* 2007; **104**: 1319–24.

37 Golding J, Pembrey M, Jones R. ALSPAC—the Avon Longitudinal Study of Parents and Children I. Study methodology. ALSPAC Study Team. *Paediatr Perinat Epidemiol* 2001; **15**: 74–87.

38 Golding J. The Avon Longitudinal Study of Parents and Children (ALSPAC)—study design and collaborative opportunities. *Eur J Endocrinol* 2004; **151** Suppl 3: U119–U123.

39 Najman JM, Bor W, O'Callaghan M, Williams GM, Aird R, Shuttlewood G. Cohort Profile: The Mater-University of Queensland Study of Pregnancy (MUSP). *Int J Epidemiol* 2005; **34**: 992–7.

40 Wadsworth M, Kuh D, Richards M, Hardy R. Cohort Profile: The 1946 National Birth Cohort (MRC National Survey of Health and Development). *Int J Epidemiol* 2006; **35**: 49–54.

41 Power C, Elliott J. Cohort profile: 1958 British birth cohort (National Child Development Study). *Int J Epidemiol* 2006; **35**: 34–41.

42 Wilson I, Huttly S, Fenn B. A case study of sample design for longitudinal research: Young Lives. *International Journal of Social Research Methodology* 2007; **9**: 351–65.

43 Bhargava SK, Sachdev HS, Fall CH, Osmond C, Lakshmy R, Barker DJ, *et al*. Relation of serial changes in childhood body-mass index to impaired glucose tolerance in young adulthood. *N Engl J Med* 2004; **350**: 65–875.

44 Chuang CH, Chang PJ, Hsieh WS, Guo YL, Lin SH, Lin SJ, *et al*. The combined effect of employment status and transcultural marriage on breast feeding: a population-based survey in Taiwan. *Paediatr Perinat Epidemiol* 2007; **21**: 319–29.

45 Yach D, Cameron N, Padayachee N, Wagstaff L, Richter L, Fonn S. Birth to ten: child health in South Africa in the 1990s. Rationale and methods of a birth cohort study. *Paediatr Perinat Epidemiol* 1991; **5**: 211–33.

46 Richter L, Norris S, Pettifor J, Yach D, Cameron N. Cohort Profile: Mandela's children: The 1990 birth to twenty study in South Africa. *Int J Epidemiol* 2007; **36**: 504–11.

47 Richter LM, Norris SA, De Wet T. Transition from Birth to Ten to Birth to Twenty: the South African cohort reaches 13 years of age. *Paediatr Perinat Epidemiol* 2004; **18**: 290–301.

48 Kramer MS, Chalmers B, Hodnett ED, Sevkovskaya Z, Dzikovich I, Shapiro S, et al. Promotion of breastfeeding intervention trial (PROBIT): a cluster-randomized trial in the Republic of Belarus. Design, follow-up, and data validation. *Adv Exp Med Biol* 2000; **478**: 327–45.

49 Kramer MS, Chalmers B, Hodnett ED, Sevkovskaya Z, Dzikovich I, Shapiro S, et al. Promotion of Breastfeeding Intervention Trial (PROBIT): a randomized trial in the Republic of Belarus. *JAMA* 2001; **285**: 413–20.

50 Bobak M, Marmot M. Alcohol and mortality in Russia: Is it different from elsewhere? *Ann Epidemiol* 1999; **9**: 335–8.

51 McKee M, Chenet L. Alcoholism and rising mortality in the Russian federation. *BMJ* 1995; **310**: 1668–9.

52 McKee M. Alcohol in Russia. *Alcohol Alcohol* 1999; **34**: 824–9.

53 McKee M, Shkolnikov V, Leon DA. Alcohol is implicated in the fluctuations in cardiovascular disease in Russia since the 1980s. *Ann Epidemiol* 2001; **11**: 1–6.

54 Kramer M, Matush L, Vanilovich I, Platt R, Bogdanovich N, Sevkovskaya Z, et al. for the Promotion of Breastfeeding Intervention Trial (PROBIT) Study Group. Effects of prolonged and exclusive breastfeeding on child height, weight, adiposity, and blood pressure at age 6.5 y: evidence from a large randomized trial. *Am J Clin Nutr* 2007; **86**: 1717–21.

55 Kramer MS, Guo T, Platt RW, Sevkovskaya Z, Dzikovich I, Collet JP, et al. Does previous infection protect against atopic eczema and recurrent wheeze in infancy? *Clin Exp Allergy* 2004; **34**: 753–6.

56 Leon AS, Connett J. Physical activity and 10.5 year mortality in the Multiple Risk Factor Intervention Trial (MRFIT). *Int J Epidemiol* 1991; **20**: 690–7.

57 Martorell R, Habicht JP, Rivera JA. History and design of the INCAP longitudinal study (1969-77) and its follow-up (1988-89). *J Nutr* 1995; **125**: 1027S–1041S.

58 Victora CG, Barros FC. Cohort profile: the 1982 Pelotas (Brazil) birth cohort study. *Int J Epidemiol* 2006; **35**: 237–42.

59 Barros FC, Victora CG, Barros AJ, Santos IS, Albernaz E, Matijasevich A, et al. The challenge of reducing neonatal mortality in middle-income countries: findings from three Brazilian birth cohorts in 1982, 1993, and 2004. *Lancet* 2005; **365**: 847–54.

60 Cardoso VC, Simoes VM, Barbieri MA, Silva AA, Bettiol H, Alves MT, et al. Profile of three Brazilian birth cohort studies in Ribeirao Preto, SP and Sao Luis, MA. *Braz J Med Biol Res* 2007; **40**: 1165–76.

61 Kuzawa CW, Adair LS. Lipid profiles in adolescent Filipinos: relation to birth weight and maternal energy status during pregnancy. *Am J Clin Nutr* 2003; **77**: 960–6.

62 Adair LS, Cole TJ. Rapid child growth raises blood pressure in adolescent boys who were thin at birth. *Hypertension* 2003; **41**: 451–6.

63 Harpham T, Huttly S, De Silva MJ, Abramsky T. Maternal mental health and child nutritional status in four developing countries. *J Epidemiol Community Health* 2005; **59**: 1060–4.

64 De Silva MJ, Huttly SR, Harpham T, Kenward MG. Social capital and mental health: a comparative analysis of four low income countries. *Soc Sci Med* 2004; **64**: 5–20.

65 Patel V, Rodrigues M, DeSouza N. Gender, poverty, and postnatal depression: a study of mothers in Goa, India. *Am J Psychiatry* 2002; **159**: 43–7.

66 Chandran M, Tharyan P, Muliyil J, Abraham S. Post-partum depression in a cohort of women from a rural area of Tamil Nadu, India. Incidence and risk factors. *Br J Psychiatry* 2002; **181**: 499–504.

67 Rahman A, Iqbal Z, Harrington R. Life events, social support and depression in childbirth: perspectives from a rural community in the developing world. *Psychol Med* 2003; **33**: 1161–7.

68 Majumder AK. Child survival and its effect on mortality of siblings in Bangladesh. *J Biosoc Sci* 1990; **22**: 333–47.

69 Grim CE, Wilson TW, Nicholson GD, Hassell TA, Fraser HS, Grim CM, *et al.* Blood pressure in blacks. Twin studies in Barbados. *Hypertension* 1990; **15**: 803–9.

70 Rao RM, Reddy GP, Grim CE. Relative role of genes and environment on BP: twin studies in Madras, India. *J Hum Hypertens* 1993; **7**: 451–5.

71 Jain S, Jain MS, Padma MV, Puri A, Sen P, Maheshwari MC. Epilepsies among twins born in families of Indian probands with epilepsy. *Seizure* 1998; **7**: 139–43.

72 Sumathipala A, Fernando DJ, Siribaddana SH, Abeysingha MR, Jayasekare RW, Dissanayake VH, *et al.* Establishing a twin register in Sri Lanka. *Twin Res* 2000; **3**: 202–4.

73 Sumathipala A, Siribaddana S, De Silva N, Fernando D, Abeysingha N, Dayaratne R, *et al.* Sri Lankan Twin Registry. *Twin Res* 2002; **5**: 424–6.

74 Anon. Sri Lankan Twin Registry. http://www infolanka com/org/twin-registry/index htm (accessed 27 September 2007).

75 Gupta PC, Ray CS. Smokeless tobacco and health in India and South Asia. *Respirology* 2003; **8**: 419–31.

76 Vineis P, Alavanja M, Buffler P, Fontham E, Franceschi S, Gao YT, *et al.* Tobacco and cancer: recent epidemiological evidence. *J Natl Cancer Inst* 2004; **96**: 99–106.

77 McKeigue PM, Shah B, Marmot MG. Relation of central obesity and insulin resistance with high diabetes prevalence and cardiovascular risk in South Asians. *Lancet* 1991; **337**: 382–6.

78 Ramachandran A, Snehalatha C, Dharmaraj D, Viswanathan M. Prevalence of glucose intolerance in Asian Indians. Urban-rural difference and significance of upper body adiposity. *Diabetes Care* 1992; **15**: 1348–55.

79 Yajnik CS, Yudkin JS. The Y-Y paradox. *Lancet* 2004; **363**: 163.

80 Yajnik CS, Lubree HG, Rege SS, Naik SS, Deshpande JA, Deshpande SS, *et al.* Adiposity and hyperinsulinemia in Indians are present at birth. *J Clin Endocrinol Metab* 2002; **87**: 5575–80.

81 Hayes RB, Yin SN, Dosemeci M, Li GL, Wacholder S, Chow WH, *et al.* Mortality among benzene-exposed workers in China. *Environ Health Perspect* 1996; **104** Suppl 6: 1349–52.

82 Stewart BW, Coates AS. Cancer prevention: a global perspective. *J Clin Oncol* 2005; **23**: 392–403.

83 Rantakallio P. The longitudinal study of the northern Finland birth cohort of 1966. *Paediatr Perinat Epidemiol* 1998; **2**: 59–88.

84 Batty GD, Der G, Deary IJ. Effect of maternal smoking during pregnancy on offspring's cognitive ability: empirical evidence for complete confounding in the US national longitudinal survey of youth. *Pediatrics* 2006; **118**: 943–50.

85 Victora CG, Barros F, Lima RC, Horta BL, Wells J. Anthropometry and body composition of 18 year old men according to duration of breast feeding: birth cohort study from Brazil. *BMJ* 2003; **327**: 901–4.

86 Araujo CL, Victora CG, Hallal PC, Gigante DP. Breastfeeding and overweight in childhood: evidence from the Pelotas 1993 birth cohort study. *Int J Obes (Lond)* 2006; **30**: 500–6.

87 Toschke AM, Martin RM, von Kries R, Wells J, Smith GD, Ness AR. Infant feeding method and obesity: body mass index and dual-energy X-ray absorptiometry measurements at 9-10 y of age from the Avon Longitudinal Study of Parents and Children (ALSPAC). *Am J Clin Nutr* 2007; **85**: 1578–85.

88 Syddall HE, Aihie SA, Dennison EM, Martin HJ, Barker DJ, Cooper C. Cohort profile: the Hertfordshire cohort study. *Int J Epidemiol* 2005; **34**: 1234–42.

89 Eriksson JG. Epidemiology, genes and the environment: lessons learned from the Helsinki Birth Cohort Study. *J Intern Med* 2007; **261**: 418–25.

90 Davey Smith G, Leary S, Ness S. Could dehydration in infancy lead to high blood pressure? *J Epidemiol Community Health* 2006; **60**: 142–3.

91 Batty GD, Davey Smith G, Fall CHD, Aihie Sayer A, Dennison E, Cooper C, *et al.* Association of diarrhoea in childhood with blood pressure and coronary heart disease in older age: analyses of two UK cohort studies. *Int J Epidemiol* 2007; **36**: 1349–55.

92 Batty GD, Davey Smith G, Cooper C, Gale C. Diarrhoea in childhood and cause-specific mortality in older age: analyses of 5,642 deaths in 33,261 individuals from the Hertfordshire studies. *Eur J Cardiovasc Prev Rehabil* 2008; **15**: 494–6.

93 Marmot MG, Adelstein AM, Robinson N, Rose GA. Changing social-class distribution of heart disease. *BMJ* 1978; **2**: 1109–12.

94 Lawlor DA, Harro M, Wedderkopp N, Andersen LB, Sardinha LB, Riddoch CJ, *et al.* Association of socioeconomic position with insulin resistance among children from Denmark, Estonia, and Portugal: cross sectional study. *BMJ* 2005; **331**: 183–7.

95 Wang Y, Monteiro C, Popkin BM. Trends of obesity and underweight in older children and adolescents in the United States, Brazil, China, and Russia. *Am J Clin Nutr* 2002; **75**: 971–7.

96 Anon. *The Tobacco Atlas*. World Health Organization, Geneva, 2002.

97 Liu BQ, Peto R, Chen ZM, Boreham J, Wu YP, Li JY, *et al.* Emerging tobacco hazards in China: 1. Retrospective proportional mortality study of one million deaths. *BMJ* 1998; **317**: 1411–22.

98 Lawlor D, Song Y, Sung J, Ebrahim S, Davey Smith G. The association of smoking and cardiovascular disease in a population with low cholesterol levels: a study of 648,346 men from the Korean National Health System prospective cohort study. *Stroke* 2008; **39**: 760–7.

99 Chen Z, Peto R. Stopping smoking works (University of Oxford Annual Review). Available at: http://www.ox.ac.uk/publicrelations/pubs/annualreview/ar98/amoking.shtml (Accessed 3rd September 2006), 1998.

100 Lawlor DA, Hubinette A, Tynelius P, Leon DA, Davey Smith G, Rasmussen F. Associations of gestational age and intrauterine growth with systolic blood pressure in a family-based study of 386,485 men in 331,089 families. *Circulation* 2007; **115**: 562–8.

101 Lawlor DA, Sterne JA, Tynelius P, Davey Smith G, Rasmussen F. Association of childhood socioeconomic position with cause-specific mortality in a prospective record linkage study of 1,839,384 individuals. *Am J Epidemiol* 2006; **164**: 907–15.

102 Batty GD, Modig Wennerstad K, Davey Smith G, Gunnell D, Deary IJ, Tynelius P, *et al.* IQ in early adulthood and later cancer risk: cohort study of one million Swedish men. *Ann Oncol* 2007; **18**: 21–8.

103 Batty GD, Deary IJ, Tengstrom A, Rasmussen F (in press). Early adult IQ and later mortality due to homicide in one million Swedish conscripts. *Brit J Psychiatry*.

104 Batty GD, Mortensen EL, Osler M. Childhood IQ in relation to later psychiatric disorder: Evidence from a Danish birth cohort study. *Br J Psychiatry* 2005; **187**: 180–1.

105 Batty GD, Mortensen EL, Nybo Andersen AM, Osler M. Childhood intelligence in relation to adult coronary heart disease and stroke risk: evidence from a Danish birth cohort study. *Paediatr Perinat Epidemiol* 2005; **19**: 452–9.

106 Hardy R, Lawlor DA, Black S, Wadsworth ME, Kuh D. Number of children and coronary heart disease risk factors in men and women from a British birth cohort. *BJOG* 2007; **114**: 721–30.

107 Victora CG, Hallal PC, Araujo CL, Menezes AM, Wells JC, Barros FC. Cohort Profile: The 1993 Pelotas (Brazil) Birth Cohort Study. *Int J Epidemiol* 2008; **37**: 704–9.

108 Leon D, Lawlor DA, Clark H, Macintyre S. Cohort Profile: The Aberdeen Children of the 1950s Study. *Int J Epidemiol* 2006; **35**: 549–52.

109 Batty GD, Morton SMB, Campbell D, Clark H, Davey Smith G, Hall M, *et al.* The Aberdeen Children of the 1950s cohort study: background, methods and follow-up information on a new resource for the study of life course and intergenerational influences on health. *Paediatr Perinat Epidemiol* 2004; **18**: 221–39.

110 US Public HS. *Smoking and Health.* Report of the advisory committee to the surgeon general of the public health service. United States department of Health, Education and Welfare, Centre for Disease Control, Washington, DC, 1964.

111 Pickles A, Maughan B, Wadsworth M. *Epidemiological Methods in Life Course Research.* Oxford University Press, Oxford, 2007.

112 Welz T, Hosegood V, Jaffar S, Batzing-Feigenbaum J, Herbst K, Newell ML. Continued very high prevalence of HIV infection in rural KwaZulu-Natal, South Africa: a population-based longitudinal study. *AIDS* 2007; **21**: 1467–72.

113 World Health Organization. *Life course perspectives on coronary heart disease, stroke and diabetes.* World Health Organization, Geneva, 2001.

114 Batty GD, Alves JG, Correia J, Lawlor DA. Examining life-course influences on chronic disease: the importance of birth cohort studies from low- and middle-income countries. *Braz J Med Biol Res* 2007; **40**: 1277–86.

115 Wadsworth ME, Butterworth SL, Hardy RJ, Kuh DJ, Richards M, Langenberg C, et al. The life course prospective design: an example of benefits and problems associated with study longevity. *Soc Sci Med* 2003; **57**: 2193–2205.

116 Wadsworth ME, Mann SL, Rodgers B, Kuh DJ, Hilder WS, Yusuf EJ. Loss and representativeness in a 43 year follow up of a national birth cohort. *J Epidemiol Community Health* 1992; **46**: 300–4.

117 Elliott J, Shepherd P. Cohort profile: 1970 British Birth Cohort (BCS70). *Int J Epidemiol* 2006; **35**: 836–43.

118 Smith K, Joshi H. The Millennium Cohort Study. *Popul Trends*, pp. 30-34, 2002.

119 Olsen J, Melbye M, Olsen SF, Sorensen TI, Aaby P, Andersen AM, et al. The Danish National Birth Cohort—its background, structure and aim. *Scand J Public Health* 2001; **29**: 300–7.

120 Martin LT, Fitzmaurice GM, Kindlon DJ, Buka SL. Cognitive performance in childhood and early adult illness: a prospective cohort study. *J Epidemiol Community Health* 2004; **58**: 674–9.

121 Silva PA. The Dunedin Multidisciplinary Health and Development Study: a 15 year longitudinal study. *Paediatr Perinat Epidemiol* 1990; **4**: 76–107.

122 Martorell R, Yarbrough C, Lechtig A, Delgado H, Klein RE. Genetic-environmental interactions in physical growth. *Acta Paediatr Scand* 1977; **66**: 579–84.

123 Horta BL, Victora CG, Menezes AM, Halpern R, Barros FC. Low birthweight, preterm births and intrauterine growth retardation in relation to maternal smoking. *Paediatr Perinat Epidemiol* 1997; **11**: 140–51.

124 Hallal PC, Wells JC, Reichert FF, Anselmi L, Victora CG. Early determinants of physical activity in adolescence: prospective birth cohort study. *BMJ* 2006; **332**: 1002–7.

125 Tome FS, Cardoso VC, Barbieri MA, Silva AA, Simoes VM, Garcia CA, et al. Are birth weight and maternal smoking during pregnancy associated with malnutrition and excess weight among school age children? *Braz J Med Biol Res* 2007; **40**: 1221–30.

126 Adair LS, Guilkey DK. Age-specific determinants of stunting in Filipino children. *J Nutr* 1997; **127**: 314–20.

Chapter 8

Using available family members as proxies to provide information on other family members who are difficult to reach

Susannah Tomkins

Abstract

In life course epidemiology studies, the use of proxy (secondary) respondents may be an integral part of the study design or a consequence of not being able to reach or obtain information from the index subject. Common situations requiring the use of proxies in life course family-based studies include a mother reporting on behalf on the father (where he is not formally recruited into the study), either parent reporting about their child (when they are too young to answer questions), or one sibling or twin reporting for the other (in situations where one or more sibling/twin is unavailable or not recruited to the study). Whilst the use of proxies allows inclusion of subjects who might otherwise be excluded from research, issues concerning the validity and reliability of data obtained must be carefully addressed. Additionally, specific issues associated with life course studies must be considered, such as the use of the index versus the proxy when the index is a child, how to treat multiple reports about one index, using the same proxy for multiple indexes, and the choice of respondent across the life course. Based on the available evidence, the main factors that increase validity and reliability of proxy responses are broad categorisation of, and focus on, directly observable characteristics and behaviours; questions requiring a binary response; recent characteristics and behaviours; face to face interviews; spouse/partner selected as proxy. Certain issues remain unaddressed by the available literature, including subject areas such as diet, the choice of proxy beyond spouse/partner, validation of responses when the index is unavailable and the effect of index characteristics on proxy responses. Finally, practical tips are presented in this chapter from a case study that successfully employed proxy respondents.

8.1 **Introduction**

An ideal family-based study design for life course epidemiology would obtain information about family members by asking them about their own characteristics via self-completed questionnaires or interviews. However, in reality there are many situations in which this might not be achievable.

Table 8.1 Life course scenarios requiring the use of proxy respondents

Family study type	Common proxy	Reasons for employing a proxy
Inter-generational studies	Mother reporting on behalf of the father (especially during pregnancy)	Father was not present at antenatal clinic or not contactable for some other reason
	Mother reporting on behalf of her parents (grand-parents of the index child)	Parents have died, are not well, or are not contactable for some other reason
	"Child" reporting on behalf of her parents	In traditional birth cohorts that enrolled the infant at birth, but did not enrol or collect data on their parents, information on the parents may subsequently be obtained from the index once they reach an age when they can act as proxy for their parents
Sibling/twin studies	One sibling reporting for the other	Temporary or permanent dropout
		Only one sibling originally recruited
Adoption	Parents report for the adopted child	Index (child) considered too young to respond themselves
Birth cohort	Parents reporting for the index child	Collection of data at birth requires the parents or medical professionals to act as proxy for the infant

For example, the subject of research (the 'index') may be unable to provide their own information due to illness, or they may be too young or not be traceable. In family-based life course studies it is possible that some family members relevant to a particular research question were never recruited to the study. One possible approach in such scenarios is to use a 'proxy informant' (secondary informant) to provide the information. For example a wife could provide information about her partner or one sibling could provide information about another sibling.

The use of proxies is particularly common in life course studies due to the inherent nature of their design. For example, a mother may complete a questionnaire about her infant's behaviour or characteristics; one twin may be recruited and may provide information about themselves and their other twin. The most common situations are summarized in Table 8.1.

The use of proxies in life course epidemiology studies addresses the problem of obtaining information from subjects who would otherwise be excluded from research. However, several issues which can affect the quality of the obtained data must be considered. For example: can a proxy ever be used to provide valid* data? What are the consequences of using different proxies during the course of a cohort? At what age should information from a child be obtained from the child themselves if a proxy has been previously used? The use of proxies necessitates careful consideration regarding these and other issues introduced here.

A review of the available literature regarding the use of proxies is presented in this chapter. This review is about proxies in general, but the findings are applicable and valuable to any studies, including life course studies, that use proxies.

---

* Valid data is data that is close to the 'truth' or gold standard. In this context, the gold standard is the index response (rather than the unknown actual behaviour of the index). So, a valid proxy response is one that most closely resembles the response that would have been obtained if the index had themselves responded. This is discussed further later in this chapter.

8.2 What are the common situations in life course epidemiology where proxy informants are likely to be required?

There are a number of situations in epidemiology in general, and family-based life course studies specifically, where one might consider using proxy informants. Three main sets of circumstances can result in the use of proxies being necessary or desirable: firstly, when the index is considered unable to respond adequately or at all; secondly, when the index cannot be found; thirdly, the use of proxies may be a specific design feature. These circumstances are detailed in Box 8.1.

8.3 How can we determine whether information from proxy informants is good enough? Validity and reliability.

In general, we can evaluate questionnaire responses in terms of validity and reliability. These terms describe the responses given by respondents *relative* to a gold standard; it is important to understand that the choice of gold standard may vary depending on the research context. In assessing the quality of information obtained from *index* respondents, one must first assume that there is a 'true' answer to every question posed (the gold standard) which may be known or, more likely, unknown. In this context, validity describes the extent to which index responses are close to the 'truth'. Responses which are close to the truth are valid. Reliability conventionally describes the extent to which repeated measurements (or responses) resemble one another, so in this context, multiple responses (provided by multiple respondents) to the same question which are similar to one another are described as reliable.

However, this chapter considers a different situation, namely the quality of responses obtained from *proxy* respondents. Proxy respondents may be unable or unwilling in specific, exaggerated (or diminished) ways to provide a valid or reliable response, compared with the index respondent. The use of proxies adds a new dimension to the evaluation of response quality, and requires consideration of the choice of gold standard. Proxy-provided data can be compared with index-provided data, thereby using the index as the standard (and disregarding the unknown 'truth'). Alternatively, proxy-provided data can be compared with that obtained from an objective, external source, e.g. cotinine levels, biomarkers of liver enzymes, anthropometric measurements rather than what the index would have responded regarding smoking, alcohol consumption, height/weight (respectively) to the relevant questions. The use of objective external data sources is discussed in the literature and is acknowledged as a reasonable method to validate proxy responses under certain conditions.[35] This latter situation is illustrated by Figure 8.1.

However, following consideration of the common situations that result in the use of proxies (**Box 8.1**), it becomes obvious that irrespective of the desirability of using such external data sources as the gold standard against which to compare proxy responses, in many situations this will not be possible. Such data may not exist or may not be accessible. Therefore, whilst recognizing that indexes themselves may be fallible sources of data, and that in some situations the proxy might actually be the better data source, this chapter is concerned with the validity and reliability of proxy responses to questions about the index in comparison to how the index themselves would answer the same questions. The use of the index as the standard is perhaps the most desirable in situations where the proxy is providing information for a proportion of the index participants, but for the majority the index themselves are providing information.

Thus, the terms validity and reliability have specific meanings when applied to the evaluation of proxy responses. Proxy responses are valid when they are similar to the relevant index responses (e.g. the proxy from each index-proxy pair reports the same number of cigarettes smoked per day as the index), and proxy responses are reliable when proxy responses over-/under-estimate by a consistent amount compared with the index (e.g. proxies consistently report five cigarettes per

Box 8.1

Three main sets of circumstances which result in the use of proxies being necessary or desirable are outlined below.

- **The index is considered unable to respond adequately or at all**—where the participant of epidemiological research is unconscious, is unable to understand or respond to questions. This can be due to dementia,[1] for example, many studies of Alzheimer's disease rely on proxy informants,[2–14] as indexes are considered unable to respond to questions validly or reliably. Other circumstances where proxies are used include studies of some conditions among the elderly[15–21] or children[22–24] where, because of age or cognitive ability, the index may be unable to provide valid or reliable responses.

- **The index cannot be found or contacted**—where contact details are not available for the index. For example, the index may be lost to follow-up but a proxy may be available and willing to provide information about the index (with ethical approval). This could also include index participants who have previously provided information about themselves but have died since the last follow-up. Indeed information on cause of death in cohort studies could be considered information from a proxy (the Doctor) who contributed to the information on a death certificate.

- **Use of proxies as a study design feature**—In the two other broad sets of circumstances described above the idea was to try and obtain information from the index but at some stage during the study this became impossible. There are also situations in which proxies are deliberately used in the study design because of cost implications of trying to collect information on all (index) family members (in family-based studies) or because it is anticipated at the start of the study that index participants will not be available for a number of reasons. The use of one family member to collect information on other family members is not unusual in family-based studies; this is often anticipated at the initial design phase of the study. For example, in the Avon Longitudinal Study of Parents and Children,[25] questionnaires were sent to partners via the mother, but mothers were also asked to provide information about their partners (and visa versa) as a validity check and also to maximize data on both parents.

In the Mater University Study of Pregnancy,[26] mothers answered questions about their partner's characteristics because resources were not available to contact them directly. In some case-control studies cases could include those who have already died if the design allows proxies to provide exposure information. For example, in the Izhevsk Family Study,[27] a case-control study of determinants of mortality among working-age men, proxies were used to obtain information about the behaviours and characteristics of both dead cases and live controls. In studies that use routine data, proxies are often used for both outcome and exposure, with this being a feature of the study design. For example, in the use of routine data sources to examine socioeconomic differentials in cause-specific mortality, where the occupation of the person who has died is obtained from the death register, despite debates regarding its validity.[28–31] This is often provided by the next of kin, so use of proxies is incorporated into the study design.[30–34]

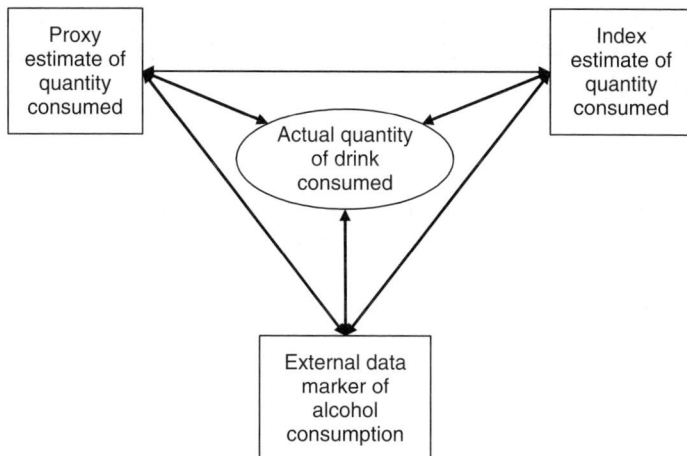

Fig. 8.1 Comparing proxy reports, index reports and external data—the example of alcohol.

day more than their index). It should be noted that validity and reliability are independent attributes. Proxy responses may therefore be reliable and simultaneously invalid with respect to the the index (or *vice versa*). These terms may also be considered in terms of misclassification of proxy relative to index responses: validity arises when there is no or little misclassification; reliability arises when there is no or differential misclassification, and non-differential misclassification results in neither valid nor reliable proxy responses.

8.3.1 Validation of proxy responses

Once we acknowledge that in most situations we are interested in trying to validate proxy responses against the index's own response, validation is problematic. As Table 8.1 and Box 8.1 illustrate proxies are usually used when it is impossible or difficult to obtain information from the index. Sometimes in life course epidemiology the proxy response is the desired response and validation is not required. For example, questioning of mothers about the characteristics of their newborn babies. Where this is not the case, it may be possible to validate proxy responses on a sub-group where information is available from the index. However, one needs to be careful that the sub-group with information from indexes as well as proxies are not importantly different from other study participants for whom it is impossible to obtain index information. In situations where internal validation of proxy responses is not possible, an alternative is to benefit from the literature on validation. Much has been researched and written about how to collect information from proxies in order to maximize the validity of obtained data. There are also analytic methods, such as incorporating weighting to adjust estimates, but the values used would be study specific. It is usually better to understand that the estimates obtained may be biased, and if so in which direction, when interpreting results, by considering the available literature on validity of data from proxies.

8.4 The current evidence base for the validity and reliability of proxy informants in epidemiological studies

The information on the evidence base for determining the validity and reliability of using proxy informants that is presented in this chapter is largely taken from a detailed systematic review that looked at this issue in relation to observational epidemiological studies in general, not specifically family-based life course epidemiological studies.[36] However, the conclusions drawn from this review, which covers all forms of observational epidemiological study, will be relevant to family-based epidemiological studies.

The majority of the papers identified in the review were based on cross-sectional surveys, with the remainder being case-control studies and one cohort study. Studies varied in size from 81 to 10,011 index-proxy pairs, with larger studies tending to use telephone or self-administered questionnaires, and smaller studies using face to face interviews as the mode of data collection. Study participants varied widely, including people with brain injury, Alzheimer's disease or dementia, men and women aged over 65 years, cancer patients and patients recovering from injuries, as well as some randomly selected population based samples. The choice of proxy also varied between studies, with some only considering specific proxy types (e.g. spouse, next of kin), some using index-nominated proxies or caregivers, and others using whoever was available. In family-based studies, the choice of proxy may also vary with the stage of life course.

The review inclusion criteria were such that only studies using Cohen's kappa coefficient or the intraclass correlation coefficient (ICC) were considered, however it was noted that only one third of the eligible studies calculated precision estimates for these parameters.[36] Where kappa values were available, degree of agreement was classified in accordance with the scheme developed by Landis and Koch:[37] <0, poor; 0.00–0.20, slight; 0.21–0.40, fair; 0.41-0.60, moderate; 0.61–0.80, substantial; >0.8, almost perfect. Some studies detailed procedures taken to avoid data contamination, which is potentially caused when index and proxy respondents have the opportunity to communicate with one another and possibly discuss their responses between interviews which may then influence responses given by the second respondent. However, many did not provide this level of detail.

Broadly speaking, four main types of characteristic have been studied: (i) health related behaviours; (ii) physical health characteristics; (iii) mental health and well-being characteristics and (iv) socioeconomic or demographic characteristics. As discussed above, responses are evaluated relative to the index's own answer to the same questions. In general proxy informants had modest levels of agreement with the index informant. However, a number of characteristics were associated with stronger levels of agreements in all four areas. Box 8.2 lists the key factors that

Box 8.2

The main factors that increase validity and reliability of proxy responses, based on the available evidence are:

- Broad categorization of characteristics and behaviours rather than more detailed categorisation (e.g. never, past, current smoking versus number of cigarettes per day or information that would enable pack years smoked to be calculated)
- Directly observable characteristics and behaviours (e.g. physical signs, behaviours occurring in the presence of the proxy)
- Questions requiring a binary yes/no answer
- Recent rather than past characteristics and behaviours
- Face to face interviews, rather than self-completed or telephone interviews
- Spouses in preference to other available proxies.

have been shown (in the available literature) to increase validity and/or reliability when using proxy informants to answer questions about the index study participant. A summary of the findings in the four main areas identified in the review is presented below.

8.4.1 Summary of findings

8.4.1.1 Studies of the validity and reliability of proxy informants reporting on alcohol, tobacco and physical activity

Studies that fulfilled the review criteria and were related to health behaviours included evaluation of validity and/or reliability of proxies for alcohol, tobacco, and physical activity behaviours of index study participants, but not of other behaviours. The key findings from studies of proxy reporting on these behaviours are summarized in Table 8.2.

These three health-related behaviours, the use of alcohol, tobacco and physical activity, may perform quite differently to one another with respect to the validity of proxy-reported data. For example, the phenomenon of under-reporting, denial, in self-reported responses on alcohol consumption and alcohol problems in particular is well-documented, although non-differential misclassification and over-reporting[38, 39] are also possible. It is important to acknowledge that over-reporting by indexes relative to proxies does not necessarily indicate that it is the proxy who is under-reporting—it may be that the index is over-reporting.[38, 40, 41] Conversely, in most societies smoking is not generally regarded as a taboo behaviour, especially among adult males, so reporting of tobacco use is likely to be free of some of the biases we would anticipate encountering with respect to alcohol reporting.[35, 38–40, 42–45] This is concordant with the consensus in the literature[46–59] as illustrated in Table 8.2.

The literature on proxy-reported alcohol consumption is wide-ranging and findings by different investigators are largely complimentary.[3, 55, 56, 60, 61] Broad indicators of alcohol consumption (average frequency, average number of drinks per occasion) show almost perfect index-proxy agreement when classified into ordinal categories,[3, 55, 60] and alcohol consumption status (yes/no) shows substantial agreement.[56] Composite measures of daily alcohol consumption (grams) show only moderate agreement[55] with considerable variability between pairs at the individual level.[60] Reliability may vary according to alcohol type: there is a suggestion it is highest for wine but only moderate for beer and hard liquor, although this could reflect differences in drinks consumed inside and outside the home, and thus whether they are directly observable by the proxy.[55] There is a suggestion that agreement for binge-and heavy drinking is moderate/good.[55]

There was a consensus in the literature regarding index-proxy agreement on cigarette use,[3, 54–56, 61, 62] whereby agreement depends on the required level of detail: there is 'good' to 'excellent' agreement about general cigarette-use (current/non/ex-smoker),[54–56] but 'poor' agreement for more detailed information, such as brand smoked and number of years of smoking. There is no clear consensus when examining agreement on amount. Some authors suggest that detail beyond that required to calculate pack-years is hard to obtain,[55] whilst others found agreement for current amount to be almost perfect.[3, 56] This lack of consensus may be due to the wide range of data collection methods and study settings which addressed this subject area.

Only two studies were identified addressing physical activity:[55, 63] little information is available on physical activity as such data tend to be collected on healthy participants, a group that do not require proxy respondents. The available literature indicates that broad indicators of physical activity level (PAL) show very good agreement, whilst detailed aspects show only moderate agreement.[55] Substantial agreement for both leisure and work-time activity was reported, using a three-point scale in one study.[63]

Table 8.2 Key findings related to index-proxy agreement on health related behaviours

Study details	Number of pairs	Outcome	Index	Proxy	Results	Comments
Demissee, S. et al., 2001.[3] Cross sectional survey. Self-administered questionnaire carried out by index and two proxies	81 indexes, 159 proxies	Medical history, medication use, health behaviour and cognitive ability	Non-demented Alzheimer sufferers	2 per index, both self-selected	'Almost perfect' agreement on overall smoking behaviour (kappa = 0.87) and pack-years (ICC = 0.90). 'Substantial' agreement on overall alcohol use (kappa = 0.74) and amount of alcohol consumed at three stages of life (ICC = 0.64). Substantial agreement found for alcohol consumption (number of drinks usually consumed) at ages 16–39 and 40–64 (kappa = 0.62 and 0.71), but only fair agreement for consumption at age 65 and older (kappa = 0.31).	Slight differences in ability of different family members to reliably report on smoking and alcohol consumption. Male proxies demonstrated almost perfect agreement, whilst female proxies demonstrated only substantial agreement for alcohol consumption. Sons and spouses as proxies provided almost perfect information on both smoking and alcohol consumption, whilst daughters provided only substantial agreement on these Authors recommend that sibs, particularly sisters, are the second ablest respondents. Also observed that spouses were able to provide information more often than other proxy informants
Graham, P. and Jackson, R. 1993.[60] Cross sectional survey. Indexes interviewed at single study centre. Proxies interviewed within	514	Alcohol consumption frequency	Myocardial infarction controls (n=456) aged 25–54 and small number of	Closest next-of-kin	No evidence that proxies systematically over- or under-reported drinking frequency (kappa = 0.79 among cases, 0.80 among controls) when examining 5 categories of alcohol	Agreement for amount of alcohol consumed lower among case-proxy pairs than control-proxy pairs (mean difference 2.25g/day, –0.77g/day). Age and sex of primary respondent and relation of proxy to the primary respondent

Study	N	Exposure	Controls	Proxy	Results	Comments
			cases (n=58) from wider case-control study (males and females)			consumption frequency.
						unrelated to the magnitude of index-proxy differences.
Graham, P. and Jackson, R. 2000.[63] Analysis of data from study that collected information on habitual physical activity. Indexes interviewed face to face using structured questionnaire, proxies interviewed 6–8 weeks later using identical questionnaire and same interviewers	456	Habitual physical activity	Controls in Auckland Heart Study, a community-based case control study of coronary heart disease	Next of kin, usually spouse	Agreement was substantial for physical activity in leisure time (kappa=0.66) and work time (kappa=0.62).	Simple 3 point scale used. Tendency observed for proxies to under-report relative to the index. Found no evidence to prefer spouse proxies when collecting information on work-time physical activity.
Hamilton, A.S. and Mack, T.M. 2000.[62] Cross-sectional study of female-female twin pairs discordant for breast cancer	671	Various, including smoking status, and number of cigarettes smoked per day	North American females who have a female twin	Index's twin	Smoking status (y/n) 'almost perfect' among monozygotic respondents (kappa=0.90–0.92) and dizygotic respondents (kappa=0.83–0.90). Agreement for number of cigarettes per day as a binary variable (<11, >11 per day) 'substantial' (kappa=0.60–0.88)	The errors were larger for number of cigarettes smoked per day but were generally nonsystematic, although dizygotic control respondents tended to underestimate the daily number of cigarettes smoked. Agreement higher between case self-report and control, than between control self-report and case, indicating the control is not as reliable a proxy respondent as the case.

Continued

Table 8.2 (continued) Key findings related to index-proxy agreement on health related behaviours

Study details	Number of pairs	Outcome	Index	Proxy	Results	Comments
Hatch, M.C. et al., 1991.[61] Cross-sectional survey of prenatal patients and their spouses/partners	136	Occupation, smoking and drinking	Women recruited from obstetric services and their spouse/ partner	N/a - the index-proxy agreement was examined in both directions	Agreement on smoking behaviour 'almost perfect' (Private patients: kappa = 0.84 for first trimester smoking, 0.95 for current smoking; public patients 0.84, 1.00 respectively). Agreement on drinking status also high (kappa = 0.57- 0.69).	Agreement was higher for smoking and drinking status, than for smoking and drinking amount, and agreement was higher for current than recent (first trimester) smoking and drinking amount. Women tended to be more reliable respondents than men. Age, level of education, marital status of the proxy did not influence validity or reliability. Found evidence of considerable misclassification with respect to alcohol use even though statistics sometimes indicated good index-proxy agreement.
Navarro, A.M. 1999.[54] Cross-sectional survey. Index and proxy completed detailed interview by telephone (n=10011)	10011	Smoking status, behaviour and attitudes, by ethnicity	Adults randomly selected as participants in California Tobacco Survey by random digit dialling	Household member aged 18 years or older	High agreement on smoking status (kappa = 0.76-0.91).	Agreement varied by ethnic group: kappa = 0.76 (Hispanics), 0.91 (Non-Hispanic whites), 0.91 (African Americans) and 0.82 (Asian Americans). Agreement hypothesised to be higher in smaller households than large households - a possible confounding factor - a proposal which could possibly be extended to a wide variety of exposures.
Nelson, L.M. et al., 1994.[55] Case control,	283 control/proxy pairs, 68 case/	Spontaneous subarachnoid haemorrhage	Live cases, healthy controls	Various, recruited in following	Alcohol consumption showed varying range of agreement depending on	Detail beyond that required to calculate pack-years thought to be hard to obtain.

	interviewer-administered interviews of all controls and their proxies and where possible of cases and their proxies.	proxy pairs	from a case-control study	order of preference: spouse, sibling, son/daughter, parent, other relative, friend.	measure. Lowest agreement was for grams per day (kappa = 0.52). Highest agreement was for amount of drinks per occasion (kappa – 0.83) and frequency of drinking (kappa = 0.82). Cigarette smoking history showed very high agreement (kappa = 0.79–0.93). Very good agreement for broad indicators of physical activity level (PAL). Only moderate agreement for detailed aspects of PAL (kappa = 0.57–0.67).	Observed that proxies tended to under-report the presence or level of exposure, meaning the specificity of proxy responses was better than the sensitivity for most exposures. Misclassification was found to be non-differential and accordingly, odds ratios computed using proxy data were similar in magnitude to those obtained using index data. The relationship of proxy to index was one reason for variation in reliability of response. Recommended order of priority for selection of proxies was spouse, sibling, child, parent, other relative and finally friend.
Passaro, K.T. et al., 1997.[56] Cross sectional study. Index and proxy both completed self-administered questionnaire	8414	Drinking and smoking habits	Husbands/ partners of pregnant women participating in Avon Longitudinal Study of Pregnancy and Childhood	Pregnant women participating in Avon Longitudinal Study of Pregnancy and Childhood	Kappa coefficient for drinking status showed 'substantial' agreement (kappa = 0.74). Kappa coefficient for smoking status 'almost perfect' (kappa = 0.90).	Agreement within one category for smoking amount = 90%, perfect agreement 81%. Percent agreement dropped dramatically when non-smokers were excluded (50%). Good agreement for alcohol amount: agreement within one category excellent (98%), and perfect agreement still good (71%). Women tended to report lower amounts of smoking and drinking compared to mens' self-reports when not in agreement.

8.4.1.2 Studies of the validity and reliability of proxy informants reporting on socioeconomic and demographic characteristics

Proxies tend to be good informants for easily observable socio-demographic characteristics including marital status, education and for body habitus measurements.[55, 61] Although there is an extensive literature examining proxy responses in studies of occupational exposures (e.g. asbestos), no studies met the inclusion criteria employed here. However, there is a suggestion that responses are more accurate when asking about current rather than past occupational exposures. Studies examining agreement between family-based indexes and proxies on socioeconomic status[64, 65] are not in agreement about the validity of such measures, although there is a suggestion that current reports are more valid than distal reports of occupation. The key findings are summarized in the Table 8.3.

8.4.1.3 Studies of the validity and reliability of proxy informants reporting on physical health

There is a lack of consensus regarding the extent of index-proxy agreement among ten studies addressing reports on physical health and symptoms.[3, 13, 16–19, 55, 66–69] There was a tendency for proxies to display moderate or better agreement when reporting overall health and easily observable, especially 'chronic physical' conditions, and for visible and unambiguous medical history items (e.g. diabetes, amputation). Agreement is lowest for conditions that are either private or very general. Agreement is generally higher for physical activities of daily living (PADL) than for instrumental activities of daily living (IADL). The former tend to be more easily observable and less subjective than IADL. The key findings are summarized in Table 8.4.

8.4.1.4 Studies of the validity and reliability of proxy informants reporting on mental health and well-being

Five reviewed studies addressed psychological state.[13, 16, 18, 70, 71] There was a consensus that index-proxy agreement was only fair for emotional states and emotional and nervous conditions and psychological well-being, since these feelings tend to be private and not well-known by proxies.[18, 69] Observable facets of social networks and social interaction are well-judged by proxies. As might be expected however, proxies are poor judges of perceived emotional support.[70] Life events are often used as indicators of exposure to stress; agreement is substantial for public and observable (e.g. death of a parent), and lower for other (e.g. serious illness of a spouse), life events.[70] There is a suggestion that proxies are not able to accurately capture a patient's own perception of their quality of life and tend towards underestimation.[13] The key findings are summarized in Table 8.5.

8.5 What the current evidence base does not cover with respect to the validity and reliability of using proxy informants

Whilst the available evidence base provides a wealth of information about the validity and reliability of proxy responses under certain circumstances, other issues remain unresolved or completely unanswered. Some of these are outlined here.

8.5.1 Areas with no or inadequate evidence base

The subject areas included in this chapter are those for which there is reasonable available evidence. Many other subject areas are of interest to epidemiology in general and life course epidemiology specifically, but the evidence base is inadequate or entirely lacking.

For example, there are only a few studies which attempt to quantitatively evaluate proxy validity and reliability for questions about diet. Those that do, tend to agree that dietary information provided by proxies is unreliable,[50, 53, 72–74] but most of these studies fail to present adequate statistics (kappa or ICC) for testing validity or reliability.

With respect to life course epidemiology there is a need for an evidence base on the use of different proxies at different ages. For example, in the 1946 birth cohort, dietary intake, child's behaviour (a marker of possible early psychological or emotional problems) and a number of other characteristics at age 4 years were obtained from the main carer (most commonly the child's mother). At age 15 the information on behaviour was obtained from the teacher[75] and for other characteristics from the index (child) themselves or from their parents. The use of these proxies is reasonable, but as we are increasingly interested in changes in behaviour and characteristics across the life course it would be useful to have some idea about how reasonable it is to use information from different proxies at different stages of the life course to measure change.

8.5.2 Choice of proxy

Whilst there are several suggestions regarding the specific selection of proxy when there is a choice available, there is no clear consensus in the literature beyond spouse/partner as the ideal proxy.[3, 17, 51, 55, 60, 61] It may be the quality and nature, rather than formal relationship (e.g. spouse, sister, etc.), which most affects the proxy response quality.[19, 68, 69, 76, 77] In family-based epidemiology studies, an understanding of the effect of using a specific proxy for a specific index is likely to be important. For example, if information on one sibling is unavailable would a parent or another sibling provide the best (most valid and reliable) proxy response? This may vary depending on the age of the index and proxy and the characteristic being asked about. However, to date, there is no strong evidence base to answer these questions.

There is some evidence that non-response rate may be affected by choice of proxy, but again, this is difficult to evaluate. Available evidence indicated that the highest response rates are achieved when spouses are proxies and lower rates are achieved when using distant relatives and friends compared with first degree relatives.[3, 16, 63, 77, 78]

8.5.3 Availability of index subject

Clearly, it is not possible to evaluate the validity and reliability of proxy responses when the index has died, or there is no available information about the index against which to compare proxy responses. Assumptions can be made regarding the extent of additional bias that would result in such situations, and attempts have been made to evaluate this to some extent,[36] but it is impossible to obtain any definitive results in this regard.

8.5.4 The effect of index attributes on proxy responses

In terms of how index attributes affect proxy responses, the available literature is sparse. The few papers that do provide evidence were broadly in agreement in their assessment of how index attributes affect proxy response quality.[19, 51, 60, 68, 79] No difference in quality of response was found by index's age or sex,[63] nor did there tend to be any difference in either quality of response or response rate by case-control status,[19, 51, 60, 68, 79, 80] other than when the examined condition was difficult to observe (e.g. back pain).[68]

8.6 Special situations in life course family-based studies

In life course studies, some particular issues associated with the use of proxies can arise.

Table 8.3 Key findings related to index-proxy agreement on socioeconomic and demographic characteristics

Study details	Number of pairs	Outcome	Index	Proxy	Results	Comments
Batty, D.G., et al., 2005.[64] Comparison of data collected in 2000–2003 in cross sectional survey, and data collected prospectively from members of Aberdeen Children of the 1950s cohort in 1962	6320	Childhood socioeconomic status retrospectively reported in adulthood	Study participants in childhood (1962)	Self, in adulthood (in 2000–2003)	Agreement between social class data based on childhood reports and adult reports 'moderate' (weighted kappa = 0.56).	Tendency to over-estimate childhood socioeconomic status (based on parental occupation) in adulthood compared to in childhood.
Hatch, M.C. et al., 1991.[61] Cross-sectional survey of prenatal patients and their spouses/partners	136	Occupation, smoking and drinking	Women recruited from obstetric services and their spouse/ partner	N/a - the index-proxy agreement was examined in both directions	Almost perfect agreement on work status. Up to 98% agreement on index's current occupation.	

Study	Design	Population	Topic	Findings	Comments
Lien N 2001 [65] Cross-sectional study using data from the Norwegian Longitudinal Health Behaviour Study. Proxies: self-completed questionnaires carried out at school at baseline, sent by mail at follow-up. Indexes: self-completed questionnaires.	924 children, 648 mothers, 735 fathers, various sets of pairings compared.	Parental education and SES. Comparisons made between parental baseline reports with both adolescent baseline and follow-up reports.	Population-based sample of Norwiegian parents	Children of index, young adolescents	Agreement on SES based on occupation 'substantial' (kappa >0.61) at proxy baseline and 'almost perfect' (kappa >0.80) at proxy follow-up, for both parents.	Agreement slightly stronger with fathers than with mothers in all instances, and agreement slightly stronger at follow-up in all instances than at baseline, although these differences were small.
Nelson, L.M. et al., 1994. [55] Case control, interviewer-administered interviews of all controls and their proxies and where possible of cases and their proxies.	283 control/proxy pairs, 68 case/proxy pairs	Spontaneous subarachnoid haemorrhage	Live cases, healthy controls from a case-control study	Various, recruited in following order of preference: spouse, sibling, son/daughter, parent, other relative, friend.	Almost perfect agreement overall (0.86–0.99%), although a tendency to underreport weight and BMI observed. Perfect or near-perfect agreement for demographic characteristics such as marital status and education (kappa >0.8).	Observed that proxies tended to under-report the presence or level of exposure, meaning the specificity of proxy responses was better than the sensitivity for most exposures. Misclassification was found to be non-differential and accordingly, odds ratios computed using proxy data were similar in magnitude to those obtained using index data. The relationship of proxy to index was one reason for variation in reliability of response.

Table 8.4 Key findings related to index-proxy agreement on physical health

Study details	Number of pairs	Outcome	Index	Proxy	Results	Comments
Demissee, S. et al., 2001.[3] Cross sectional survey. Self-administered questionnaire carried out by index and two proxies	81 indexes, 159 proxies	Medical history, medication use, health behaviour and cognitive ability	Non-demented Alzheimer sufferers	2 per index, both self-selected	Overall agreement 'almost perfect' for diabetes and heart disease (kappa = 0.89, 0.82), 'substantial' for thyroid disease, hypertension, cancer and arthritis (kappa = 0.75, 0.72, 0.72, 0.68) and 'moderate' for head injury (0.43).	High non-response rate when proxies asked about medication history. Authors recommend that sibs, particularly sisters, are the second ablest respondents. Also observed that spouses were able to provide information more often than other proxy informants.
Farrow, D.C. and Samet, J.M. 1990.[16] Cross sectional survey. In-person interview of index and abbreviated interview of proxy	622	Health status, major life events, social network and functional status	Elderly cancer patients, 65 years or older	Spouse if available, then friend, adult relative or child	Overall agreement ranged widely (kappa = 0.33–0.67). For medical conditions, including high blood pressure, heart problems, bronchitis/emphysema, asthma, agreement was usually 'moderate' (kappa >0.61) or 'almost perfect' (kappa >0.8) diabetes, when reported by spouses.	Agreement higher when factual information solicited rather than personal information or attitudes, and almost always higher when spouse was the respondent, rather than child or friend. Lowest non-response rate observed among spouses as proxies.
Halabi, S. et al., 1992.[68] Case control. Face to face interviews carried out with cases and their proxies and controls and their proxies. Physical examination carried	100 case/proxy pairs, 100 control/proxy pairs	Heart disease, back pain, rheumatoid arthritis, hypertension or pulmonary disease	Adults from a sample of screened households reporting themselves to have one	Spouse if available, otherwise randomly selected household member	Level of agreement varied between conditions, and for case-proxy versus control-proxy pairs. Agreement best for heart disease: 'substantial' for cases (0.79).	Results suggest that health interview surveys are accurate for data collection of well defined chronic conditions.

				out on all indexes to confirm presence/absence of disease	of 5 chronic diseases	'almost perfect' for controls (1.00). Agreement for hypertension 'substantial' for cases, (0.65), 'fair' for controls (0.50). Agreement for back pain 'fair' for both cases and controls (0.49, 0.50 respectively).	
Long, K. et al., 1998.[17] Cross-sectional survey. Telephone interviews of indexes and their proxies	340	Functional status and medical history	People aged 65 and older	Index's caregiver		Percentage agreement for difficulty of carrying out some activities of daily living ranged were as high as 99.7% (kappa = 0.856) for 'toileting' - although some categories elicited much lower agreement, e.g. bathing, kappa = 0.17 - with an overall kappa for ADL of 0.66. Agreement on medical history was sometimes as low as 78%, although kappas ranged widely from 'slight' for Alzheimer's (kappa = 0.28) to 'almost perfect' for easily observable medical items diabetes (kappa = 0.85) and amputation (0.83).	Very wide range of kappa values with respect to medical history items. Highest concordance for visible and unambiguous conditions. Observed increased index-proxy agreement when the issues being addressed were readily observable. An association was observed between the index-proxy relationship and the extent of medical history agreement. The self-reported burden of the caregiver was associated with the extent to which they overestimated the disability of the index.

Continued

Table 8.4 (continued) Key findings related to index-proxy agreement on physical health

Study details	Number of pairs	Outcome	Index	Proxy	Results	Comments
Maziner, J. et al., 1996.[69] Health survey. Face to face interviews carried out with indexes, and with proxies 3 weeks later.	538	Physical health and physical and instrumental functioning	Women aged 65 years and older, participating in the third home interview of the health survey	Self-selected	Substantial to almost perfect agreement for most physical activities of daily living (PADL) and for all instrumental activities of daily living (IADL) (kappa >0.6). Almost perfect agreement observed for some easily observable chronic conditions (diabetes, kappa=0.86; thyroid or other glandular disorders, kappa=0.74; heart trouble, kappa=0.76).	Observed that proxies are more likely to report the presence of, or to over-report the level of a condition, symptom or functional problem than indexes. Proxies living with the index demonstrate better agreement for chronic conditions, physical symptoms and PADL. Among proxies not living with the index, those who visited the index more frequency demonstrated greater agreement for physical symptoms, PADL and IADL.
Maziner, J. et al., 1997.[18] Cross sectional study. Indexes interviewed at place of residence, proxies interviewed by phone within 1 month.	233	Functional status	Patients aged 65 years or older participating in 12 month follow-up study of hip fracture recovery	Self-selected	Agreement highest for easily observable measures of independence of instrumental functioning (handling money, kappa=0.81; taking medications, kappa=0.81), and lower for less easily observable measures of dependence of physical activities of daily living (taking a shower, bath or sponge bath, kappa=0.18; climbing five stairs, kappa=0.18).	Proxies tend to report more disability than indexes.

Nelson, L.M. et al., 1994.[55] Case control, interviewer-administered interviews of all controls and their proxies and where possible of cases and their proxies.	283 control/proxy pairs, 68 case/proxy pairs	Spontaneous subarachnoid haemorrhage	Live cases, healthy controls from a case-control study	Various, recruited in following order of preference: spouse, sibling, son/daughter, parent, other relative, friend.	Very good agreement for broad indicators of physical activity level (PAL). Only moderate agreement for detailed aspects of PAL (kappa = 0.57–0.67).	Observed that proxies tended to under-report the presence or level of exposure, meaning the specificity of proxy responses was better than the sensitivity for most exposures. Misclassification was found to be non-differential and accordingly, odds ratios computed using proxy data were similar in magnitude to those obtained using index data. The relationship of proxy to index was one reason for variation in reliability of response. Recommended order of priority for selection of proxies was spouse, sibling, child, parent, other relative and finally friend.
Novella, J.L. et al., 2001.[13] Cross sectional survey. Self-administered questionnaire carried out by index and two proxies	148	Assessment of quality of life using Duke Health Profile	Patients with mild to moderate Alzheimer's disease	Two proxies - (1) family member (2) care provider	Agreement between index and family proxy 'moderate' for directly observable measures of function such as physical health (ICC = 0.44) or disability (ICC = 0.61), which was higher when examining only spouses as proxies (ICC = 0.66 and 0.80 respectively).	Similar agreement observed when using health professionals as proxies: physical health ICC = 0.69 disability ICC = 0.53 when excluding nurses' aides. Agreement was worse for more subjective measures. Similar agreement observed when using health professionals as proxies: physical health ICC = 0.69 disability ICC = 0.53 when excluding nurses' aides. Proxies tended to underestimate quality of life as reported by index case. Agreement was especially weak for Duke subscales such as perceived health or social health.

Continued

Table 8.4 (continued) Key findings related to index-proxy agreement on physical health

Study details	Number of pairs	Outcome	Index	Proxy	Results	Comments
Ostbye, T. et al., 1997.[19] Cross sectional survey. General survey of indexes, face to face interview of proxies	800	Activities of daily living	People aged 65 and older with or without dementia, part of a larger case control study of dementia and health	Caregivers	Agreement for PADL (kappa = 0.26–0.81) with the majority of values in the 'moderate' category) is generally higher than for IADL (kappa = 0.18–0.61 with the majority of values in the 'fair' category).	Found proxies to be a reasonable source of data. Agreement decreases as severity of dementia increases. Caregivers as proxies are not as reliable as other proxies, possibly because their judgement is impaired by their burden with respect to the index. The relationship of the caregiver to the subject did not appear to make an important difference to index-proxy agreement. Authors suggested that it is specific characteristics of the proxy such as amount of time spent with subject, or the 'quality' of the relationship, rather than their formal relationship to the subject, that affects quality of response.
Shaw, C. et al., 2000.[66] Cross sectional survey. Face to face interview of index and their proxy within a few days	140	Functional ability	Women aged 65 years and older, part of a larger study of outcomes of fractured	Self-selected	Concordance was 'substantial' for several categories, including cutting food (kappa = 0.68), bathing (kappa = 0.75), washing clothes (kappa = 0.72) and cooking (kappa = 0.70).	Proxy responses tend to be biased in the direction of overestimation of incapacity, with more proxies reporting that the index needed help for ¾ of the questions asked. The authors observed a tendency for improved agreement with more distant

				neck of femur post-surgery	relationships and contact with the proxy. This is contrary to other findings, but may be because in the specific study population used, which was used to examine functional ability and continence in older people, the mood of the proxy who was frequently a caregiver, affected the quality of the proxy responses. Observed increased index-proxy agreement when the issues being addressed were readily observable.
Tepper et al., 1996.[67] Cross-sectional survey. Interviews of indexes and proxies	148	Agreement between index and proxy on a number of exposures related to recovery after traumatic brain injury	Traumatic brain injury patients	'Significant others'	Agreement substantial for ulcers (kappa=0.91), cancer (0.89), diabetes (0.84) and lung disease (0.77). Moderate agreement (kappa <0.6) observed for less easily observable medical conditions heart disease, stroke, liver disease and high blood pressure.

8.6.1 The use of the index versus a proxy when the index is a child

The inclusion of infants and children as index subjects is a common feature of life course studies. At very young ages, children are unable to provide information about themselves and the use of proxies is essential. As they become older, the decision to use a proxy requires greater consideration. At some point a child becomes able to provide their own information, and the benefits of collecting data from a young index may outweigh the issues introduced by using a proxy respondent. So, at what age would we consider that a child is able to answer for themselves? Once this point is reached, an additional consideration is whether information should additionally, or only, be collected from the previously used proxy. Related to these points is the question of whether it is appropriate to assess change in characteristics across the life course using proxy measurements in early life and own measurements in later life without some adjustment for the change in informant. A good practice (if resources are available) might be to collect information from both the index and proxy from an age at which the index is considered able to provide information on that proxy and to use differences between the two to 'correct' previous proxy reports. However, this assumes that any difference between proxy and index at a later age of the index, represents a difference (under or over estimation) that has been constant since the child's younger age.

8.6.2 Obtaining dual or multiple reports about one index

In family-based studies, reports can sometimes be obtained from both the index and the proxy, resulting in dual reports that may then differ. Careful consideration must then be given as to how to treat these measurements. For example, both the child and carer might be asked to complete a standard behaviour questionnaire that is used to determine emotional problems and to describe the child's personality (e.g. as 'internalizing' or 'externalizing'). Since these questionnaires would be collecting information about internal psychological states, the child's own completion of such a questionnaire and the carer's completion could be treated as two separate characteristics which would not necessarily be expected to agree. Alternatively, one report (the child's own or the carers) might be considered the gold-standard against which to validate the other report. Similarly in measuring diet and physical activity in children/young people, separate responses from the child and the carer could be seen as jointly providing a more complete picture (with the child knowing better what they ate for lunch on school days and what activity they have done outside the home and the carer perhaps knowing better about food and activity in the home). Conversely this could be treated as an attempt to measure the same thing in two different ways or one measure may be validated against the other. The key thing is that researchers consider *a priori* how they will use measurements that are reported by an index and one or more proxies and justify their decisions.

8.6.3 Using a proxy who is a cohort participant and asking them to report for themselves and another index

In life course family-based studies, the situation may arise where one family member responds about themselves, and also acts as proxy for other family members. For example, in the intergenerational studies the mother could be also be reporting for the father. In twin/sibling studies, one could be reporting on behalf of the other(s) as well as themselves. This could result in clustering of responses beyond that expected due to similarities between family members. For example, if one sister is asked to report the smoking behaviour of another sister, whilst also reporting her own smoking behaviour, she may be more likely to make the two responses similar to each other than if she were only responding for herself or only responding for her sister. The studies that have, to date, assessed validity and reliability of proxies have not considered whether the proxy also reporting on their own behaviours influences their proxy response, but clearly for family-based life course studies this is an important issue to consider.

8.6.4 Proxy information across life course may vary

In life course studies the challenges of using proxies can be compounded by the use of different proxies at different life stages. In the 1946 birth cohort, for example, information about the subjects' childhood and adolescence was obtained from the carer, subsequently from school doctors and their teachers and ultimately from the index themselves.[75] In most life course studies we are interested in measuring change in an outcome/exposure of interest. The use of different proxies at different times may introduce additional bias due to over/under reporting or reduced validity due to the choice of respondent, and as with other specific aspects of using proxies in life course epidemiology, there is as yet no strong evidence base on which to assess the likely extent of any such bias.

8.7 Practical experience of using proxy informants

A recent example of use of proxies in a family-based epidemiological study is the Izhevsk Family Study.[27] This was a case-control study of the determinants (alcohol consumption and other) of premature mortality among men of working age (25–54) resident in Izhevsk, Russia. Proxies were interviewed about 1,750 cases (men who had died). Proxies were also used for 1,750 live controls to ensure comparable assessments. In addition, all controls were interviewed themselves, and a number of external data sources were also employed to assess proxy validity. An extensive analysis of the validity and reliability of the proxy responses obtained in this study was therefore possible.[36]

Because of the specific circumstances giving rise to use of proxies in this study, interviewers reported that some of the interviews were very traumatic to carry out, since they were with recently bereaved family members.

Levels of validity between interviews with control proxies and controls were explored using kappa statistics and other methods.[36] There was wide variability, but it was reassuring that the specific findings were largely in accordance with what was expected based on the available evidence base. High index-proxy agreement was obtained when asking about directly observable behaviour, and lower agreement was obtained when asking questions about subjective, detailed, or private behaviours.[36] Use of an external data source to validate proxy-obtained data indicated that proxy reported alcohol use may actually be more valid with respect to the 'truth' than self reported, a finding which may also apply to other parallel behaviours (those implicated in poor health/death tend to be underestimated by the index relative to the proxy).

The use of proxies was successful in many regards. The response rate was good, especially among case proxies (62%) but also among control proxies (59%). It is likely that case proxies were especially motivated to participate because of a recent death in the family. Selection of the most appropriate proxy was carried out by interviewers asking for the household composition and then selecting the best available proxy using an order of preference derived from the available evidence (wife, sister, mother, brother, father, child over 18). This was time consuming for the interviewers and reported to be an awkward exercise, since it was carried out at first contact with the household. However, the results suggested that this was a worthwhile exercise, since index-proxy agreement among controls was often high, suggesting valid proxy responses.

The Izhevsk Family Study demonstrates that provided a study is carefully designed and implemented, proxy respondents can be successfully used in family-based epidemiological studies to obtain valid and reliable information on index respondents.

Table 8.5 Key findings related to index-proxy agreement on mental health and well-being

Study details	Number of pairs	Outcome	Index	Proxy	Results	Comments
Conner, K.R., et al., 2001a.[71] Cross sectional survey. Structured interview of index and their proxy.	80	Stressful life event, social support and suicidal behaviour	Psychiatric in-patients aged 50–91 who attempted suicide	Mainly women, including spouses, partners, children, other relatives, friends and caregivers	'Good' agreement for social interaction (ICC = 0.61), but not for perceived emotional support (ICC = 0.28).	When examining life events, agreement was substantial for public and observable events ('death of a parent, child, sibling or spouse', kappa=0.70, employment/business disruption, kappa=0.61), but lower for more ambiguous events ('disruption of spousal relationships', kappa = 0.48, 'serious illness of parent, child, sibling or spouse', kappa=0.38).
Conner, K.R., et al., 2001b.[70] Cross sectional survey. Structured interview of index and their proxy	80	Psychiatric diagnosis	Psychiatric in-patients aged 50–91 who attempted suicide	Mainly women, including spouses, partners, children, other relatives, friends and caregivers	Agreement 'substantial' for dependence (kappa = 1), but 'poor' for substance abuse disorders (values not reported).	
Farrow, D.C. and Samet, J.M. 1990.[16] Cross sectional survey. In-person interview of index and abbreviated interview of proxy	622	Health status, major life events, social network and functional status	Elderly cancer patients, 65 years or older	Spouse if available, then friend, adult relative or child	Overall agreement ranged widely (kappa = 0.33–0.67). Agreement was 'almost perfect' for easily observable major life events when reported by spouses (moved during year prior to diagnosis, kappa=0.85, number of	Agreement was especially low for Duke subscales such as perceived health or social health. Agreement inconsistent for questions on social network and major life events. Agreement higher when factual information solicited rather than personal information or attitudes, and almost always higher when spouse was the respondent, rather than child or friend.

					children visited at least monthly, kappa=0.89, but much lower for questions about social contact when reported by any respondent and was either 'moderate' or 'almost perfect' when reported by child/friend proxies.	Lowest non-response rate observed among spouses as proxies.
Magaziner, J. et al., 1997.[18] Cross sectional study. Indexes interviewed at place of residence, proxies interviewed by phone within 1 month.	233	Functional status	Patients aged 65 years or older participating in 12 month follow-up study of hip fracture recovery	Self-selected	Agreement lowest for a subjective measure of depression (ICC=0.38).	Proxies tend to report more disability than indexes.
Novella, J.L. et al., 2001.[13] Cross sectional survey. Self-administered questionnaire carried out by index and two proxies	148	Assessment of quality of life using Duke Health Profile	Patients with mild to moderate Alzheimer's disease	Two proxies - (1) family member (2) care provider	Agreement was weak Duke subscales such as mental health (ICC=0.24) and self-esteem (ICC=0.19). Agreement was especially weak for perceived health (ICC=0.00) and social health (ICC=0.06).	Proxies tended to underestimate quality of life as reported by index case. Agreement was worse for more subjective measures.

8.8 Conclusions

Using proxies is likely to be important for family-based life course epidemiology studies because there will be many situations in which obtaining relevant information from the index participant will not be possible. In these situations excluding the informants for whom it is not possible to obtain information could result in selection bias and/or not being able address some research questions. Using proxy informants is one solution, and currently available evidence suggests that in many situations these can provide valid and reliable information. However, it would be useful to have more information on the validity of non-spousal informants, more information on the validity of using proxies for some common health related behaviours, such as diet and illicit drug use, for which the evidence base is currently very thin and information on the effects of using different proxies at different stages of the life course and using study participants to provide proxy information at the same time as providing their own information on validity and reliability.

References

1 **Nelson LM, Longstreth WT, Jr., Koepsell TD, van Belle G.** Proxy respondents in epidemiologic research. *Epidemiologic Reviews* 1990; **12**: 71–86.

2 **Burgio L and Leon J.** Using patient and proxy reports as outcome measures in Alzheimer disease research. *Alzheimer's Disease and Associated Disorders* 1997; **11**: 179–80.

3 **Demissie S et al.** Reliability of information collected by proxy in family studies of Alzheimer's disease. *Neuroepidemiology* 2001; **20**: 105–11.

4 **Debanne SM et al.** On the use of surrogate respondents for controls in a case-control study of Alzheimer's disease. *Journal of the American Geriatrics Society* 2001; **49**: 980–4.

5 **Heyman A et al.** Alzheimer's disease: a study of epidemiological aspects. *Annals of Neurology* 1984; **15**: 335–41.

6 **Friedland RP et al.** Patients with Alzheimer's disease have reduced activities in midlife compared with healthy control-group members. *Proceedings of the National Academy of Sciences of the United States of America* 2001; **98**: 3440–5.

7 **Korten AE, Jorm AF, Henderson AS, McCusker E, Creasey H.** Control-informant agreement on exposure history in case-control studies of Alzheimer's disease. *International Journal of Epidemiology* 1992; **21**: 1121–31.

8 **Kukull WA et al.** Solvent exposure as a risk factor for Alzheimers disease - a case-control study. *American Journal of Epidemiology* 1995; **141**: 1059–71.

9 **Chong JP et al.** Concordance of occupational and environmental exposure information elicited from patients with Alzheimer's disease and surrogate respondents. *American Journal of Industrial Medicine* 1989; **15**: 73–89.

10 **Logsdon RG and Teri L.** Depression in Alzheimer's disease patients: caregivers as surrogate reporters. *Journal of the American Geriatrics Society* 1995; **43**: 150–5.

11 **Petot GJ et al.** Use of surrogate respondents in a case control study of dietary risk factors for Alzheimer's disease. *Journal of the American Dietetic Association* 2002; **102**: 848–50.

12 **Loewenstein DA et al.** Caregivers' judgments of the functional abilities of the Alzheimer's disease patient: a comparison of proxy reports and objective measures. *Journal of Gerontology: Psychological Sciences* 2001; **56**: 78–84.

13 **Novella JL et al.** (2001). Agreement between patients' and proxies' reports of quality of life in Alzheimer's disease. *Quality of life research* **10**, 443-452.

14 **Weiss A, Fletcher AE, Palmer AJ, Nicholl CG, Bulpitt CJ.** Use of surrogate respondents in studies of stroke and dementia. *Journal of Clinical Epidemiology* 1996; **49**: 1187–94.

15 **Dewey ME, Parker CJ, Analysis group of the MRC CFA STUDY.** Survey into health problems of elderly people: multivariate analysis of concordance between self-report and proxy information. *International Journal of Epidemiology* 2000; **29**: 698–703.

16 Farrow DC and Samet JM. Comparability of information provided by elderly cancer patients and surrogates regarding health and functional status, social network, and life events. *Epidemiology* 1990; **1**: 370–6.

17 Long K, Sudha S, Mutran EJ. Elder-proxy agreement concerning the functional status and medical history of the older person: the impact of caregiver burden and depressive symptomatology. *Journal of the American Geriatrics Society* 1998; **46**: 1103–11.

18 Magaziner J, Zimmerman SI, Gruber-Baldini AL, Hebel JR, Fox KM. Proxy reporting in five areas of functional status. Comparison with self-reports and observations of performance. *American Journal of Epidemiology* 1997; **146**: 418–28.

19 Ostbye T, Tyas S, McDowell I, Koval J. Reported activities of daily living: Agreement between elderly subjects with and without dementia and their caregivers. *Age and Ageing* 1997; **26**: 99–106.

20 Pierre U, Wood-Dauphinee S, Korner-Bitensky N, Gayton D, Hanley J. Proxy use of the Canadian SF-36 in rating health status of the disabled elderly. *Journal of Clinical Epidemiology* 1998; **51**: 983–90.

21 Sitoh YY *et al.* Proxy assessment of health-related quality of life in the frail elderly. *Age and Ageing* 2003; **32**: 459.

22 Rajmil L *et al.* Influence of proxy respondents in children's health interview surveys. *Journal of Epidemiology and Community Health* 1999; **53**: 38–42.

23 Ravelli A *et al.* Discordance between proxy-reported and observed assessment of functional ability of children with juvenile idiopathic arthritis. *Rheumatology.(Oxford)* 2001; **40**: 914–19.

24 Ronen GM, Streiner DL, Rosenbaum P. Health-related quality of life in children with epilepsy: development and validation of self-report and parent proxy measures. *Epilepsia* 2003; **44**: 598–612.

25 Golding J, Pembrey M, Jones R. ALSPAC—the Avon Longitudinal Study of Parents and Children. I. Study methodology. *Paediatr.Perinat.Epidemiol* 2001; **15**: 74–87.

26 Najman JM *et al.* Cohort Profile: The Mater-University of Queensland Study of Pregnancy (MUSP). *Int J Epidemiol* 2005; **34**: 992–7.

27 Leon DA *et al.* Hazardous alcohol drinking and premature mortality in Russia: a population based case-control study. *Lancet* 2007; **369**: 2001–9.

28 Gute DM and Fulton JP. Agreement of occupation and industry data on Rhode Island death certificates with two alternative sources of information. *Public Health Rep* 1985; **100**: 65–72.

29 Schumacher MC. Comparison of occupation and industry information from death certificates and interviews. *American Journal of Public Health* 1986; **76**: 635–7.

30 Schade WJ and Swanson GM. Comparison of death certificate occupation and industry data with lifetime occupational histories obtained by interview: variations in the accuracy of death certificate entries. *American Journal of Industrial Medicine* 1988; **14**: 121–36.

31 Turner DW, Schumacher M.C., West DW. Comparison of occupational interview data to death certificate data in Utah. *American Journal of Industrial Medicine* 1987; **12**: 145–51.

32 Gute G and Fulton J. Agreement of occupation and industry data on Rhode Island death certificates with two alternative sources of information. *Public Health Rep* 1985; **100**: 65–72.

33 Schumacher M.C. Comparison of occupation and industry information from death certificates and interviews. *American Journal of Public Health* 1986; **76**: 635–7.

34 Swanson GM, Schwartz AG, Burrows RW. An assessment of occupation and industry data from death certificates and hospital records for population-based cancer surveillance. *American Journal of Public Health* 1984; **74**: 464–7.

35 Midanik LT. Validity of self-reported alcohol use: a literature review and assessment. *British Journal of Addiction* 1988; **83**: 1019–30.

36 Tomkins, S. Proxy respondents in a case-control study: validity, reliability and impact. PhD thesis, London School of Hygiene & Tropical Medicine, University of London; 2006.

37 Landis JR and Koch GG. The measurement of observer agreement for categorical data. *Biometrics* 1977; **33**: 159–74.

38 Midanik LT. Perspectives on the validity of self-reported alcohol use. *British Journal of Addiction* 1989; **84**: 1419–23.

39 Midanik LT. The validity of self-reported alcohol consumption and alcohol problems: a literature review. *British Journal of Addiction* 1982; **77**: 357–82.

40 Midanik LT. Over-reports of recent alcohol consumption in a clinical population: a validity study. *Drug and Alcohol Dependency* 1982; **9**: 101–10.

41 Pernanen, K. Validity of survey data on alcohol use in Research advances in alcohol and drug problems, R. J. Gibbens, Ed. John Wiley & Son, Inc, New York, vol. 1, 1974.

42 Midanik LT. Drunkenness, feeling the effects and 5+ measures. *Addiction* 1999; **94**: 887–97.

43 Midanik LT and Clark WB. The demographic distribution of US drinking patterns in 1990: description and trends from 1984. *American Journal of Public Health* 1994; **84**: 1218–22.

44 Midanik LT. Reliability of self-reported alcohol consumption before and after December. *Addictive Behaviour* 1992; **17**: 179–84.

45 Midanik LT, Klatsky AL, Armstrong MA. A comparison of 7-day recall with two summary measures of alcohol use. *Drug and Alcohol Dependency* 1984; **24**: 127–34.

46 Barnett T, O'Loughlin J, Paradis G, Renaud L. Reliability of proxy reports of parental smoking by elementary schoolchildren. *Annals of Epidemiology* 1997; **7**: 396–9.

47 Gilpin EA *et al.* Estimates of population smoking prevalence: self-vs proxy reports of smoking status. *American Journal of Public Health* 1994; **84**: 1576–9.

48 Greenberg RS, LIFF JM, Gregory HR, Brockman JE. The use of interviews with surrogate respondents in a case-control study of oral cancer. *The Yale Journal of Biology and Medicine* 1986; **59**: 497–504.

49 Kolonel LN, Hirohata T, Nomura AM. Adequacy of survey data collected from substitute respondents. *American Journal of Epidemiology* 1977; **106**: 476–84.

50 Lerchen ML and Samet JM. An assessment of the validity of questionnaire responses provided by a surviving spouse. *American Journal of Epidemiology* 1986; **123**: 481–9.

51 McLaughlin JK, Mandel JS, Mehl ES, Blot WJ. Comparison of next-of-kin with self-respondents regarding questions on cigarette, coffee, and alcohol consumption. *Epidemiology* 1990; **1**: 408–12.

52 McLaughlin JK, Dietz MS, Mehl ES, Blot WJ. Reliability of surrogate information on cigarette smoking by type of informant. *American Journal of Epidemiology* 1987; **126**: 144–6.

53 Metzner HL, Lamphiear DE, Thompson FE, Oh MS, Hawthorne VM. Comparison of surrogate and subject reports of dietary practices, smoking habits and weight among married couples in the Tecumseh Diet Methodology Study. *Journal of Clinical Epidemiology* 1989; **42**: 367–75.

54 Navarro AM. Smoking status by proxy and self report: rate of agreement in different ethnic groups. *Tobacco Control* 1999; **8**: 182–5.

55 Nelson LM, Longstreth WT, Jr., Koepsell TD, Checkoway H, van Belle G. Completeness and accuracy of interview data from proxy respondents: demographic, medical, and life-style factors. *Epidemiology* 1994; **5**: 204–17.

56 Passaro KT, Noss J, Savitz DA, Little RE. Agreement between self and partner reports of paternal drinking and smoking. *International Journal of Epidemiology* 1997; **26**: 315–20.

57 Pickle LW, Brown LM, Blot WJ. Information available from surrogate respondents in case-control interview studies. *American Journal of Epidemiology* 1983; **118**: 99–108.

58 Thorogood M and Vessey M. The reliability of surrogate information about oral contraceptive use, smoking, height and weight collected from men about their wives. *Contraception* 1989; **39**: 401–8.

59 Woo JG and Pinney SM. Retrospective smoking history data collection for deceased workers: completeness and accuracy of surrogate reports. *Journal of Occupational and Environmental Medicine* 2002; **44**: 915–23.

60 Graham P and Jackson R. Primary versus proxy respondents: comparability of questionnaire data on alcohol consumption. *American Journal of Epidemiology* 1993; **138**: 443–52.

61 Hatch MC, Misra D, Kabat GC, Kartzmer S. Proxy respondents in reproductive research: a comparison of self- and partner-reported data. *American Journal of Epidemiology* 1991; **133**: 826–31.

62 Hamilton AS and Mack TM. Use of twins as mutual proxy respondents in a case-control study of breast cancer: effect of item nonresponse and misclassification. *Am J Epidemil* 2000; **152**: 1093–1103.

63 Graham P and Jackson R. A comparison of primary and proxy respondent reports of habitual physical activity, using kappa statistics and log-linear models. *Journal of Epidemiology and Biostatics* 2000; **5**: 255–65.

64 Batty GD, Lawlor DA, Macintyre S, Clark H, Leon DA. Accuracy of adults' recall of childhood social class: findings from the Aberdeen children of the 1950s study. *J.Epidemiol.Community Health* 2005; **59**: 898–903.

65 Lien N, Friestad C, Klepp KI. Adolescents' proxy reports of parents' socioeconomic status: How valid are they? *Journal of Epidemiology and Community Health* 2001; **55**: 731–7.

66 Shaw C, McColl E, Bond S. Functional abilities and continence: the use of proxy respondents in research involving older people. *Quality of Life Research* 2000; **9**: 1117–26.

67 Tepper S, Beatty P, DeJong G. Outcomes in traumatic brain injury: self-report versus report of significant others. *Brain Injury* 1996; **10**: 575–81.

68 Halabi S, Zurayk H, Awaida R, Darwish M, Saab B. Reliability and validity of self and proxy reporting of morbidity data: a case study from Beirut, Lebanon. *International Journal of Epidemiology* 1992; **21**: 607–12.

69 Magaziner J, Bassett SS, Hebel JR, Gruber-Baldini A. Use of proxies to measure health and functional status in epidemiologic studies of community-dwelling women aged 65 years and older. *American Journal of Epidemiology* 1996; **143**: 283–92.

70 Conner KR, Conwell Y, Duberstein PR. The validity of proxy-based data in suicide research: a study of patients 50 years of age and older who attempted suicide. II. Life events, social support and suicidal behavior. *Acta Psychiatrica Scandinavia* 2001; **104**: 452–7.

71 Conner KR, Duberstein PR, Conwell Y. The validity of proxy-based data in suicide research: a study of patients 50 years of age and older who attempted suicide. I. Psychiatric diagnoses. *Acta Psychiatrica Scandinavia* 2001; **104**: 204–9.

72 Herrmann N. Retrospective information from questionnaires. I. Comparability of primary respondents and their next-of-kin. *American Journal of Epidemiology* 1985; **121**: 937–47.

73 Hislop TG, Coldman AJ, Zheng YY, Ng VT, Labo T. Reliability of dietary information from surrogate respondents. *Nutr Cancer* 1992; **18**: 123–9.

74 Humble CG, Samet JM, Skipper BE. Comparison of self- and surrogate-reported dietary information. *American Journal of Epidemiology* 1984; **119**: 86–98.

75 Wadsworth M, Kuh D, Richards M, Hardy R. Cohort Profile: The 1946 National Birth Cohort (MRC National Survey of Health and Development). *International Journal of Epidemiology* 2006; **35**: 49–54.

76 Magaziner J, Simonsick EM, Kashner TM, Hebel JR. Patient-proxy response comparability on measures of patient health and functional status. *Journal of Clinical Epidemiology* 1988; **41**: 1065–74.

77 The Medical Research Council Cognitive Function and Ageing Study. Survey into health problems of elderly people: multivariate analysis of concordance between self-report and proxy information. *International Journal of Epidemiology* 2000; **29**: 698–703.

78 Boyle CA and Brann EA. Proxy respondents and the validity of occupational and other exposure data. The Selected Cancers Cooperative Study Group. *American Journal of Epidemiology* 1992; **136**: 712–21.

79 Marshall J, Priore R, Haughey B, Rzepka T, Graham S. Spouse-subject interviews and the reliability of diet studies. *American Journal of Epidemiology* 1980; **112**: 675–83.

80 Mills KM *et al.* Reliability of proxy-reported and self-reported household appliance use. *Epidemiology* 2000; **11**: 581–8.

Chapter 9

Discussant chapter—the practicalities of undertaking family-based studies

Rebecca Hardy and Diana Kuh

Abstract

The three chapters in this section address topics related to the practicalities of undertaking family-based studies. Chapter 6 discusses the methodological and practical issues involved in carrying out intergenerational cohort studies, Chapter 7 the undertaking of family-based life course studies in low and middle income countries, and Chapter 8 the issues related to the use of proxy informants in family-based studies. We summarize the origins of some of the existing life course studies and the current potential for using these studies to address family-based life course questions. We also highlight important methodological and practical issues for the future conduct of such studies. It has to be considered carefully whether it is worth collecting more prior generation and/or offspring generation data in these established cohorts given the practical difficulties and costs associated with such an undertaking as detailed in Chapters 6, 7, and 8. We conclude that there is a growing need to build infrastructure across cohort studies to encourage and support collaborative research. It is also clear that there is a great need to value and support the lifelong volunteers and the researchers who initiate and run longitudinal studies in order to realize the full scientific potential of life course research.

9.1 Introduction

The authors of the three preceding chapters provide excellent reviews of their respective topics: methodological and practical issues in carrying out intergenerational cohort studies (Chapter 6); an overview of the potential for family-based life course studies in low and middle income countries (LMIC) (Chapter 7); and the validity and reliability of proxy informants and their use in family-based studies (Chapter 8).

We summarize the origins of some of the existing life course studies and the current potential for using these studies to address family-based life course questions. We highlight important methodological and practical issues for the future conduct of such studies raised in Chapters 6, 7, and 8.

9.2 The developmental origins of life course studies matters

Kuh and Ben-Shlomo define life course epidemiology as the study of the long term impacts on adult disease of social, biological, behavioural and psychological processes operating during gestation, childhood, adolescence, adulthood, and between generations.[1] Life course epidemiology therefore is specifically interested in how the characteristics of one generation influence those of the next, either through genetics, behaviour, and social characteristics or through biological programming at critical or sensitive developmental stages. While we agree with the authors of Chapter 7 that the term 'life course epidemiology' is recent (coined in 1997[2]), ideas of intergenerational and early life effects on adult health and vitality are not new, indeed were seen as conventional wisdom in the early 20th century.[3, 4] For example, Kermack and colleagues (1934) interpreted their cohort analysis of age-specific death rates that showed that mortality risk of each successive generation was lower at each 5 year age group from age 10–14 years as evidence that 'the expectation of life was determined by the conditions which existed during a child's earlier years' (p.703).[5] They suggested that the delay in the reduction in the infant mortality rate that lagged behind by a generation was due to infant health being dependent on the health of the mother. The post war revival in these ideas has been due to growing empirical evidence from maturing birth cohort studies and revitalized historical cohort studies that early life experience matters for later health. Within chronic disease epidemiology, testing the fetal origins of adult disease hypothesis[6] has been a major catalyst for this research. Distinguishing the biological, social, and psychological pathways that link childhood exposures and experiences and adult health has drawn heavily on the theoretical strengths of other disciplines, particularly developmental psychology,[7] that recognize that we need a combination of research strategies, including family-based studies to address such questions.[8]

Chapter 7 questions whether the term 'life course study' is redundant. We believe it is a useful generic term to distinguish those cohort studies that have information from at least one stage of development (gestation, childhood or adolescence) and in adult life. The developmental stage at which a life course study begins depends on the underlying research questions and the hypotheses to be tested; these are influenced by the social context at the time, as well as by scientific understanding. The initial research questions for the older national birth cohorts did not focus on long-term outcomes. For the 1946 British birth cohort (the Medical Research Council (MRC) National Survey of Health and Development (NSHD)), information was first collected from the mother when her baby was about eight weeks old and the focus was on the social and economic costs of pregnancy and birth and standards of health care received. Dr James Douglas, who directed the maternity survey, seized the opportunity of following a subset of this nationally representative sample to observe their health, growth and development.[9] Douglas was aware of the research emanating from the US child development studies of the 1920s–1940s. The initial research questions for the birth cohorts set up in the 1950s and 1960s (such as the UK 1958 birth cohort, the US Perinatal Collaborative Cohorts 1958–76, the Helsinki cohort 1955, the Danish Prospective Perinatal project 1959 and the North Finland cohort 1966) concerned the 'continuum of reproductive wastage.' These cohort studies focused on fetal and obstetric influences on pregnancy outcome, and perinatal and social determinants of subsequent neurological and neurosensory childhood conditions associated with later handicap. There was active collaboration between the investigators of some of these US and UK birth cohort studies.

Understanding childhood mental retardation and learning difficulties was also the catalyst for the Scottish mental health surveys where the entire Scottish population aged 11 in 1932 and 1947 were tested for mental ability; they have become the basis for historical cohort studies in Aberdeen and Edinburgh.[10] In the US, the other main source for historical cohort studies has been the pre-war studies of child growth and development that grew out of the new discipline of developmental psychology.[11] In the UK in contrast, the historical cohorts, such as the Hertfordshire birth cohorts of 1921–30 and 1935–39 have been based on birth and infant records where the initial aim was to provide information that could lead to improvements in the health of the mother and her baby.[6] The origins of these records lay in concerns about the high infant mortality rates in the early twentieth century. In Aberdeen, the presence of the Maternal and Neonatal Databank established by Dugald Baird in 1948, together with the US-funded Aberdeen 1964 reading survey of schoolchildren born 1950–56, which included a number of siblings, and linkage to Scottish school and health records, has made the Aberdeen Children of the 1950s study a particularly valuable resource.[12–15] As Chapter 6 points out there were active collaborations between the investigators on these surveys and similar surveys being carried out in Denmark at the same time (e.g. Metropolit cohort).

For the British birth cohorts the rationale for following participants into adulthood and thus becoming 'life course studies' evolved over time. During the childhood and adolescent years the focus was on the effects of the home and the school on educational and cognitive development, and later on early adult work and fertility outcomes. In adult life, the UK birth cohorts have had diverging interests: the 1946 birth cohort study funded by the Medical Research Council (MRC) has had a greater focus on testing life course hypotheses that link earlier exposures to adult health, biological function and disease; in contrast, the 1958 (NCDS) and 1970 birth cohort studies, funded by the Economic and Social Research Council (ESRC), have maintained a greater focus on social and economic outcomes and have become a general resource for social scientists.

In the US, funding for the Perinatal Collaborative Cohorts did not continue beyond seven years, they were casualties of the prevailing climate in the late 1960s and 1970s which questioned the value of longitudinal studies[16] and the attention placed on critical development periods at the expense of attention on risk factors at later life stages.[17] Criticisms of the pre-war US child development studies included the fact that they were unrepresentative and ungeneralizable, had collected unanalysable or inappropriate data, and had made serious errors in measuring individual change over time. Even Dr James Douglas was affected by the climate of opinion. In his evidence to the review of longitudinal studies[16] he noted in relation to the NHSD: 'I find it difficult to know what will happen after these young people are 25. The problems of keeping contact with them are certain to increase, and from many points of view the sample becomes in any event unsatisfactory. For example, marriages and births are so widely spread that it would be very many years before we would have an adequate return, and it would be a complex and rather messy administrative problem to arrange, for example, that the mothers were seen and the infants assessed at a specific date after confinement and thereafter at various intervals. I think it is likely that after these young people are 25 we will be content to get as much information fed back to us as possible from official sources …. While it is unlikely that we will keep close personal touch with all the individual members of the sample after 25 there may well be some special groups that we will follow'.(pp. 196–7)

Despite this climate, well-designed and pioneering life course studies in the 1970s showed that children of below-average weight who became overweight as adults were more likely to suffer from hypertensive vascular disease and cardiovascular renal disease,[18] and investigated the long-term effects of famine exposure *in utero* on mental performance.[19] In epidemiology from the 1980s, the scientific rationale for the revitalisation of many historical cohort studies, was the growing research interest in the effects of prenatal and postnatal factors on adult disease, largely inspired by the Barker hypothesis of the fetal origins of cardiovascular disease. The blossoming theories of the developmental origins of adult health and disease have also led to continued MRC funding for the 1946 birth cohort and for the biomedical sweep of the 1958 cohort, and encouraged investigators on many of the new cohort studies to start collecting information during pregnancy or before conception (see Chapter 6). One exception is the UK Millennium Cohort which did not collect its initial information until the index child was nine months old. Although this was driven by logistic and financial considerations, the questions that UK social scientists wish to address using data from this cohort are less focused on investigating the effect of fetal exposures on offspring health, putting a greater emphasis on socioeconomic data.[20]

Chapter 7 documents a number of birth cohort studies of reasonable size in low and middle income countries. Most of these are recent but some started as early as the 1970s. It would be fascinating to learn where the origins of those studies lay and their original justification.

Despite the varied origins and histories of birth and historical cohort studies there is a need to exploit the overlapping areas of these studies for cross-cohort comparisons and harmonize core measures wherever possible for future comparative study, including cohorts from LMICs. Some of the reasons proposed in Chapter 7 in support of conducting studies in LMICs are relevant when considering the value of cross-cohort comparisons in general. Inter-cohort comparisons are a useful way of testing the robustness of findings. Collaboration between cohorts allows for an immediate replication of a finding and tests its robustness to different populations (with different composition of exposures and potential confounding structures as pointed out in Chapter 7), different measurement and study design. When results vary by cohort, bias or confounding are difficult to rule out as potential explanations (see Chapter 6). However, by understanding the socioeconomic environment that each cohort experienced during childhood, there may be instances where prediction of differences and the testing of these is possible and informative.

9.3 Incorporating family-based designs into life course studies: current potential in the older life course studies

All three chapters in this section acknowledge the importance of intergenerational studies. Chapter 6 highlights the impact of maternal characteristics and behaviours before and during pregnancy and how often they influence the health of offspring; Chapter 7 highlights the importance of maternal under-nutrition and exposure to toxins in LMIC; and Chapter 8 provides a useful reminder of the necessity of using proxy informants across generations (parents reporting for children in the child's early life and vice versa when parents have aged). What we consider as intergenerational information, what intergenerational information has already been collected, and what intergenerational hypotheses can be tested in the mature cohort studies using this information are questions worth further discussion.

9.3.1 Parents and grandparents

Birth cohorts must, by the nature of the early childhood follow-ups, be 'family-based'. As discussed in Chapter 8, information in infancy and early childhood is provided by a parent or guardian, most often the mother. Most birth cohorts collect information about the family home and environment in which the cohort member is growing up. Some have also collected data relating to parents such as their education, occupation, and heights and weights, generally without explicit inter-generational hypotheses in mind. Once the cohort members reach adulthood, studies may collect information from cohort members on parental morbidity and death. While the role of a proxy informant is problematic (Chapter 8) some of these data can be confirmed through death registrations and hospital records.

Almost all cohort studies collect information on parental social class when the cohort members were children, often describing this as 'childhood social class' losing sight of the fact it is a parental characteristic. Considerable research has shown that low childhood social class (i.e. parental social class) is associated with increased risk of later mortality and morbidity over and above the association with own adult social class.[21–23] Potential mechanisms or pathways by which childhood social class influences health may be either through intergenerational continuity of social class, education, and health behaviours or through accumulation of biological insults to the individual throughout life. Epidemiologists are generally more concerned with elucidating biological rather than social or psychological pathways so often view family characteristics as 'noise' that needs to be controlled for. Sociologists and economists have explicitly investigated the impact of intergenerational social mobility on adult health. Competing hypotheses are that downward social mobility is the cause of additional damage to health or the consequence of poor prior health.[24] Such social mobility hypotheses do not require birth cohorts, but ideally require follow-up from childhood that can identify the health and social characteristics of the individual, their family and the wider social context that influence adult socioeconomic destinations. These studies have their origins in the intergenerational social class and income mobility studies that were a feature of the 1970s and 1980s.[25, 26]

Investigators on the Aberdeen Children of the 1950s cohort study have been able to exploit the unique data that Baird recorded to investigate the influence of grandparent characteristics on the health of grandchildren. For example, they showed that the effects of the social class of grandparents influenced the birth weight of their grandchildren through influencing the childhood growth of the mother (see Chapters 2 and 10). As well as considering how maternal characteristics influence offspring health (Chapter 6), reproductive characteristics may serve as sentinels of later chronic disease (See Chapter 15 for a detailed discussion). Further, by assessing the relative strengths of the association between offspring birth weight and maternal and paternal mortality, the relative contribution of genetic and intrauterine factors can be investigated (see Chapters 2 and 13). The 1958 British birth cohort carried out such an analysis, using mortality registrations obtained after tracing the parents of the cohort members,[27] showing stronger associations with maternal mortality consistent with the fetal origins hypothesis.[28] However, such comparisons can be hampered by the greater missing data and measurement error in the paternal information (as discussed in all three chapters). The Mater-University Study of Pregnancy in Australia[29] and ALSPAC[30] have two parallel cohorts having followed up the offspring through childhood and adolescence and their mothers from pregnancy and are thus also able to investigate the associations between pregnancy characteristics and later maternal health.

Developmental and life span psychologists and psychiatrists have also made use of these broad based birth cohort studies to study continuity and discontinuity in psychopathology between childhood and adulthood.[31–33] In addition, they have used more focused longitudinal studies, and a range of family-based and genetic study designs to identify potential causal factors or processes that may be amenable to intervention.[7] Intergenerational factors, whether parental behaviour or genetic predisposition, are major features of these studies.

9.3.2 Offspring

Basic information on the offspring of the index cohort members, such as the date of birth and sex of each child, has also been collected in existing cohort studies, where the cohort member is generally the proxy informant (Chapter 8) for this next generation and even the one after that (i.e. reporting on birth of grandchildren). Some cohort studies, including the British 1946 and 1958 cohort studies, carried out special offspring studies, collecting data from offspring and not simply relying on maternal reports. Collecting data on offspring of the index cohort is difficult (Chapter 7) as children are born over 20–30 years. This means that findings based on this information do not become available until long after the data collection has been initiated. More restrictive designs may be necessary in practice but these may limit the generalisability of the findings. For example, the NSHD conducted a sub-study on the first born offspring of the cohort members, but only offspring that were born when mothers were aged 20–25 years. The offspring were followed up at 4 and 8 years, with the initial aim being to compare generation differences in child rearing, pre-school education, and verbal attainment.[34, 35] Similarly for the 1958 cohort study more detailed information was recorded on the offspring of a randomly selected sub-sample of one third of the cohort members who had children by 1991.[27, 36]

Such data are now being used to assess the link between pregnancy outcomes and subsequent maternal health in midlife.[37, 38] to address hypotheses similar to those investigated when linking birth weight of the cohort members themselves with parental mortality (see Section 9.3.1). When the mother is the cohort member, more detailed information on health outcomes and potential confounding variables are available. This work has shown that mothers who have had a low birth weight or pre-term baby are more likely to develop diabetes and cardiovascular disease in later life.[28, 38] These studies have also been used to assess life course maternal influences, such as growth, on the birth weight of her offspring.[39]

9.3.3 Siblings

All three chapters in this section discuss sibling studies. As detailed in Chapters 3 and 4, sibling and twin studies are a valuable resource for life course studies as they can help disentangle the effects of nature and nurture. The US collaborative cohorts collected birth information over a number of years and thus their samples contain a fairly high proportion of siblings and the follow-up of these cohorts is making use of this as a design feature (http://www.cumc.columbia.edu/dept/imprints/index.html). Similarly, the Aberdeen Children of the 1950s study has sibling pairs as it was based on a cohort of children born between 1950 and 1956 who had been included in a reading survey in 1962. The lack of any association between birth weight and childhood intelligence within sibling pairs from this study,[13] and also a recent analysis of the US National Longitudinal Study of Youth,[40] suggests that the association is largely explained by fixed family effects that are constant from one pregnancy to the next. In studies that do not explicitly collect information on siblings, information on, for example, number of siblings is collected so as to relate family size and birth order to later health outcomes.[41, 42]

9.4 Incorporating family-based designs into new birth cohorts

As discussed in Chapter 6, many new birth and pre-conceptual cohorts have recently started or are currently being planned. Those investigating the impact of fetal exposures on offspring health have to be started during pregnancy and, as yet, have only followed participants into childhood (the cohorts on http://www.birthcohorts.net are mostly young, born around the year 2000). The long term consequences on adult health in these studies will not be known for 50 years. Chapter 6 rightly makes the point that the new birth cohorts should avoid being a 'source for self-perpetuating research on fetal exposures'.

As detailed in Chapter 6, some of these new birth cohort studies are much larger than the older cohorts (including 100,000 pregnancies) and come with a biobank containing samples from the mothers and sometimes the fathers as well as from the infants. The benefits of these large prospective cohorts, detailed elsewhere,[43] include the ability to test genetic as well as environmental risk factors and their interaction, or to use genetic factors to elucidate environmental causes of disease through Mendelian Randomisation. The debate regarding the benefits of 'large thin' as opposed to 'small thick' cohorts is ongoing, but there is a general consensus that massive sample sizes are gained at the expense of quality and richness of the phenotypic and environmental measures[43–45] which may limit their usefulness for some other research questions. It clearly helps when these cohorts are set up in countries, such as Norway and Denmark, where there is excellent linkage of electronic health records.

9.5 Running a long term study: example of the MRC National Survey of Health and Development

In this section, we use our experience on the 1946 British birth cohort (MRC NSHD) to discuss some of the challenges of running a long-term prospective study. Decisions about study design and focus do not end with enrolment of a new birth cohort. The MRC NSHD, the oldest birth cohort study with an original sample size of 5,362, and more than 20 follow-ups on the whole sample, has inevitably changed its scientific focus as it addresses the issues of each life stage and incorporates advances in scientific knowledge (Section 9.2).[46] In the 1980s the second director, Professor Michael Wadsworth, influenced by the new cohort studies of ageing in North America and Europe, was responsible for the decision to train research nurses to undertake home visits at 36, 43, and 53 years to measure health in terms of biological function, such as blood pressure, lung function, memory and concentration, and strength and balance. This gave the NSHD its unique value, not foreseen at initiation of the study in 1946, namely the ability to trace the influence of physical and cognitive developmental trajectories from birth through to adolescence, and lifetime health and social circumstances, on these adult quantitative traits. Despite the richness of the dataset, there is information it might seem astonishing that the study did not collect. As in the Aberdeen Children of the 1950s study (Chapter 7), the NSHD did not collect information on parental smoking habits at the birth of the cohort as this was prior to Doll and Hill's publications on smoking and lung cancer and mortality.[47, 48]

Study members are now 62 years old and the new MRC-funded five year research programme is designed to capitalize on the study's strengths as a life course study of ageing. A new clinic data collection will enrich NSHD by not only repeating measures of social environment and biological function but also by establishing new baseline measures of cardiac and vascular structure and function, bone density and body composition, and a wide range of metabolic factors and other biochemical markers.

Thus, the size, scientific strengths, and national representativeness of NSHD encourages a 'small thick' study design that focuses on intensively phenotyping the cohort member. The rationale for collecting information on parental and offspring circumstances is to understand the health of cohort members. Other cohorts will have a different balance of strengths, depending on size, geographical distribution of the sample, and age, and some may be more appropriate for family-based designs described in other chapters of this book. Cohorts based in a restricted geographical area are able to carry out clinic measurements more easily as only a single central clinic is required. The NSHD, and the other British birth cohorts, have previously used home visits by interviewers or nurses so it has been important to demonstrate in a feasibility study that NSHD cohort members are prepared to travel some distance to attend clinics.

We wholeheartedly agree with Chapter 6 in highlighting the need for dedication, documentation, and data sharing. One challenge to researchers running a study is to balance immediate aims of the study with data necessary for longer term goals. Funding bodies will want to see an immediate return on their investment, and research careers are dependent on publications. There is no agreed system for rewarding investigators for the time and effort given to running studies, maintaining response rates and collecting high quality data. Jones *et al.* warned in 1960 that 'the scientific worker who likes to move swiftly from one hypothesis to the next may feel frustrated in such a slow research milieu'.[49] Garn (1965), in a presentation to a Colloquium on Longitudinal Studies organised by the National Institute of Child Health and Development in Bethesda in 1965 had argued that what he called 'someday' or 'Methuselah' research forces a worker to choose between professional immobility or the abandonment of many years of work without evident result. Some believed it was only the mediocre that would accept the restriction of their professional interests to collect similar kinds of data on the same individual; this was contested by Wall and Williams,[16] although they recognized that particular difficulties arose where the programme of data collection is so considerable that no time is allowed for concurrent analysis and feed-back. We hope that in 2008, with the maturing of a number of life course studies, the revival of life course epidemiology, the richness of life course hypotheses and analysis, and the growing cross-cohort collaborations that this work is more highly valued.

Many of the practical issues raised in the previous three chapters have arisen in the NSHD. To maintain attachment of the cohort members to the study, a birthday card with a letter giving recent research findings is sent to each cohort member each year. It is, however, difficult to assess the success of different strategies to improve response rates in long-running cohorts. Feedback of information may help to maintain the participation of cohort members and must be undertaken when duty of care issues exist. In the NSHD, a plethora of ethically approved strategies detail how clinically relevant results are fed back to the cohort members directly or via GPs, and immediate action is taken where necessary. By necessity this means that the cohort study is no longer completely observational in design, but the health of cohort members must be the primary concern. Medical Research Ethics Committees are increasingly involved in approving research strategies for informed consent in situations where the cohort member no longer has the capacity to give consent. This is one of the situations, as detailed in Chapter 8, in which a proxy respondent is then required. Documentation in long term studies is of paramount importance for future researchers and for data sharing. It would be helpful to have an agreed classification system for storing variables and classifying metadata within life course studies that integrate biomedical and social data. Data sharing systems are evolving to meet the needs of both biomedical and social scientists and to ensure data security and participant confidentiality for the lifelong volunteers on whom these longitudinal studies depend.

9.6 Conclusions and lessons for the future

All birth cohort studies and many other life course cohorts have at least some inter-generational information, either on parents, siblings and/or offspring. It has to be considered carefully whether it is worth collecting more prior generation and/or offspring generation data in these established cohorts given the practical difficulties and costs associated with such an undertaking as detailed in Chapters 6, 7, and 8. As described in Chapter 8, if proxies are used, careful consideration of the questions asked, the mode of data collection and the selection of the proxy are required. More evidence on which to base such decisions is clearly required (Chapter 8).

Chapters 6 and 7 touch on the question of what the ideal family-based study would be. Chapter 7 suggest that the ideal intergenerational study will have information on two or more generations—grandparents, parents, and offspring- and in addition the ideal family-based study would have data on siblings and cousins. This is not necessarily needed to answer every type of intergenerational and family-based hypothesis and different academic disciplines will have different priorities for life course research. Both chapters focus on studies which start from birth or before. However, the decades required for these studies to mature means that studies starting at other phases of the life course to address current inter-generational hypotheses should also be considered.

There is a growing need to build infrastructure across cohort studies to encourage and support collaborative research. Cross-cohort comparisons require data-sharing and collaboration between cohorts to harmonize data. In order to obtain funding for a cohort, however, there needs to be unique aspects of each study, while still collecting a common core of measures to assist comparative research. In order for future inter-generational and cross-cohort comparison to continue, building capacity for life course research is vital. Training of future generations of researchers should include the practicalities of data collection and running studies as well as the analytical and epidemiological techniques. There is a great need to value and support the lifelong volunteers and the researchers who initiate and run longitudinal studies in order to realize the full scientific potential of life course research.

References

1 **Kuh D, Ben-Shlomo Y.** *A Life Course Approach to Chronic Disease Epidemiology.* Oxford, Oxford University Press, 2004.
2 **Kuh D, Ben-Shlomo Y.** *A Life Course Approach to Chronic Disease Epidemiology; tracing the origins of ill-health from early to adult life.* Oxford, Oxford University Press, 1997.
3 **Kuh D, Davey Smith G.** When is mortality risk determined? Historical insights into a current debate. *Soc Hist Med* 1993; **6**: 101–23.
4 **Kuh D, Davey Smith G.** The life course and adult chronic disease: an historical perspective with particular reference to coronary heart disease. In: Kuh D, Ben-Shlomo Y, eds. *A life course approach to chronic disease epidemiology*. Oxford, Oxford University Press, pp. 15–37, 2004.
5 **Kermack WO, McKendrick AG, McKinlay PL.** Death rates in Great Britain and Sweden: Some general regularities and their significance. *Lancet* 1934; **226**: 698–703.
6 **Barker DJP.** *Mothers, Babies and Health in Later Life.* Edinburgh, Churchill Livingstone, 1998.
7 **Rutter M, Kim-Cohen J, Maughan B.** Continuities and discontinuities in psychopathology between childhood and adult life. *J Child Psychol Psychiatry* 2006; **47**: 276–95.
8 **Rutter M, Pickles A, Murray R, Eaves L.** Testing hypotheses on specific environmental causal effects on behavior. *Psychol Bull* 2001; **127**: 291–324.
9 **Douglas JWB.** *Children under five.* London, Allen & Unwin, 1958.
10 **Deary IJ, Whiteman MC, Starr JM, Whalley LJ, Fox HC.** The impact of childhood intelligence on later life: following up the Scottish mental surveys of 1932 and 1947. *J Pers Soc Psychol* 2004; **86**: 130–47.
11 **Cravens H.** Behaviorism Revisited: Developmental Science, the Maturation Theory, and the Biological Basis of the Human Mind, 1920s-1950s. In: Benson KR, Maienschein J, Rainger R, eds. *The Expansion of American Biology*. New Brunswick, Rutgers University Press, pp. 133–63, 1991.
12 **Batty GD, Morton SMB, Campbell D et al.** The Aberdeen Children of the 1950s cohort study: background, methods, and follow-uo information on a new resource for the study of life course and intergenerational influences on health. *Paediatr Perinat Epidemiol* 2004; **18**: 221–39.
13 **Lawlor DA, Clark H, Davey Smith G, Leon DA.** Intrauterine growth and intelligence within sibling pairs: findings from the Aberdeen children of the 1950s cohort. *Pediatrics* 2006; **117**: e894–e902.
14 **Leon DA, Lawlor DA, Clark H, MacIntyre S.** Cohort profile: the Aberdeen children of the 1950s study. *Int J Epidemiol* 2006; **35**: 549–52.
15 **Nitsch D, Morton S, DeStavola BL, Clark H, Leon DA.** How good is probabilistic record linkage to reconstruct reproductive histories? Results from the Aberdeen Children of the 1950s study. *BMC Med Res Methodol* 2006; **6**: 15.
16 **Wall WD, Williams HL.** *Longitudinal Studies and the Social Sciences.* London, Heinemann Educational Books Ltd, 1970.
17 **Clarke AM, Clarke ADB.** The formative years? In: Clarke AM, Clarke ADB, eds. *Early Experience: Myth and Evidence*. New York, The Free Press, 1976.
18 **Abraham S, Collins G, Nordsieck M.** Relationship of childhood weight status to morbidity in adults. *HSMHA Health Reports* 1971; **86**: 273–84.
19 **Stein Z, Susser M.** The Dutch famine, 1944-1945, and the reproductive process. I. Effects on six indices at birth. *Pediatric Research* 1975; **9**(2): 70–6.

20 Smith K, Joshi H. The millennium cohort study. *Pop Trends* 2002; **107**: 30–4.
21 Davey Smith G, Lynch J. Life course approaches to socioeconomic differentials in health. In: Kuh D, Ben-Shlomo Y, eds. *A Life Course Approach to Chronic Disease Epidemiology*. Oxford, Oxford University Press, 2004.
22 Lawlor DA, Sterne JA, Tynelius P, Davey Smith G, Rasmussen F. Association of childhood socioeconomic position with cause-specific mortality in a prospective record linkage study of 1,839,384 individuals. *Am J Epidemiol* 2006; **164**: 907–15.
23 Power C, Kuh D. Life course development of unequal health. In: Siegrist J, Marmot M, eds. *Social Inequalities in Health. New Evidence and Policy Implications*. New York, Oxford University Press, pp. 27–54, 2006.
24 Chandola T, Bartley M, Sacker A, Jenkinson C, Marmot M. Health selection in the Whitehall II study, UK. *Soc Sci Med* 2003; **56**: 2059–72.
25 Atkinson AB, Maynard AK, Trinder GG. *Parents and Children: incomes in two generations*. London, Heinemann Educational Books, 1983.
26 Goldthorpe JH. *Social Mobility and Class Structure in Modern Britain*. Oxford, Clarendon Press, 1980.
27 Hypponen E, Davey Smith G, Shepherd P, Power C. An intergenerational and lifecourse study of health and mortality risk in parents of the 1958 birth cohort: (I). methods and tracing. *Public Health* 2005; **119**: 599–607.
28 Davey Smith G, Hypponen E, Power C, Lawlor DA. Offspring birth weight and parental mortality: prospective observational study and meta-analysis. *Am J Epidemiol* 2007; **166**: 160–9.
29 Najman JM, Bor W, O'Callaghan M, Williams GM, Aird R, Shuttlewood G. Cohort Profile: The Mater-University of Queensland Study of Pregnancy (MUSP). *Int J Epidemiol* 2005; **34**: 992–7.
30 Golding J, Pembrey M, Jones R. ALSPAC—the Avon Longitudinal Study of Parents and Children. I Study methodology. *Paediatr Perinat Epidemiol* 2001; **15**: 74–87.
31 Clark C, Rodgers B, Caldwell T, Power C, Stansfeld S. Childhood and adulthood psychological ill health as predictors of midlife affective and anxiety disorders: the 1958 British Birth Cohort. *Arch Gen Psychiatry* 2007; **64**: 668–78.
32 Colman I, Ploubidis GB, Wadsworth ME, Jones PB, Croudace TJ. A longitudinal typology of symptoms of depression and anxiety over the life course. *Biol Psychiatry* 2007; **62**: 1265–71.
33 Rutter M, Kim-Cohen J, Maughan B. Continuities and discontinuities in psychopathology between childhood and adult life. *J Child Psychol Psychiatry* 2006; **47**: 276–95.
34 Wadsworth MEJ. Effects of parenting style and preschool experience on children's verbal attainment: a British longitudinal study. *Early Childhood Res Quarterly* 1986; **1**: 237–48.
35 Wadsworth MEJ. Social class and generation differences in pre-school education. *British Journal of Sociology* 1981; **32**: 560–82.
36 Li L, Power C. Influences on childhood height: comparing two generations in the 1958 British birth cohort. *Int J Epidemiol* 2004; **33**: 1320–8.
37 Hypponen E, Davey Smith G, Power C. Parental diabetes and birth weight of offspring: intergenerational cohort study. *BMJ* 2003; **326**: 19–20.
38 Kuh D, Mishra GD, Black S *et al*. Offspring birth weight, gestational age and maternal characteristics in relation to glucose status at age 53 years: evidence from a national birth cohort. *Diabet Med* 2008; **25**: 530–5.
39 Hypponen E, Power C, Davey Smith G. Parental growth at different life stages and offspring birthweight: an intergenerational cohort study. *Paediatr Perinat Epidemiol* 2004; **18**: 168–77.
40 Yang S, Lynch J, Susser ES, Lawlor DA. Birthweight and Cognitive Ability in Childhood among Siblings and Non-siblings. *Pediatrics* 2008; **122**: e350–e358.
41 Li L, Dangour AD, Power C. Early life influences on adult leg and trunk length in the 1958 British birth cohort. *Am J Hum Biol* 2007; **19**: 836–43.

42 **Rudnicka AR, Owen CG, Richards M, Wadsworth ME, Strachan DP.** Effect of breastfeeding and sociodemographic factors on visual outcome in childhood and adolescence. *Am J Clin Nutr* 2008; **87**: 1392–9.

43 **Stoltenberg C, Pickles A.** Designs for large life course studies of genetic effects. In: Pickles A, Maughan B, Wadsworth M, eds. *Epidemiological Methods in Life Course Research*. Oxford, Oxford University Press, pp. 81–109, 2007.

44 **Foster MW, Sharp RR.** Will investments in large-scale prospective cohorts and biobanks limit our ability to discover weaker, less common genetic and environmental contributors to complex diseases? *Environ Health Perspect* 2005; **113**: 119–22.

45 **Wong MY, Day NE, Luan JA, Chan KP, Wareham NJ.** The detection of gene-environment interaction for continuous traits: should we deal with measurement error by bigger studies or better measurement? *Int J Epidemiol* 2003; **32**: 51–7.

46 **Wadsworth M, Kuh D, Richards M, Hardy R.** Cohort Profile: The 1946 National Birth Cohort (MRC National Survey of Health and Development). *Int J Epidemiol* 2006; **35**: 49–54.

47 **Doll R, Hill AB.** Smoking and carcinoma of the lung: preliminary report. *Br Med J* 1950; 739–48.

48 **Doll R, Hill AB.** The mortality of doctors in relation to their smoking habits; a preliminary report. *Br Med J* 1954; **1**: 1451–5.

49 **Jones HE, Macfarlane JW, Eichorn DH.** A progress report on growth studies at the University of California. *Vita Hum Int Z Lebensalterforsch* 1960; **3**: 17–31.

Part III

Statistical methods in family-based studies

Chapter 10

Statistical considerations in intergenerational studies

Dorothea Nitsch and Gita D Mishra

Abstract

Intergenerational data necessarily reflect the time and place that the different generations of participants were living in. This chapter describes some of the statistical issues that arise specifically from analysing data over several generations of individuals. It aims first to introduce simple concepts to provide an understanding of the founding assumptions and principles, before moving on to more complex analytic methods. As the objectives of analyses may vary substantially across intergenerational studies, there is no easy guideline for analyses, except perhaps that some *a priori* clarity on the main associations of interest is crucial. Since parents and their offspring are genetically related, intergenerational studies are to some extent genetically informative even if no genotyping was performed. Much of the analyses are concerned with identifying or unravelling the relationship between outcomes and genetic and environmental factors. Ways of handling missing data as well as approaches to deal with non-paternity will also be discussed. Illustrative examples are drawn from the Aberdeen *Children of the 1950s* cohort study and from the MRC National Survey of Health and Development (NSHD) birth cohort study.

10.1 **Introduction**

Intergenerational studies, as defined here, hold data on familial related participants from more than one generation, for example data on parents and their children. In life course epidemiology the interest lies usually in the long term effects of being raised in a certain environment. In such a setting, intergenerational studies may be helpful to distinguish familial effects from a range of non-familiar factors, such as the effects of particular life events, secular change, specific risk factors, and exposures at a given particular age/developmental stage (Figure 10.1).

Everyone will be familiar with the notion that relatives are more likely to have certain features in common than other unrelated people. Mendelian laws govern the inheritance of traits in families, so that for each pair of chromosomes present in the offspring one chromosome is received from the father and the other from its mother. It follows that a child inherits 50% of its genes from each parent (Figure 10.2). In most cases this holds true even if the genetic variation itself that gives rise to the trait of interest is not measured (genotyped). This in turn means that the correlation of a trait between parent and offspring provides a measure for the expression of the extent of shared inherited information. It was this topic that helped establish the important

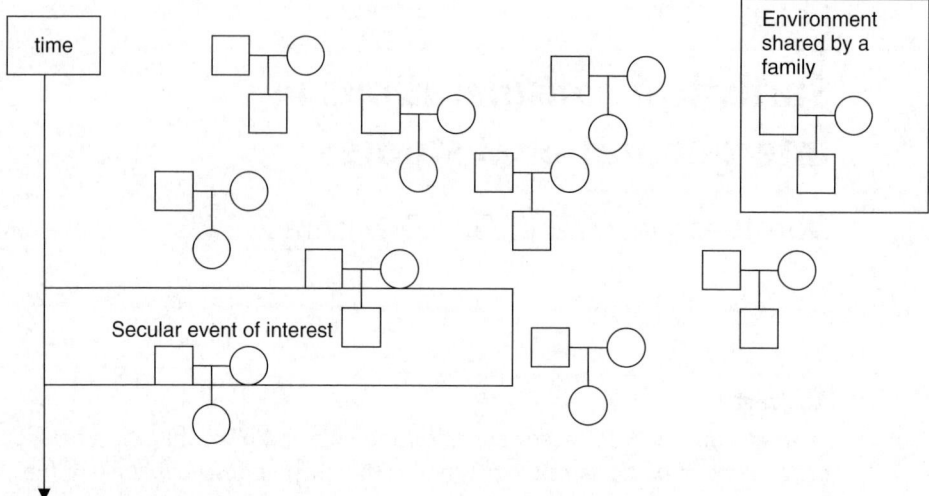

Fig.10.1 Intergenerational studies and different variables of interest.

Circles denote women, squares denote men. The vertical connections denote the child of the parents (circles and squares joined by a horizontal line), i.e. the genetic relation amongst family members.

Some major event of interest, for example a famine, or an earthquake, may affect some, but not all members of families at a given point in time. There may be some families where all members are sharing a given environment, as opposed to other families who share a different environment.

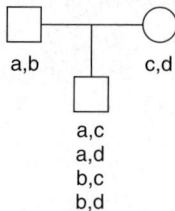

Fig. 10.2 Pedigree showing a trio of two parents (father: box; mother: circle) and their offspring, with all possible genotype combinations for the offspring given the parental genotypes under Mendelian inheritance.

principles of linear regression analysis by examining if the height of a son was a function of the height of the father.[1] Studies of those with a disease and their parents have also been used to identify potential genes causing disease.[2]

Similarities amongst family members may not only be due to shared genetic information but they can also be described as a function of shared behavioural characteristics and/or shared external influences. The tension between what is perceived as behavioural, or modifiable, versus genetic or heritable effects is often parameterized at its most simplest, in statistical modelling terms, as a dichotomy of 'genetic' (G) and 'environmental' (E) effects that determine the trait or phenotype of interest (Y) in the offspring.

$$Y = G + E \tag{10.1}$$

Depending on the study question, the aim of analysis may be to separate out different parts of equation (10.1) whilst controlling for, but not necessarily estimating, the effect of the other.

In an extreme case this may lead to treating the whole family as a single unit for comparisons of the effects of other environmental exposures. One classic example from life course epidemiology is the comparison of rates of mental illness in offspring of migrant families with rates in offspring of local resident families to determine the extent that social stressors related to migration cause mental disease, as opposed to the hypothesis that the presence of mental disease leads to subsequent social decline.[3]

After a brief excursion on possible data sources for intergenerational studies, simple analyses on data from two generations (parents and offspring) will be described to illustrate the main points that extend to analytical approaches for data on three generations. Ways of handling missing data, as well as possible approaches to deal with non-paternity, are also discussed briefly. At the end of the chapter (after the references) we provide complete Stata codes for all of the examples in the chapter. They do require anyone wanting to use them to be familiar with the statistical software.

10.2 Design features of intergenerational studies

Recent years have seen vast developments in terms of setting up large population based cohort studies. Some countries have a long tradition in standardized recording of health data, for example the Scandinavian Countries, Canada, and Scotland. The simultaneous existence of a national identification number opens the possibility to assemble in a short period of time large datasets spanning several generations and to link various characteristics of individuals across generations.[4] In some countries, large scale birth cohort studies have been conducted that also include data on the parents of participants (see Chapter 6 for more details). Examples of such studies include the Avon Longitudinal Study on Parents and Children (ALSPAC), the MRC National Survey of Health and Development (NSHD) or the 1946 British birth cohort, and the National Child Development Study (NCDS) or the 1958 British birth cohort.[5–7]

If individuals of a given age were sampled at random from a general population at a given point in time and subsequently linked to data on their offspring, it is assumed that all of the index participants (parents and 'non-parents') are representative of the general population of their age, as well as their offspring being representative of offspring of such a cohort as a whole at that time and place. An example of this type of study is the Southampton Women's survey, which recruited a random sample of women of reproductive age and plans to collect data on all offspring of these women.[8] A more common study design in life course epidemiology, however, involves sampling children from births in a given country or population, in a given year to form a birth cohort (for example, the British 1946 (known as NSHD),[5] 1958 (NCDS)[7] or 1970s birth cohort[9]), or sampling pregnant women from a given population at a given time (for example, ALSPAC[6] or Mater University Study of Pregnancy (MUSP)[10]), with the subsequent gathering of information on both parents and offspring. Such parents of a birth/pregnancy cohort may represent a selected group of individuals who reflect the social determinants of starting a family at that given point in time. For example, Hypponen E *et al.* showed that mortality rates of parents of the 1958 birth cohort were lower than for the general population of the same age.[11]

In times of rising general mobility, the long term follow up of members of a family is an increasingly complex task. This need not be seen as a drawback—rather, if it is possible to follow up participants who have migrated, it may provide a unique opportunity to perform within cohort comparisons of the longitudinal effect of migration on outcomes.

In contrast to population based intergenerational datasets, there have been several large disease oriented studies where the main aim was the identification of genetic variants causing disease.

In such family-based studies, in order to minimize costs and to maximize power to detect genetic effects, the sampling of families is usually predicated on some extremes of a trait/disease of interest in a given proband, a term that refers to the person who was sampled first with the subsequent identification of their other family members.[12] For example, for a study of hypertension only families with children displaying hypertension at an early age may have been recruited. When only sampling families from the extremes of a trait distribution, such as childhood hypertension, analyses and interpretation have to be conditional on the disease status in the proband, i.e. the hypertensive child.[2, 13, 14]

10.3 Analyses of data collected on two generations

The outcome of interest Y may be measured once or several times during follow-up of the family, both on parents and offspring (see detailed example of intergenerational studies of birth weight in Chapter 2). It may be normally distributed, or binary, or categorical. First, the situation of a single measurement of a normally distributed Y is considered—generalizations to other types of outcome are straightforward, with commands readily available in Stata[15] (Table 10.1). A general notation is used here, whereby suffixes p, m, and o represent paternal, maternal, and offspring values respectively, so for Y, the outcome trait of interest, becomes Y_p, Y_m, Y_o. Variables that refer to other (exposure and covariate) traits or characteristics are denoted by X with the same respective suffixes.

Depending on the study question, the outcome of interest may be a parental feature and/or a feature of the offspring. Due to the temporal ordering across generations (parents being born before their offspring) data on the subsequent generation are often treated as the outcome of the analyses. However, as discussed in detail in Chapter 2, this may not always be the case. For instance, Davey Smith *et al.* analyzed parental mortality as a function of offspring birth weight to quantify indirectly the extent that the relation between low birth weight and cardiovascular disease may be a genetic feature rather than due to early intrauterine environment predetermining later cardiovascular outcome.[16, 17]

Table 10.1 Variables and simple analysis methods for offspring outcome and parental data

Distribution of variable (one single measure of outcome per person)		Only offspring data as outcome	Stata command	Modeling jointly parental and offspring data as outcome	Stata command
Normal		Linear regression	regress	Multilevel model	xtmixed xtpcse
Binary	Without censoring	Logistic regression	logit logistic	Multilevel model	xtmelogit
	With censoring	Survival analysis, for example Cox regression	stcox	See text section 10.3.4.3.	See text
Categorical		Proportional odds model	ologit, omodel	See text section 10.3.4.1.	gllamm

10.3.1 Similar traits collected on two generations

We first introduce a few important concepts from quantitative genetics. Following on from the model given in the introduction, we can parameterize the variability of a trait Y, denoted as V_Y, as a function of

(i) the variability of the genes V_G that determine Y
(ii) the variability of other environmental variables V_E that may influence Y,

where both are features of a given population. Most analytic approaches assume that environmental variables are independent from the genetic background of a person, in which case both components of variability simply add together.

If a given characteristic is more similar for members of a family than in unrelated individuals, then shared variation amongst family members will tend in similar directions, a notion that is captured statistically by covariance. The degree to which the total variability of Y, V_Y, is then determined by the underlying genetic variation V_G has been defined in a broad sense as 'heritability':

$$h^2 = V_G / V_Y \quad (10.2)$$

The following simplified example illustrates this using childhood height at age of 6 years as a function of paternal and maternal height (Table 10.2). The data derive from the MRC NSHD, a birth cohort study consisting of a socially stratified sample of 2,547 women and 2,815 men born during one week in March 1946.[5] The analysis only includes participants who have complete data on parental information that were collected for both parents at the same visit in 1952. It is assumed that the adult height of the parents remains stable during adulthood and that childhood height of the offspring is a proxy of their later adult height.

Outcome: $Y_o \sim N(\mu_o, \sigma_o^2)$, where Y_o is childhood height at 6 years, one offspring per family
Exposure: $Y_{p,m}$ adult height collected on both parents

To quantify the extent of shared variation in height between parents and offspring, the first approach might be the correlation coefficient between offspring height and the paternal height, which is a function of their covariance, cov_{op}:

$$r_{op} = cov_{op} / [\sigma_o \sigma_p] \quad (10.3)$$

As can be seen, the correlation coefficient is dependent on the variance of the offspring height, σ_o^2, which in turn is affected by the number of offspring. The variance of paternal height, σ_p^2, is less problematic, as each child only has one biological father. Here we are interested in familial similarities, and the measure of heritability should not be influenced by number of offspring in a given family. Therefore, a simple correlation coefficient is not the ideal tool to capture similarities amongst familial relatives unless outcome variables are first standardised to family size.

A linear regression analysis is an extension of finding correlation. Indeed the regression coefficient derived from the linear regression of offspring trait on paternal trait has more favourable features because:

$$E(Y_o) = \alpha + \beta_{op} Y_p \quad \text{where algebraically } \beta_{op} = cov_{op} / \sigma_p^2;$$
$$\text{with the assumption: } \beta_{op} = [\tfrac{1}{2} V_G] / V_Y = \tfrac{1}{2} h^2 \quad (10.4)$$

Table 10.2 Results of analysis of childhood height (offspring) at age 6 as a function of maternal and paternal height in the MRC NSHD study

	Parents	(n = 3212)			Correlation of height between parents (p-value)
	Fathers		Mothers		
Mean height in cm (sd)	173.4(8.1)		161.4(6.4)		0.248
Offspring					(p <0.001)
Female					
(n=1524)	113.9(5.4)	173.4(8.2)	161.4(6.5)		
Male					
(n=1688)	114.7(5.2)	173.3(8.0)	161.4(6.3)		
Correlation between parents and offspring by sex (p-value)					
Female	0.333	(p<0.001)	0.362	(p<0.001)	
Male	0.312	(p<0.001)	0.380	(p<0.001)	
Regression coefficients of offspring height on parental height with standard errors and adjustment factors for unequal parental variance of trait					
Female	0.221	±0.016 × 1.259	0.302	±0.020	
	=0.278	±0.020			
Male	0.206	±0.015	0.315	±0.019 × 0.794	
			= 0.250	±0.015	
Heritabilities, per cent, with standard errors					
Female	56	±4	60	±4	
Male	41	±3	50	±3	

In particular, if height is assumed to be determined only by genes, which means that no shared environmental effects within a family additionally influenced height of the offspring, then due to 50% sharing of genes between father and child, the covariance cov_{op} captures 50% of the effect of genetic variability (denoted by V_G) of the offspring height. If it is also assumed that the paternal variability of height represents the variability of height in the population, denoted by V_Y, then it follows that β_{op} capturing 50% of the heritability h^2 of childhood height. If an equivalent assumption is made regarding mothers and the childhood height of their offspring, then a similar estimate can be obtained for h^2 by regressing childhood height, Y_o, on maternal height, Y_m. If variances of the trait are unequal between fathers and mothers, the heritability estimates need to be adjusted for the different variances of height in boys and girls. The regression coefficient of the height of the daughter on paternal height β_{op} is then adjusted by multiplying by $[\sigma_p/\sigma_m]$, and likewise the regression coefficient of the son's height on maternal height β_{om} is multiplied by $[\sigma_m/\sigma_p]$.[18]

In theory, if both fathers and mothers had equal and independent variances of height, then a regression of childhood height on the mean parental value of height, $\{½(Y_p+Y_m)\}$, would give a direct estimate of the heritability of height.[18]

$$E(Y_o) = \alpha + \beta_{o\_mean}\{\tfrac{1}{2}(Y_p + Y_m)\} \qquad \text{where, algebraically } \sigma_{mean}^2 = \tfrac{1}{2}\sigma_p^2.$$
$$\text{Thus } \beta = cov_{o\_mean}/\sigma_{mean}^2 = V_G/V_T = h^2. \tag{10.5}$$

However, the analysis used for the results shown in Table 10.2 is unrealistic for several reasons. The example does not use adult height of the offspring and therefore does not model identical traits in offspring and parents. Further, intrauterine growth of a child is affected by several maternal features including height, leading to closer correlations between maternal and offspring anthropometric values than for fathers (see Table 10.2[16]). The method for formally testing for this is given in Section 10.3.2.

At first glance, it appears reasonable to assume that the population of mothers and the population of fathers are genetically independent, unless there is some form of inbreeding, such as first cousin marriages or culturally restricted marriages within a clan or geographically isolated populations. However, even if we assume negligible genetic correlation between parents, some correlation of heights between parents is usually observed. Human couples may consciously or unconsciously self-select each other based on trait similarity and/or similarity of life-style. This phenomenon, referred to by geneticists as 'assortative mating', leads to higher heritability estimates than under the assumption of random mating.[19] Based on experimental data and some preliminary human data, this is unlikely to alter heritability estimates by more than 10%.[20, 21]

10.3.2 Differences between maternal and paternal effects

Differences between maternal and paternal effects on outcomes can arise due to several reasons. As mentioned above, the maternal intrauterine environment may have a specific effect on outcome and we will show a possible example of this below. However, differences between maternal and paternal effects on an offspring trait can also arise due to parent-of-origin effects'. A parent-of-origin effect on transcription, or genomic imprinting, results from epigenetic modification of the genome which, in turn, results in unequal transcription of parental alleles. For these imprinted genes, expression of the alleles is dependent upon the sex of the parent from which they were inherited.[13, 22]

We illustrate how to test for a difference in effects between parents with the classic example of birth weight as a function of both paternal and maternal height (Table 10.3). Again the data are sourced from the NSHD cohort.[5]

Outcome: $Y_o \sim N(\mu_o, \sigma_o^2)$, where Y_o is the birth weight of one offspring per family
Exposure: $X_{p,m}$ adult height collected on both parents

Since birth weight was a normally distributed outcome, a conventional linear regression approach was taken. There are various parameterizations possible, including modelling birth weight as a function of both maternal and paternal height. This is algebraically identical to having birth weight as a function of average parental height and the extent to which the father is taller than the average parental height.

$$E(Y_o) = \alpha + \beta_p X_p + \beta_m X_m \tag{10.6}$$
$$= \alpha + \beta_{mean}\{\tfrac{1}{2}(X_p + X_m)\} + \beta_{diff}\{\tfrac{1}{2}(X_p - X_m)\}$$
$$\text{where } \beta_p = \{\tfrac{1}{2}(\beta_{mean} + \beta_{diff})\} \text{ and } \beta_m = \{\tfrac{1}{2}(\beta_{mean} - \beta_{diff})\} \tag{10.7}$$

From this follow two possibilities to test for a difference in the effects between maternal and paternal height on offspring birth weight. A model with both coefficients β_p and β_m as outlined

Table 10.3 Difference between paternal and maternal effects: Regression of birth weight in male offspring on parental height in various parameterisations with corresponding F-statistics. The data stem from the NSHD study

	Male offspring (n=1786)		
Mean birth weight in g (sd)	3322.4 493.3		
Regression on	Regression coefficient (g/cm height) with corresponding standard error	F-statistic for regression	F-statistic for difference between maternal and paternal effects
paternal height alone: β_p	3.9 1.5	6.2	
maternal height alone: β_m	14.4 1.9	56.85	
paternal and maternal height adjusting for each other as in equation (10.6)			
β_p	0.9 1.6	28.57	21.7
β_m	14.1 2.0		
mean parental height and half parental difference in height adjusting for each other as in equation (10.7)			
β_{mean}	15.0 2.2	28.57	
β_{diff}	−13.2 2.8		(t-statistic of β_{diff})^2 = 21.7
mean parental height alone: β_{mean}	12.7 2.1	35.05	

in equation (10.6) can be compared to a model with the effects of maternal and paternal height on birth weight constrained to be equal, i.e. $\beta_p = \beta_m$. This is equivalent to, the second possibility for testing for a parental difference, modelling birth weight directly as a function of mean parental height and half the difference in height between the parents as in equation (10.7). In contrast to both these approaches, one could compare models with both parental heights to those where one of the two was left out. However, this would be misleading because of the correlation in parental heights (see Table 10.2).

In the parameterization used here a negative sign for this highly significant coefficient (β_{diff}) indicates a stronger association of maternal height with offspring birth weight than paternal height with offspring birth weight (Table 10.3), suggesting, in line with previous data, that maternal height may be more important for birth weight than paternal height even in these crude, unadjusted analyses.[23–25] Apart from the possibility that these differences are due to intrauterine environment, if one wanted to interpret this in terms of a possible difference in genetic effects, the same assumptions as outlined above, including the importance of standardization of parental height (Section 10.3.1), apply. It is straightforward to extend this analysis to other non-anthropometric traits.

10.3.3 A few comments on gene-environment interaction

A great deal of literature on mathematical models already exists for how environmental selection affects the gene-pool of a population—which among others has practical applications in animal breeding.[18, 20] It should be kept in mind that such theoretical models encompass hundreds or more generations—as opposed to the type of datasets dealt with in this chapter, and common in life course epidemiology, that cover at maximum three or four generations.

There has been a long-running discussion on whether the statistical assumption that genes and environment act independently on outcome holds for all situations, for instance regarding the heritability of intelligence or behavioural traits.[26–28] Some findings in this area suggest that the genetic background of a family may be correlated with a certain behaviours which in turn acts synergistically on behaviour of offspring.[29, 30] However, what is more commonly being referred to as 'interaction' is the departure from a pre-specified statistical model which is sometimes only a function of scale. Statistical interaction is equivalent to the need of an additional statistical term to model joint presence of two covariates. Observing such an interaction between two variables may be dependent on the type of link function. For example, if effects of two covariates are modelled on a log-scale, these are assumed to multiply on their original scale. Any departure of effect of covariates from that scale will need to be taken account of by adding an interaction term. A change in scale for the model may obviate the need of such a term. In life course epidemiology, 'gene-environmental' effects often refer to this more general statistical phenomenon and are discussed in more detail in Chapter 4. In genetic epidemiology there is the specific situation where an effect can only be present when both covariates are jointly present. This corresponds to a two-by-two table where three cells of the table are empty and only one cell representing the joint presence of both variables has observations. However, this rarely applies to life course epidemiology because most exposures that are tested have an effect on their own. Therefore, for most problems in family studies, it seems appropriate to assume that genes and environment act independently—as parameterized in all the statistical models that are presented in this chapter.

10.3.4 More complex problems

10.3.4.1 Clustering in families—multilevel models and variance components

So far analytic methods reduced the family structure of data collected on at least three individuals (father, mother, child) to a simple problem of looking at a single individual (offspring) by conditioning on the parental data as exposures. But there may also be interest in assessing the effects of the same exposure variable X on a given outcome trait Y in all family members simultaneously whilst taking account of families as units.

A possible approach is to use a multilevel model.[31] In most instances, the family can be seen as a level 2 unit ($j=1, 2, ..., J$ family), and family members (parents, offspring) as level 1 unit ($i=1, 2, ..., I$ family members in family j).[32, 33] For example, suppose a normally distributed trait Y_{ij} was measured once on I individuals in J families, then:

$$Y_{ij} = \beta_{0j} + \beta_1 X_{1ij} + \beta_2 X_{2ij} + \varepsilon_{ij}, \tag{10.8}$$

where β_{0j} are family specific intercepts for joint factors within a family, and ε_{ij} are residual error terms. The β_{0j} are modeled as:

$$\beta_{0j} = \beta_0 + \xi_{0j} \tag{10.9}$$

where β_0 is the mean intercept across the whole sample of families and ξ_{0j} is the deviation of the family specific intercept from the mean. In matrix notation this corresponds to stacking the values for each family j in matrices, with each line denoting an individual in that family.

$$\underbrace{\begin{bmatrix} y_{1j} \\ y_{2j} \\ y_{3j} \end{bmatrix}}_{y_j} = \underbrace{\begin{bmatrix} 1 & x_{11j} & x_{21j} \\ 1 & x_{12j} & x_{22j} \\ 1 & x_{13j} & x_{23j} \end{bmatrix}}_{X_j} \underbrace{\begin{bmatrix} \beta_0 \\ \beta_1 \\ \beta_2 \end{bmatrix}}_{\beta} + \underbrace{\begin{bmatrix} 1 \\ 1 \\ 1 \end{bmatrix}}_{Z_j} \underbrace{[\xi_{0j}]}_{\xi_j} + \underbrace{\begin{bmatrix} \varepsilon_{1j} \\ \varepsilon_{2j} \\ \varepsilon_{3j} \end{bmatrix}}_{\varepsilon_j} \tag{10.10}$$

Defining σ_ε^2 as the variance of the ε_{ij} and σ_ξ^2 as the variance of ξ_{0j} it is typically assumed that
(i) the families are independent,
(ii) given the covariates (the Xs), the ε_{ij} follow a Normal distribution $\varepsilon_{ij} \sim N(0, \sigma_\varepsilon^2)$, where the errors for two family members within the same family are assumed to be independent,
(iii) given the covariates (the Xs), the ξ_{0j} follow a normal distribution $\xi_{0j} \sim N(0, \sigma_\xi^2)$ being independent from the individual errors ε_{ij}, i.e. $\text{Cov}(\xi_{0j}, \varepsilon_{ij}) = 0$.

In the setting of intergenerational data, the $\xi_{0j} \sim N(0, \sigma_\xi^2)$ may be interpreted as the sum of family specific genetic and shared environmental effects, and the $\varepsilon_{ij} \sim N(0, \sigma_\varepsilon^2)$ may be interpreted as residual environmental variation of the trait for each individual that is not explained by explanatory variables in the model.

Usually, assumption (i) can be easily satisfied via an appropriate study design. Assumption (ii) states that data within a family need to be explained by covariates sufficiently well so that no residual correlation between family members remains and such that covariates are not correlated with residual errors. For example, in any given family it is desirable to avoid residual errors between parent and child that are systematically more similar to each other than those between the parents. Taking the example of height—modelling adult height in a family, observed on both parents and their two children a function of age and sex, means that according to assumption (ii) height should not be more correlated in the siblings than it is for their parents. In genetic terms a violation of assumption (ii) may well happen, because parents are genetically unrelated, whilst siblings are related. However, in reality, the presence of phenotypic correlations between parents due to assortative mating poses less of a problem than one would anticipate based on theory.[19, 34]

From assumption (iii), the degree of deviation from the overall mean of all family means for a specific family should not imply any given degree of residual environmental error. Hence, in order for assumptions (ii) and (iii) to hold, it is crucial to have an appropriate linear predictor and always to model explicitly the age, generation, and gender of individuals—with interaction terms if necessary. If covariates and family specific errors remain associated, a full variance components model may be necessary (as described below). Another solution may be to extend the models to include random slope effects, for example a dependence on age or sex.[35] Simple 2-level random intercept multilevel models may be implemented with standard software, including Stata.[15]

A crude measure for heritability that may be obtained from random intercept analysis is the intra class correlation coefficient:

$$r_I = \sigma_\xi^2 / [\sigma_\varepsilon^2 + \sigma_\xi^2]. \qquad (10.11)$$

This relation holds only under the assumption that no unmeasured shared environmental variable explains correlations amongst family members. A full random coefficients model, with random intercepts and random slopes, implies a dependence of family specific effects on the covariate and its scale. In such models there is no direct output of an intra class correlation coefficient. It is possible to estimate the degree of correlation amongst family members holding the covariate determining random slopes constant, for example estimating the correlation amongst family members of a defined age and sex. For other covariates apart from age and sex, the interpretation in terms of heritability may not be as straightforward.

If one aim of the analysis was the estimation of heritability, then an explicit partitioning of variances and co-variances of phenotype data between siblings and their parents is required: into the shared genetic background between siblings, siblings and parents, and into the shared environment and other main effects.[36–38] The correlation matrix $Cov(A)$ given in equation (10.12) is what would be expected for genetic correlations between parents and their offspring, and between their two children (siblings)—assuming genes do not have a dominant effect. The genetic correlation between family members is therefore called *Cov(A)*, and the correlation matrix for common shared environment within a family, is denoted by *Cov(C)*. The first two columns and rows represent the individual parents, the third and fourth columns and rows represent a sibling pair (children of those parents).

$$Cov(A) = \sigma_A^2 \begin{bmatrix} 1 & 0 & \frac{1}{2} & \frac{1}{2} \\ 0 & 1 & \frac{1}{2} & \frac{1}{2} \\ \frac{1}{2} & \frac{1}{2} & 1 & \frac{1}{2} \\ \frac{1}{2} & \frac{1}{2} & \frac{1}{2} & 1 \end{bmatrix}$$

$$Cov(C) = \sigma_c^2 \begin{bmatrix} 1 & 0 & 0 & 0 \\ 0 & 1 & 0 & 0 \\ 0 & 0 & 1 & 1 \\ 0 & 0 & 1 & 1 \end{bmatrix}$$

(10.12)

For the genetic correlation matrix denoted in *Cov(A)*, parents are assumed not to share any genes, hence the factor zero multiplied with the genetic variance σ_A^2 to obtain correlations between the first two columns and rows. Parents share half of their genes with their children so the co-variance between mothers and children (the first and the third and fourth column/rows) is set to half of σ_A^2, similarly for the fathers and their children (second and the third and fourth column/row). In addition, full siblings share on average half of their genes across the full range of genetic loci, so that 50% of the correlation between siblings (in the third and fourth column) is assumed to be genetic. With regards to environmental correlations denoted in the matrix for *Cov(C)*, it is expected that siblings have shared their environment since birth and hence the remaining correlation between siblings is set to 1.

Traditionally, such variance components models have been applied for the analysis of twin studies, and have been also called 'structural' models or path analysis models (discussed later in Section 10.4.3). The difference between structural models and other statistical approaches is that rather starting with specifying direct fixed effects with a series of equations and then extending the models to incorporate random effects to allow for hierarchy, structural models start with specification of the covariance structure of the data and then are extended to allow fixed effects. The error structure that is assumed to give rise to the observed data is represented by what is termed 'latent' quantities. In this example the latent quantities are the shared environmental effects and the shared genetic effects of members within a family which we only observe indirectly by comparing similarity of family members.

These variance components models can be implemented by introducing additional levels and new dummy variables for additive genetic variance into a multilevel model, in software such as Stata.[15, 39] The re-parameterization involves the sum of three random effects, ξ_{1j}, ξ_{2j}, and ξ_{3j}, which capture the family specific genetic correlations. For families with more than one child there is an additional level *l* to explicitly model correlations between siblings. Within a family, *l* is set to be equal for two siblings and to differ for parents. A random effect c_{lj} is introduced to capture shared environmental effects between siblings. Dummy variables for each person in a family are set to *M=1* for mothers, *P=1* for fathers and *O=1* for offspring, and otherwise to zero.

These dummy variables are used to rescale the random effects in terms of genetic and environmental correlations within a given family:[39]

$$y_{ilj} = \beta_0 + \beta_1 x_{1ij} + \beta_2 x_{2ij} + \varsigma_{1j}^{(4)}\left[M_i + O_i/2\right] + \varsigma_{2j}^{(4)}\left[P_i + O_i/2\right] + \varsigma_{ilj}^{(2)}\left[O_i/\sqrt{2}\right] + c_{lj}^{(3)} + \varepsilon_{ilj} \quad (10.13)$$

For a given family characteristic involving a mother y_1, father y_2, and their children y_3, y_4, the random effects have the following scaling:

$$\underbrace{\begin{bmatrix} y_{1j} \\ y_{2j} \\ y_{3j} \\ y_{4j} \end{bmatrix}}_{y_j} = \underbrace{\begin{bmatrix} 1 & x_{11j} & x_{21j} \\ 1 & x_{12j} & x_{22j} \\ 1 & x_{13j} & x_{23j} \\ 1 & x_{14j} & x_{24j} \end{bmatrix}}_{X_j} \underbrace{\begin{bmatrix} \beta_0 \\ \beta_1 \\ \beta_2 \end{bmatrix}}_{\beta} + \underbrace{\begin{bmatrix} 1 \\ 0 \\ \frac{1}{2} \\ \frac{1}{2} \end{bmatrix}}_{Z_3}\varsigma_{1j}^{(4)} + \underbrace{\begin{bmatrix} 0 \\ 1 \\ \frac{1}{2} \\ \frac{1}{2} \end{bmatrix}}_{Z_4}\varsigma_{2j}^{(4)} +$$

$$\underbrace{\begin{bmatrix} 0 & 0 & 0 & 0 \\ 0 & 0 & 0 & 0 \\ 0 & 0 & \sqrt{\frac{1}{2}} & 0 \\ 0 & 0 & 0 & \sqrt{\frac{1}{2}} \end{bmatrix} \begin{bmatrix} \varsigma_{11j}^{(2)} \\ \varsigma_{22j}^{(2)} \\ \varsigma_{33j}^{(2)} \\ \varsigma_{44j}^{(2)} \end{bmatrix}}_{Z_2} + \begin{bmatrix} 1 & 0 & 0 \\ 0 & 1 & 0 \\ 0 & 0 & 1 \\ 0 & 0 & 1 \end{bmatrix}\begin{bmatrix} c_{1j}^{(3)} \\ c_{2j}^{(3)} \\ c_{3j}^{(3)} \end{bmatrix} + \underbrace{\begin{bmatrix} \varepsilon_{1j} \\ \varepsilon_{2j} \\ \varepsilon_{3j} \\ \varepsilon_{4j} \end{bmatrix}}_{\varepsilon_j} \quad (10.14)$$

From the above covariance matrices $Cov(A)$ and $Cov(C)$ in (10.12), this then leads to:

$$Cov(y_j) = \sigma_A^2(Z_3 Z_3' + Z_4 Z_4' + Z_1 Z_1') + \sigma_C^2 Z_2 Z_2' + \sigma_\varepsilon^2 I. \quad (10.15)$$

The assumption of such a model is that genetic effects σ_A^2 act on an additive scale, and that these are conditionally independent from common and residual environmental variation, σ_C^2 and σ_ε^2. It is also assumed that paternal and maternal influence on offspring characteristics are of similar strength.

As an example for this approach adult height of members and parents of the NSHD cohort were used. The data only involve trios (one offspring, two parents), which leads to an unidentified common environment (i.e. that between siblings). The model above then reduces to a simple two level model:

$$y_{ilj} = \beta_0 + \beta_1 x_{1ij} + \beta_2 x_{2ij} + \varsigma_{1j}^{(2)}\left[M_i + O_i/2\right] + \varsigma_{2j}^{(2)}\left[P_i + O_i/2\right] + \varsigma_{ij}^{(2)}\left[O_i/\sqrt{2}\right] + \varepsilon_{ilj} \quad (10.16)$$

The heritability estimated in this model for un-standardized adult height is estimated to be 63% (95% CI: 59%–67%). After standardising adult height by sex in order to remove differences in variance between parents (see Section 10.3.1 and Table 10.2) the estimated heritability of adult height increases to 68% (95% CI: 64%–71%).

The advantage of multilevel models, including those for binary data,[39, 40] is that they can be applied in readily available software. If more than two levels are needed for binary applications, the software needs appropriate maximization routines (adaptive quadrature) and not just penalized quasi-likelihood,[41] which may have poor performance in the current setting.[42, 43]

Also, the fit of any variance components models tends to be much poorer for case-based sampling than for population based data.[44] As mentioned before—for some analysts a specification of the correlation matrices between family members as outlined in equation (10.12) may be conceptually much easier than fitting multilevel models.[45] Then, specialist applications such as Mplus can be used to fit these structural models[46]. Within Stata the command gllamm can be used after having specified the matrix for latent quantities.[15,45]

All of the above models can be directly implemented using a Bayesian formulation in WinBUGS.[47] Here again there are convergence problems for modelling variance components for binary outcome traits in nuclear families, which may require a complex parameterization of the variance components to be generated.[48] Inevitably, the larger the datasets, the longer the computational time needed for Bayesian approaches.

A crude way to deal with clustered outcome data is to fit simple one-level models and then use adjusted variance estimates with robust standard errors. This will, however, only provide population averaged effects and may lead to wrong conclusions if effects within a family work in opposite directions to what is observed for the whole sample—analogous to the way that the ecological fallacy may arise from analyses from aggregate data. There have been attempts to overcome this by using generalized estimating equations (GEEs) that explicitly specify the form of correlations amongst family members. Their performance is less satisfactory when compared to the classical variance components and multilevel models.[49]

Although in theory fitting proportional odds models for categorical data collected across generations is possible, in reality researchers often face the difficulty that the meaning and categorization of a variable, and indeed its associations with other exposures, may change from one generation to another. In the setting of multilevel models, this leads to highly complex model structures with many un-testable underlying assumptions regarding measurement errors.

10.3.4.2 Tetrachoric correlation analyses for binary data

Having an observation coded as disease in a dataset may only capture the extremes above a certain threshold, for example getting diagnosed by a doctor, whilst other data may suggest an underlying continuum. In this context, a tetrachoric correlation is defined as the correlation coefficient computed for in truth two normally distributed variables that are both expressed as a dichotomy. The two normally distributed variables A and B would be liabilities to get the disease A (variable A) or disease B (variable B).

In the setting of family studies, it is possible to use tetrachoric correlation in order to estimate the overall odds of having a disease, given that another family member has the same disease whilst individually adjusting for individual covariates.

The relative recurrence risk is:

$$\lambda_R = \frac{\text{Probability of disease given that a relative is affected}}{\text{Overall probability of getting the disease}} \quad (10.17)$$

In reality the probability of disease is a function of environmental and genetic variables that vary between individuals. If all environmental variables that are associated with disease were measured and included in the statistical model, then the relative recurrence risk λ_R would be a measure of the strength of genetic effect on disease in that particular population.

The following simplified example uses data on pregnancy related hypertension collected from mothers and daughters participating in the Aberdeen study.[50] Covariates of interest include maternal age when giving birth (centred on its mean), manual social class coded as one, and parity greater than zero coded as one. Here a global cross ratio model is used that simultaneously models the odds of disease in two relatives in a bi-variate logistic regression, which also gives an overall estimate of the odds ratio of having disease given that a relative has disease and after adjusting for covariates.[51] This global odds ratio approximates λ_R for rare chronic diseases. The results of the global cross ratio model are shown in Table 10.4. These results are very similar to a simple logistic regression analysis with outcome maternal pregnancy related hypertension and after adjusting for the same covariates (shown in Table 10.5). Thus, both suggest that the risk of having pregnancy induced hypertension is increased by 54% (both odds ratios = 1.54) if one's mother had pregnancy induced hypertension when she was pregnant with the daughter, after controlling for other covariates.

As outlined in more detail in Section 10.4.1 below, the covariates in the logistic regression model have to be interpreted as the effect of changes between generations conditional on

Table 10.4 Global cross ratio model for the association between maternal pregnancy related hypertension and daughters pregnancy related hypertension. Individual logistic model for mothers and daughters pregnancy related hypertension adjusting for the covariates as displayed in the table. The data derive from the Aberdeen *Children of the 1950's* study

Effect of co-variates on		Odds ratio	(95% CI)
pregnancy related hypertension (mother)			
	parity greater than 1 child (mother)	0.20	(0.16, 0.25)
	per 5 years of age (mother)	1.16	(1.05, 1.28)
	manual social class (mother)	0.94	(0.74, 1.19)
pregnancy related hypertension (daughter)			
	parity greater than 1 child (daughter)	0.42	(0.32, 0.57)
	per 5 years of age (daughter)	1.12	(1.03, 1.22)
	manual social class (daughter)	0.98	(0.83, 1.16)
Global odds ratio for pregnancy related hypertension in daughters given that the mother is affected		1.54	(1.26, 1.88)

Table 10.5 Effects of maternal pregnancy related hypertension on daughters pregnancy related hypertension (logistic regression) adjusting for covariates as displayed in the table. The data derive from the Aberdeen *Children of the 1950's* study

Effect of	on daughters pregnancy related hypertension	
	odds ratio	(95% CI)
maternal pregnancy related hypertension	1.54	(1.26, 1.89)
parity greater than 1 child (mother)	0.95	(0.79, 1.14)
per 5 years of age (mother)	1.13	(1.03, 1.23)
manual social class (mother)	1.15	(0.94, 1.40)
parity greater than 1 child (daughter)	0.42	(0.31, 0.57)
per 5 years of age (daughter)	0.97	(0.90, 1.05)
manual social class (daughter)	0.97	(0.82, 1.15)

the baseline. The main advantage of using a tetrachoric approach lies in the possibility to formally test for equality of co-variate effects between generations. Here, there is some evidence for parity having a different effect between generations (Wald test for difference of effects: p = 0.0001), being more strongly protective of pregnancy induced hypertension in earlier (mothers, G1) compared with more contemporary (daughters, G0) generations. It also provides a slightly more precise estimate of the global relative recurrence odds ratio if more covariates have to be adjusted for per generation.

10.3.4.3 Censored (survival) data on two generations

Dealing with survival data collected on two generations may be problematic. The inherent age-difference between offspring and parents will lead to more events in the parental generation (particularly for conditions that are more prevalent at older ages) and more censoring in the offspring generation. There has to be also a careful consideration on when time at risk starts for given exposure variables. Bayesian implementations already exist for analysis of nuclear family survival data.[52]

In a simple hypothetical example, using parental and offspring educational and social class data with outcome parental survival, it becomes apparent that there may be time-dependent confounding between predictor variables (Figure 10.3). Adult social class of the offspring may be a function of the adult social class of the parent, both may be a function of the respective educational variables and all these variables may have an effect on survival of the parent. Age-differences between parents and offspring may also mean that exposure-time to (un-) observed confounding variables is fundamentally different and this may lead to biases. Marginal structural models may help to deal with time-dependent confounding, however, these models are unable to disentangle genetic and environmental components.[53]

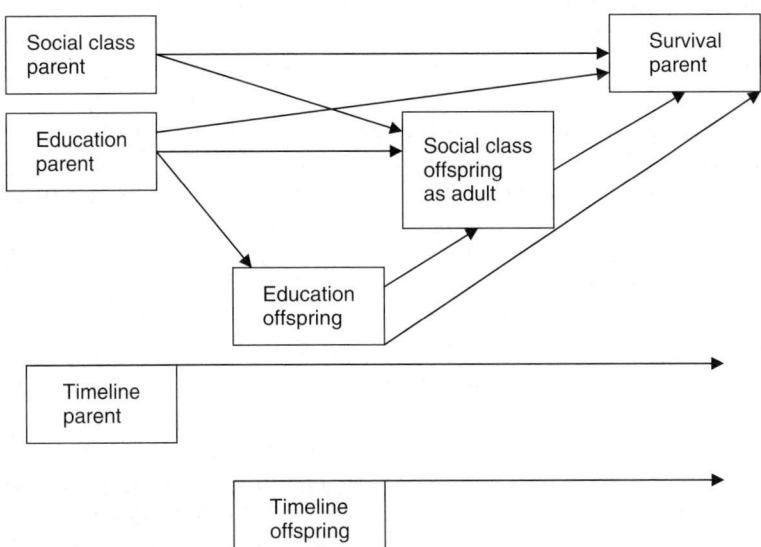

Fig. 10.3 Time dependent confounding for survival data collected on two generations in a simplistic example (Section 10.3.4.3).

10.3.4.4 Repeated measurements over the life course

Analyses methods that deal with repeated measures on offspring in classical life-course epidemiology have been described in great detail elsewhere.[54, 55] With regards to testing for a difference in parental effects, the considerations above apply equally to the situation of repeated measurements on offspring. Apart from measurements within a person being correlated, it should also be noted that the measurement error of the outcome variable may change with the data collection time point. For example, height may be directly measured on some visits and later self-reported on questionnaires. The presence of such measurement error may lead to inflated estimates for the parental effects on outcome. For linear repeated outcomes of this kind, a ready programmed tool exists in Stata (xtpcse, Table 10.1).[15]

In the same way, variance components analysis on longitudinal data can be performed for single measurements that are clustered in families by simply adding a further level for the repeated measurements.[35, 39] There are also readily available implementations in WinBugs.[47, 56]

10.4 Analysis of more than two generations

Intergenerational studies can present further research opportunities since they can simultaneously provide information on micro social data for individuals in families, as well as encompassing a long time frame with a changing macro social context (Figure 10.1). The next example considers different analytic approaches for determining the impact of changes of social class across generations on birth weight, and in a second step assesses the extent to which this relation may be mediated via the final adult height reached by a given woman. The data are a subset from the Aberdeen *Children of the 1950s* cohort study, described in detail elsewhere,[50] which was conducted during a time of major economic change. Results from this particular example are also discussed in Chapter 2. Findings of oil in the Northern Sea transformed the local economy in Aberdeen in 1971, making the city the most affluent city in Scotland, whereas prior to this time Aberdeen was one of the more deprived cities in Scotland. This study collected, via questionnaires and record linkage, anthropometric and social data on three generations of women; where G0 denotes the grand maternal generation, G1 the maternal, and G2 the offspring generation (Figure 10.4).[57] For the sake of simplicity, at this point the correlations between sibling girls in the last generation are disregarded—full models that take account of correlations amongst siblings would need to be fitted as outlined in previous sections, which then requires specialist software. In this example ignoring the clustering of siblings in a family affects the standard errors of the point estimates for the intergenerational effects, but does not change the main conclusions.

It is of considerable advantage to have all anthropometric measurements standardized, rather than having to deal with various correction factors for changes in variance across generations. Foetal growth scores (z-scores) were calculated by subtracting the sex specific mean birth weight for each completed week of gestation from the individual's absolute birth weight and dividing by the standard deviation of all the sex specific birth weights for that gestational age. The first generation foetal growth scores were calculated using an internal standardization process, whereas the second generation are standardized using the population all Scottish singleton live born births between 1975 and 1990 as a reference. In order to interpret changes in height across generations independent of changes in height between reference populations at different times, maternal and grand maternal height were also transformed to z-scores using the population means at given time points. Social class (SC) was based on the occupations of fathers at the time of the participant's and their offspring's birth. Both grand paternal and paternal social class were collapsed into two categories non-manual (I-IIINM), coded as zero, and manual (IIIM to V and unemployed), coded as one. Parity was coded as binary variable, with zero denoting a mother who had never

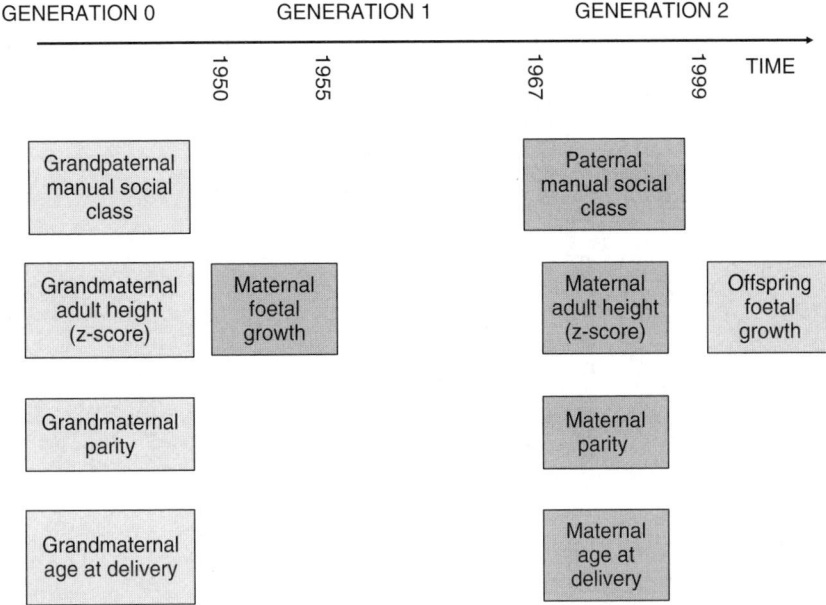

Fig. 10.4 The Aberdeen *Children of the 1950s* study. Temporal ordering of variables used for the present analysis. The arrow denotes time and the generations on which we observed the displayed variables.

given birth before, and the value of one for a mother who had previously given birth. Age at delivery was a continuous variable in years, centred on its mean.

10.4.1 Linear and multivariate linear regression models

Before attempting any data analyses, it is worthwhile to clarify the temporal ordering and causal relationships between exposures of interest and confounders.[58, 59] In order to address the first question, separate linear regressions for the G1 birth weight and G2 birth weight could be run by using the same predictor variables collected in the study:

$$E(Y_{o,G1}) = \alpha_{G1} + \beta_{1,G0} SC_{G0} + \beta_{2,G0}\, parity_{G0} + \beta_{3,G0}\, adult\ height_{G0} + \beta_{4,G0}\, age_{G0}$$
$$E(Y_{o,G2}) = \alpha_{G2} + \beta_{1,G1} SC_{G1} + \beta_{2,G1}\, parity_{G1} + \beta_{3,G1}\, adult\ height_{G1} + \beta_{4,G1}\, age_{G1} \quad (10.18)$$

The regression coefficients between generations appear similar except the regression coefficient associated with social class, which suggest a weaker association of father's social class on birth weight in more contemporary (G2) generations than earlier (G1) generations (Table 10.6). The confidence intervals of the coefficients, however, are not directly comparable, as separate regressions ignore the significant correlation (0.26, $p < 0.0001$) between birth weights of mothers and daughters (i.e. between $Y_{o,G1}$ and $Y_{o,G2}$), and, moreover, they use different samples of women since the model for birth weight in the daughters ($Y_{o,G2}$) will only include participants where the mother had a linked offspring, whereas the model for birth weight in the mothers ($Y_{o,G1}$) is a random sample of females born in Aberdeen in the 1950s. A possible solution is a multivariate model in which both $Y_{o,G1}, Y_{o,G2}$ are modelled simultaneously as correlated outcomes—it is then possible to formally test for equality of effects between equations (Table 10.6). In this case, there was evidence for significant differences between manual social class on birth weight between

Table 10.6 Separate linear regressions of determinants of foetal growth in girls and subsequently joint model. All effects are adjusting for variables displayed and for maternal age at birth. Data derive from the Aberdeen *Children of the 1950's* study

Explanatory variables		Dpendent variables: Direct effects				Joint model: Direct effects			
	units	G2 foetal growth (n=2879)*		G1 foetal growth (n=3377)		G2 foetal growth (n=2878)		G1 foetal growth (n=2878)	
		β	(95% CI)	β	(95% CI)	β	(95% CI)	β	(95% CI)
G1 adult height	1 SD (=6.0cm)	0.24	(0.20, 0.27)			0.20	(0.16, 0.23)		
G1 parity >0	0 or >0	0.19	(0.12, 0.27)			0.18	(0.11, 0.26)		
G1 manual social class	vs non-manual	−0.04	(−0.12, 0.03)			−0.05	(−0.12, 0.03)		
G0 adult height	1 SD (=5.6cm)			0.20	(0.16, 0.23)			0.20	(0.16, 0.23)
G0 parity >0	0 or >0			0.17	(0.10, 0.25)			0.18	(0.10, 0.26)
G0 manual social class	vs non-manual			−0.22	(−0.30, −0.14)			−0.21	(−0.30, −0.12)

generations within girls (p = 0.007) (as noted above this association appears weaker in the daughter's than in the mother's generation).

At this stage the change in social class between generations may still have been disregarded, as well as correlations between grand maternal and maternal height. As a first easy analytic approach, sequential regression models can be applied to each outcome in turn. To test for the effects of both grand paternal social class and maternal social class, both can be fitted as predictors in a model for foetal growth (G2):

$$\begin{aligned} E(Y_{0,G2}) &= \alpha_{G2} + \beta_{1,G1} SC_{G1} + \beta_{2,G0} SC_{G0} + \Sigma \beta_i X_i \\ &= \alpha + (\beta_0 + \beta_1) SC_{G0} + \beta_1 (SC_{G1} - SC_{G0}) + \Sigma \beta_i X_i \\ &= \alpha + (\beta_0 + \beta_1) SC_{G1} + \beta_0 (SC_{G0} - SC_{G1}) + \Sigma \beta_i X_i \end{aligned} \qquad (10.19)$$

A model with simultaneous adjustments for social class over two generations corresponds to modelling the change from non-manual to manual social class over generations, adjusting for baseline (Table 10.7). The process for dealing with more than one social class variable has been described elsewhere.[60]

10.4.2 Path analysis: direct and indirect effects

Previous analyses elucidate patterns within the data, but do not provide a comprehensive picture of all the relations present. For example, it is difficult to estimate the extent that an adverse social environment affects birth weight indirectly, for example, via its impact on anthropometric variables in previous generations. One way to obtain estimates of both direct and indirect effects of selected variables is path analysis. This uses simultaneous regression models, whereby exposure variables for one regression may be outcome variables for another simultaneous regression, for example.

$$\begin{aligned} y_{ij} &= \beta_0 + \beta_1 x_{1i} + \beta_2 x_{2i} + \beta_2 x_{2i} + \beta_3 x_{3i} + \varepsilon_{1i} \\ x_{3i} &= \delta_0 + \delta_1 x_{1i} + \delta_2 x_{2i} + \varepsilon_{2i} \end{aligned} \qquad (10.20)$$

Y and x_3 are modelled as a function of other variables and are therefore called *endogenous* variables, while x_1 and x_2 are *exogenous* since they are not outcomes. These path models may be rewritten in matrix notation as:

$$\underbrace{\begin{bmatrix} x_{1i} \\ x_{2i} \\ x_{3i} \\ y_i \end{bmatrix}}_{Z_i} = \underbrace{\begin{bmatrix} 0 \\ 0 \\ \delta_0 \\ \beta_0 \end{bmatrix}}_{a} \underbrace{\begin{bmatrix} 0 & 0 & 0 & 0 \\ 0 & 0 & 0 & 0 \\ \delta_1 & \delta_2 & 0 & 0 \\ \beta_1 & \beta_2 & \beta_3 & 0 \end{bmatrix}}_{B} \underbrace{\begin{bmatrix} x_{1i} \\ x_{2i} \\ x_{3i} \\ y_i \end{bmatrix}}_{z_i} + \underbrace{\begin{bmatrix} x_{1i} \\ x_{2i} \\ \varepsilon_{2i} \\ \varepsilon_{1i} \end{bmatrix}}_{u_i} \qquad (10.21)$$

The expression $Z_i = (1-B)^{-1}(a+u_i)$ is used for parameter estimations in computational routines.

In the current example, the endogenous variables all represent anthropometric data on G1 and G2 (Table 10.8). By simultaneously estimating several linear regressions, the co-variances between anthropometric measures are partitioned into direct and indirect effects.[61, 62] The indirect effect of exposures upon foetal growth of the second generation can then be estimated

Table 10.7 Direct effects of separate linear regressions of determinants of foetal growth and maternal adult height of the first and foetal growth of the girls in the second generation. All continuous variables are standardised z-scores. Total numbers quoted related to the number of births in G2. Effects are adjusting for variables displayed and for (grand-*) maternal† age at birth. Data derive from the Aberdeen *Children of the 1950's* study

Explanatory variables		Dependent variables: Direct effects						
		G2 foetal growth† (n = 2879)			G1 adult height (n = 3318)		G1 foetal growth* (n = 3377)	
	units	β	(95% CI)		β	(95% CI)	β	(95% CI)
G1 adult height	1 SD (=6.0cm)	0.17	(0.13, 0.22)					
G1 parity >0	0 or >0	0.18	(0.11, 0.26)					
G1 manual social class	vs non-manual	−0.05	(−0.12, 0.03)					
G1 foetal growth	1 SD	0.21	(0.18, 0.25)		0.21	(0.18, 0.24)		
G0 adult height	1 SD (=5.6cm)	−0.01	(−0.05, 0.03)		0.48	(0.45, 0.51)	0.20	(0.16, 0.23)
G0 parity >0	0 or >0	−0.09	(−0.17, −0.02)		−0.14	(−0.20, −0.09)	0.17	(0.10, 0.25)
G0 manual social class	vs non-manual	0.06	(−0.03, 0.15)		−0.05	(−0.12, 0.03)	−0.22	(−0.30, −0.13)

Table 10.8 Path analysis of determinants of foetal growth (ZscoreG1) and maternal adult height of the first and foetal growth of the girls in the second generation (ZscoreG2, n=2878). Data derive from the Aberdeen *Children of the 1950's* study

Explanatory variables		Dependent variables: Total, indirect and direct effects			
		G2 foetal growth		G1 adult height	
	Type of effect	β	(95% CI)	β	(95% CI)
G0 adult height	total	0.12	(0.09, 0.16)	0.51	(0.48, 0.54)
[1 SD (=5.6cm)]	indirect	0.12	(0.09, 0.16)	0.15	(0.06, 0.25)
	direct	0	(not fitted)	0.36	(0.26, 0.46)
G0 parity>0	total	−0.08	(−0.16, 0.00)	−0.15	(−0.22, −0.08)
[0 or >0]	indirect	−0.01	(−0.13, 0.15)	0.13	(0.02, 0.23)
	direct	−0.09	(−0.27, 0.09)	−0.28	(−0.41, −0.14)
G0 manual social class	total	0.01	(−0.09, 0.10)	−0.05	(−0.13, 0.03)
[vs non-manual]	indirect	−0.05	(−0.16, 0.06)	−0.15	(−0.27, −0.04)
	direct	0.06	(−0.10, 0.21)	0.10	(−0.03, 0.23)

by multiplying the standardised partial coefficients along the relevant pathways. Note that this is possible by directly using the regression coefficients since in our example all anthropometric variables were pre-standardised. Direct effects of the path model correspond to a simple linear regression model on all variables with available data (compare Table 10.8 with Table 10.7). For continuous outcomes such a model is most easily implemented in Stata with the command reg3, which uses an ordinary least squares approach.[15,63,64] More complex models that take account of correlations within siblings in each generation can be run in specialized software, such as Mplus.[46]

In our example, grand maternal (G0) parity had a strong indirect effect on their daughters' adult height (Table 10.8). There was an estimated negative indirect effect of grand paternal manual social class on the foetal growth of their grand children, mainly through its influence on mother's birth weight and adult height. However, a woman's marriage to a socially more advantaged husband than her own father may have a positive effect on the foetal growth of her children. Of note, that here the results from path model for adult maternal height do appear slightly different compared to those from simple regression. As path analysis utilizes data over three generations on women who reproduced only, mothers appeared different from women without offspring.

All these observations should be interpreted in terms of the local context of the Grampian – specifically the changing economic conditions following the discovery of oil—and findings from this study may not be directly generalizable to another population in another period of time. Great care has also to be taken in interpreting the effect of socio-economic variables, as their association with general life-style may well change within a given population from generation to generation.

10.5 **Non-paternity**

Estimates of non-paternity in the general population vary, ranging from 1% to as high as 20%.[65] Non-paternity leads to an underestimation of the genetic portion of the covariance between fathers and offspring. In classical genetic studies, offspring with non-paternity pedigrees are found by genotyping and are excluded from analyses.

If no genotyping is available, and no other information on whether the fathers were biological fathers, then adjustments for non-paternity depend on the original sampling frame of the study. If families are sampled based on the disease status of the child, and assuming that the disease is genetic and recessive, then its biological parents will be genetically more similar to each other than parents from a general population—over and above the presence of assortative mating based on phenotype values. Studies in animal breeding show that the presence of non-biological fathers will then increase the genetic portion of the phenotype variance of fathers, and hence decrease correlation between fathers and offspring, leading to an over-estimation of the maternal effect.[66] The statistical consideration above and the biological knowledge gained in animal breeding experiments suggest that for comparisons of paternal and maternal effects on outcomes, adjustments for non-paternity have to be made if we believe that the outcome is under strong genetic influence as well as affected by considerable assortative mating. In such a situation, sensitivity analyses can be applied over a range of probabilities for non-paternity, p, and used to adjust directly the partial maternal and paternal regression coefficients by the factor $(1-p)$ to inflate paternal variance and respective co-variances.[67, 68]

If the precise genetic correlations for a given trait are unknown such adjustments for non-paternity may lead to the wrong conclusions. Especially with regards to the effect of life-style factors, non-biological fathers living in the same household may have comparable correlations with offspring when compared to the biological father. However, the sensitivity analyses describe above assume that the covariance between father and offspring is genetic, and thus the effects of environmental co-variance are adjusted away. Shared familial environmental factors are less likely to be affected by non-paternity than genetic estimates would be. It follows, therefore, that if social effects across generations are of particular interest, all fathers should be kept in the analysis irrespective of his genetic relation with the child.

A far more crude approach is to perform structured sensitivity analyses for different percentages of assumed non-paternity and without assuming any fixed effects on correlations or paternal variance. In a number of simulated datasets, say 100, a given percentage of fathers is set as missing, with subsequent repeating of the original analyses. Of these 100 sets of estimates, it is possible then to calculate ranges of uncertainty (lowest 95%CI limit of those datasets up to highest 95%CI limit of those datasets). As for the example above, one can then plot ranges of possible results for different percentages of non-paternity. If the bounds of uncertainty cross the null point for a specific level of non-paternity, then at least one of the simulated data sets contained an estimated confidence interval that overlapped with the null point. Such sensitivity analyses enable one to quantify the uncertainty of the initial results from the data by providing a range of possible values under varying degrees of missing paternal information.[69] These sensitivity analyses were carried out for the results displayed in Table 10.3, with the finding that the stronger association of maternal height with offspring birth weight, compared with the association of paternal height with offspring birth weight, remained even under high percentages of assumed non-paternity levels (Figure 10.5).

10.6 Missing data

In the setting of intergenerational data, due to the long follow up time involved in such studies, it is very common to have missing information on parents, and/or on several covariates within the whole dataset.

With regard to missing information on covariates, readily implemented tools are now available to perform multiple imputation, or an EM (expectation maximization) routine for mixed models

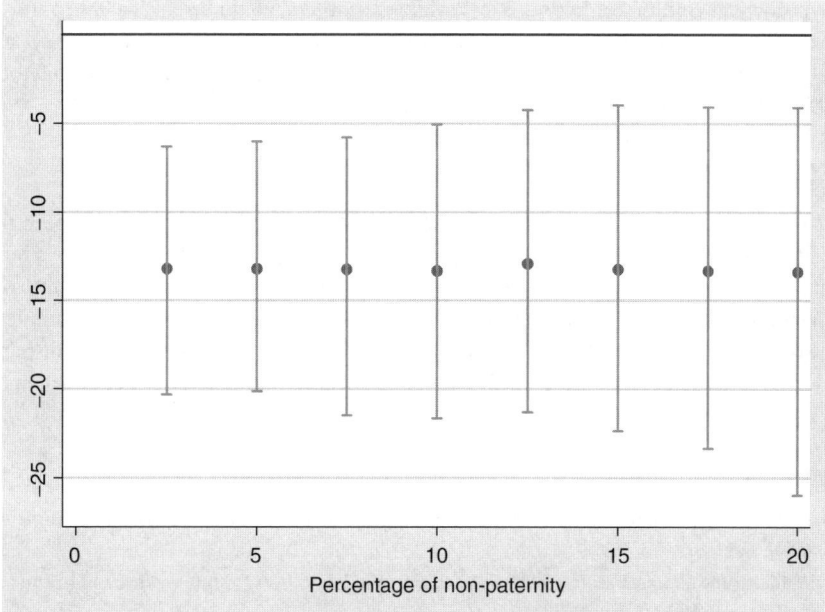

Fig. 10.5 Ranges of uncertainty for a maternal parent of origin effect on birth weight assuming varying portions of non-paternity. Corresponding analyses on the full data are displayed in table 10.3. The horizontal line on top denotes zero (no effect).

so as to deal with missing data under a missing at random (MAR) assumption.[45, 46, 70, 71] Other longitudinal imputation methods include the use of WinBUGS to compensate for missing data using multiple imputations, and to incorporate longitudinal structure using random effects.[47, 72] Again these methods assume MAR. This MAR assumption means that the occurrences of missing data are assumed to be a function of the collected data and their interdependencies, only. For genetic data collected within a genetic study of a complex trait this assumption is often defensible, because classical statistical models used for the genetic analysis familial association studies are conditioning on proband status. Whether the MAR assumption for missing data in any life course epidemiological study is upheld will depend upon the study design, the particular research question being addressed, what type of data are missing and the mechanisms that have resulted in these data being missing. It is beyond the scope of this chapter to discuss these in detail and readers are referred to detailed texts on dealing with missing data.[73] Here we describe a particular situation, that is relevant to intergenerational studies where records are linked between generations but information on those who migrate in anyone generation is incomplete. In this situation the assumption of MAR is unlikely to hold.

Apart from migration leading to missing covariate information on study participants, the issue also arises that intergenerational data are by definition dependent on the reproduction of individuals. For example, it may make sense to impute the missing covariates on maternal age within the Aberdeen dataset. On the other hand, it does not appear sensible to impute responses for the missing grandchildren in G2 for all those women in G1 who did not bear children. Of course this would assume that all the women who were recorded as not having children in fact bore offspring, but simply migrated prior to giving birth. Thus the relations between variables for these hypothetical children of hypothetical migrant mothers would be equivalent to those who remained in the Grampian. In summary any form of dealing with missing data under a MAR assumption must be viewed as a form of more sophisticated sensitivity analysis. For the Aberdeen study this is discussed in more detail in Nitsch et al.[69]

10.7 Conclusion

A range of statistical models from simple linear regression to multilevel models to path models can be fitted to data collected from intergenerational studies. Each of these models relies on implicit assumptions about the form and nature of the intergenerational relationship. Missing data is a common problem in any longitudinal studies and ignoring them by using complete case analysis may or may not produce biased results. On the other hand, any method of handling missing data such as multiple imputations for missing individuals must in the setting of be viewed as a form of sensitivity analysis.

References

1. Fisher, R. The correlation between relatives on the supposition of Mendelian inheritance. *Trans R Soc Edinburgh* 1918; **52**: 399–433.
2. Spielman, RS and Ewens, WJ. The TDT and other family-based tests for linkage disequilibrium and association. *Am J Hum Genet* **59**, 983-9.
3. Dohrenwend, B. P., Levav, I., Shrout, P. E., Schwartz, S., Naveh, G., Link, B. G., Skodol, A. E., and Stueve, A. Socioeconomic status and psychiatric disorders: the causation-selection issue. *Science* 1996; **255**: 946–52.
4. Sweden, S. Bakgrundsfakta till befolknings-och valfardsstatistik (The Multi-Generation Registry). Statistika Centralbyran, Orebro, 2001.
5. Wadsworth, M. E., Mann, S. L., Rodgers, B., Kuh, D. J., Hilder, W. S., and Yusuf, E. J. Loss and representativeness in a 43 year follow up of a national birth cohort. *J Epidemiol Community Health* 1992; **46**: 300–4.
6. Golding, J., Pembrey, M., and Jones, R. ALSPAC—the Avon Longitudinal Study of Parents and Children. I. Study methodology. *Paediatr Perinat Epidemiol* 2001; **15**: 74–87.
7. Peckham, C. S. A national study of child development (NCDS 1958 cohort). Preliminary findings in a national sample of 11-year-old children. *Proc R Soc Med* 1973; **66**: 701–3.
8. Harvey, N. C., Poole, J. R., Javaid, M. K., Dennison, E. M., Robinson, S., Inskip, H. M., Godfrey, K. M., Cooper, C., and Sayer, A. A. Parental determinants of neonatal body composition. *J Clin Endocrinol Metab* 2007; **92**: 523–6.
9. Golding, J., and Peters, T. J. The epidemiology of childhood eczema: I. A population based study of associations. *Paediatr Perinat Epidemiol* 1987; **1**: 67–79.
10. Bor, W., Najman, J. M., Andersen, M., Morrison, J., and Williams, G. Socioeconomic disadvantage and child morbidity: an Australian longitudinal study. *Soc Sci Med* 1993; **36**: 1053–61.
11. Hypponen, E., Davey Smith, G., Shepherd, P., and Power, C. An intergenerational and lifecourse study of health and mortality risk in parents of the 1958 birth cohort: (II) mortality rates and study representativeness. *Public Health* 2005; **119**: 608–15.
12. Cannings, C., and Thompson, E. A. Ascertainment in the sequential sampling of pedigrees. *Clin Genet* 1977; **12**: 208–12.
13. Weinberg, C. R., Wilcox, A. J., and Lie, R. T. A log-linear approach to case-parent-triad data: assessing effects of disease genes that act either directly or through maternal effects and that may be subject to parental imprinting. *Am J Hum Genet* 1998; **62**: 969–78.
14. Self, S., Longton, G., Kopecky, K., *et al.* On estimating HLA/disease association with application to the study of aplastic anaemia. *Biometrics* 1991; **47**: 53–61.

15 StataCorpLP. Stata Statistical Software: Release 10.0. Stata Corporation, College Station, TX, 2007.
16 Davey Smith, G., Hart, C., Ferrell, C., Upton, M., Hole, D., Hawthorne, V., and Watt, G. Birth weight of offspring and mortality in the Renfrew and Paisley study: prospective observational study. *Bmj* 1997; **315**: 1189–93.
17 Davey Smith, G., Hypponen, E., Power, C., and Lawlor, D. A. Offspring birth weight and parental mortality: prospective observational study and meta-analysis. *Am J Epidemiol* 2007; **166**: 160–9.
18 Falconer, D., and Mackay, T. *Introduction to Quantitative Genetics*, 4th ed., Pearson Education Limited, 1996.
19 Rao, D. C., Morton, N. E., and Cloninger, C. R. Path analysis under generalized assortative mating. I. Theory. *Genet Res* 1979; **33**: 175–88.
20 Hasstedt, S. J. Phenotypic assortative mating in segregation analysis. *Genet Epidemiol* 1995; **12**: 109–27.
21 McBride, G., and Robertson, A. Selection using assortative mating in Drosophila melanogaster. *Genet Res* 1963; **4**: 356–69.
22 Reik, W., and Walter, J. Genomic imprinting: parental influence on the genome. *Nat Rev Genet* 2001; **2**: 21–32.
23 Alberman, E., Filakti, H., Williams, S., Evans, S. J., and Emanuel, I. Early influences on the secular change in adult height between the parents and children of the 1958 birth cohort. *Ann Hum Biol* 1991; **18**: 127–36.
24 Morrison, J., Williams, G. M., Najman, J. M., and Andersen, M. J. The influence of paternal height and weight on birth-weight. *Aust N Z J Obstet Gynaecol* 1991; **31**: 114–6.
25 Kramer, M. Determinants of low birth weight: methodological assessment and meta-analysis. *Bull World Health Organ* 1987; **65**: 663–737.
26 Cloninger, C. R., Rice, J., and Reich, T. Multifactorial inheritance with cultural transmission and assortative mating. II. a general model of combined polygenic and cultural inheritance. *Am J Hum Genet* 1979; **31**:176–98.
27 Layzer, D. (1974). Heritability analyses of IQ scores: science or numerology? *Science* **183**, 1259-66.
28 Rao, D. C., Morton, N. E., and Yee, S. Resolution of cultural and biological inheritance by path analysis. *Am J Hum Genet* 1976; **28**: 228–42.
29 Button, T. M., Lau, J. Y., Maughan, B., and Eley, T. Parental punitive discipline, negative life events and gene-environment interplay in the development of externalizing behavior. *Psychol Med* 2008; **38**(1): 29–39, Epub 2007.
30 Eaves, L., Heath, A., Martin, N., Maes, H., Neale, M., Kendler, K., Kirk, K., and Corey, L. Comparing the biological and cultural inheritance of personality and social attitudes in the Virginia 30,000 study of twins and their relatives. *Twin Res* 1999; **2**: 62-80.
31 Goldstein, H. Multilevel mixed linear model analysis using iterative generalised least squares. *Biometrika* 1986; **73**: 43–56.
32 Burton, P. Applications in genetic epidemiology: modelling correlations in nuclear families using multilevel modelling. *Multilevel Modelling Newsletter* 1995; **7**: 5–8.
33 Elston, R. C., and Stewart, J. A general model for the genetic analysis of pedigree data. *Hum Hered* 1971; **21**: 523–42.
34 Rice, J., Cloninger, C. R., and Reich, T. Multifactorial inheritance with cultural transmission and assortative mating. I. Description and basic properties of the unitary models. *Am J Hum Genet* 1978; **30**: 618–43.
35 Goldstein, H., Healy, M. J., and Rasbash, J. Multilevel time series models with applications to repeated measures data. *Stat Med* 1994; **13**: 1643–55.
36 Boyle, C., and Elston, R. Multifactorial genetic models for quantitative traits in humans *Biometrics* 1979; **35**: 55–68.
37 Hopper, J. L. Variance components for statistical genetics: applications in medical research to characteristics related to human diseases and health. *Stat Methods Med Res* 1993; **2**:199–223.

38. Morton, N. E., and MacLean, C. J. Analysis of family resemblance. 3. Complex segregation of quantitative traits. *Am J Hum Genet* 1974; **26**: 489–503.
39. Rabe-Hesketh, S., Skrondal, A., and Gjessing, H. K. Biometrical Modeling of Twin and Family Data Using Standard Mixed Model Software. *Biometrics* 2008; **64**(1): 280–8, Epub 2007 May.
40. Pawitan, Y., Reilly, M., Nilsson, E., Cnattingius, S., and Lichtenstein, P. Estimation of genetic and environmental factors for binary traits using family data. *Stat Med* 2004; **23**: 449–65.
41. Breslow, N. E., and Clayton, D. Approximate inference in generalized linear mixed models. *J Am Stat Ass* 1993; **88**: 9–25.
42. Rodriguez, G., and Goldman, N. An assessment of multilevel models with binary responses. *Journal Royal Statistical Society, Series A* 1995; **158**: 73–89.
43. Rodriguez, G., and Goldman, N. Improved estimation procedures for multilevel models with binary response: A case study. *Journal Royal Statistical Society, Series A* 2001; **164**: 339–55.
44. Boehnke, M., and Lange, K. Ascertainment and goodness of fit of variance component models for pedigree data. *Prog Clin Biol Res* 1984; **147**: 173–92.
45. Skrondal, A., and Rabe-Hesketh, S. *Generalized Latent Variable Modeling: Multilevel, Longitudinal and Structural Equation Models*, Chapman & Hall/CRC, Boca Raton, Florida, 2004.
46. Muthen, L., and Muthen, B. *Mplus. Statistical analyses with latent variables. Version 3.0. User's Guide.* Muthen & Muthen, Los Angeles: CA, 2004.
47. Spiegelhalter, D., Thomas, A., Best, N., and Lunn, D. Winbugs Version 1.4. User Manual. MRC Biostatistics Unit, Cambridge, 2003.
48. Burton, P. R., Tiller, K. J., Gurrin, L. C., Cookson, W. O., Musk, A. W., and Palmer, L. J. Genetic variance components analysis for binary phenotypes using generalized linear mixed models (GLMMs) and Gibbs sampling. *Genet Epidemiol* 1999; **17**: 118–40.
49. Lee, H., and Stram, D. O. Segregation analysis of continuous phenotypes by using higher sample moments. *Am J Hum Genet* 1996; **58**: 213–24.
50. Batty, G. D., Morton, S. M., Campbell, D., Clark, H., Davey Smith, G., Hall, M., Macintyre, S., and Leon, D. A. The Aberdeen Children of the 1950s cohort study: background, methods and follow-up information on a new resource for the study of life course and intergenerational influences on health. *Paediatr Perinat Epidemiol* 2004; **18**: 221–39.
51. Wallace, C., and Clayton, D. Estimating the relative recurrence risk ratio using a global cross-ratio model. *Genet Epidemiol* 2003; **25**: 293–302.
52. Scurrah, K. J., Palmer, L. J., and Burton, P. R. Variance components analysis for pedigree-based censored survival data using generalized linear mixed models (GLMMs) and Gibbs sampling in BUGS. *Genet Epidemiol* 2000; **19**: 127–48.
53. Robins, J. M., Hernan, M. A., and Brumback, B. Marginal structural models and causal inference in epidemiology. *Epidemiology* 2000; **11**: 550–60.
54. Pickles, A., Wadsworth, M., and Maughan, B. *Epidemiological Methods in Life Course Research*, Oxford University Press, Oxford, 2007.
55. De Stavola, B. L., Nitsch, D., dos Santos Silva, I., McCormack, V., Hardy, R., Mann, V., Cole, T. J., Morton, S., and Leon, D. A. Statistical issues in life course epidemiology. *Am J Epidemiol* 2006; **163**: 84–96.
56. Burton, P. R., Scurrah, K. J., Tobin, M. D., and Palmer, L. J. Covariance components models for longitudinal family data. *Int J Epidemiol* 2005; **34**:1063–77; discussion 1077–9.
57. Morton, S. Lifecourse determinants of offspring size at birth: An intergenerational study of Aberdeen women. University of London, 2005.
58. Greenland, S., and Brumback, B. An overview of relations among causal modelling methods. *Int J Epidemiol* 2002; **31**:1030–7.
59. Greenland, S., Pearl, J., and Robins, J. Causal diagrams for epidemiologic research. *Epidemiology* 1999; **10**: 37–48.

60 Mishra, G., Nitsch, D., Black, S., DeStavola, B. L., Kuh, D. J., and Hardy, R. A structured approach to modelling the effects of socioeconomic status over the life course. *International Journal of Epidemiology*. 2008; doi:10.1093/ije/dyn229

61 Aitken, A. On least squares and linear combination of observations.. *Proceedings, Royal Society of Edinburgh* 1935; **55**: 42–8.

62 Wright, S. On the method of path coefficients. *Ann Math Statistics* 1934; **5**: 161–215.

63 Kline, T. J., and Klammer, J. D. Path model analyzed with ordinary least squares multiple regression versus LISREL. *J Psychol* 2001; **135**: 213–25.

64 Zellner, A., and Theil, H. Three stage least squares: simultaneous estimate of simultaneous equations. *Econometrica* 1962; **29**: 63–8.

65 Allison, D. The use of discordant sibling pairs for finding genetic loci linked to obesity: practical considerations. *Int J Obes* 1996; **20**: 553–60.

66 Senneke, S. L., MacNeil, M. D., and Van Vleck, L. D. Effects of sire misidentification on estimates of genetic parameters for birth and weaning weights in Hereford cattle. *J Anim Sci* 2004; **82**: 2307–12.

67 Davey Smith, G., Steer, C., Leary, S., and Ness, A. Is there an intra-uterine influence on obesity? Evidence from parent-child associations in ALSPAC. *Arch Dis Child* 2007; **92**(10): 876–80, Epub 2007 Jun 26.

68 Clemons, T. A look at the inheritance of height using regression toward the mean. *Hum Biol* 2000; **72**: 447–54.

69 Nitsch, D., DeStavola, B. L., Morton, S. M. B., and Leon, D. A. Linkage bias in estimating the association between childhood exposures and propensity to become a mother: an example of simple sensitivity analyses. *Journal Royal Statistical Society, Series A* 2006; **169**: 493–505.

70 Royston, P. Multiple Imputation of Missing Values: Update. *The Stata Journal* 2005; **5**: 1–14.

71 SASInstituteInc. SAS/STAT software, Version 9.1. Cary, NC, 2003.

72 Carrigan, G., Barnett, A., Dobson, A., and Mishra, G. Compensating for Missing Data from Longitudinal Studies Using WinBUGS. *Journal of Statistical Software* 2007; **19**: 1–17.

73 Little, R., and Rubin, D. *Statistical Analysis with Missing Data*, John Wiley & Sons, Inc, New York, 1987.

Appendix: Stata code for examples
Table 10.2: Heritability, simple linear regression
```
use heightage6.dta
*mmht: maternal height in cm, fmht: paternal height in cm, height6: childhood
height at age 6,
*sex=1: male, sex=2: female
bysort sex: summ mmht fmht height6 if mmht<. & fmht <. & height6<.
summ mmht fmht if mmht<. & fmht <. & height6<.
pwcorr mmht fmht if  height6<., sig
bysort sex: pwcorr mmht fmht height6 if mmht<. & fmht <. & height6<.
bysort sex: regress height6 mmht if mmht<. & fmht <.& height6<.
bysort sex: regress height6 fmht if mmht<. & fmht <.& height6<.
*to obtain heritabilities multiply regression coefficients with correction
factors as indicated in table as well as the factor 2.
```

Table 10.3: parent of origin effect, simple linear regression
```
use pateffect.dta
*mmht: maternal height in cm, fmht: paternal height in cm, mbwt: offspring birth
weight
summ mbwt fmht mmht if mbwt<. & fmht<. & mmht<.
regress mbwt fmht if mmht<.
regress mbwt mmht if fmht<.
regress mbwt fmht mmht
test fmht=mmht
egen meanheight= rowmean(fmht mmht)
gen diffheight= 0.5*(fmht-mmht)
regress mbwt meanheight diffheight
di (-4.66)^2
regress mbwt meanheight if mbwt<. & fmht<. & mmht<.
```

Variance components model and heritability estimate (taken from[39])
```
version 9.2
set more off
set mem 100m
set matsize 500

use adultheight.dta

** reshape to long
gen y1=heightm
gen y2=heightp
gen y3=heighto
gen family=_n
drop height*
reshape long y, i(family) j(member)
```

```
** transform variables
*sex = 1 = male and 2 = female
replace sex=1 if member==2
replace sex=2 if member==1

gen M = member==1
gen P = member==2
gen O = member==3

gen var1 = M+O/2
gen var2 = P+O/2
gen var3 = O/sqrt(2)

** Estimate model

xtmixed y sex    || family: var1 var2 var3, ///
   nocons cov(ident) mle

**** get heritability and confidence interval

** confidence interval for heritability
** using standard error of heritability
** (delta method used once)

nlcom (heritability: exp(2*[lns1_1_1]_b[_cons]) /  ///
     ( exp(2*[lns1_1_1]_b[_cons]) + exp(2*[lnsig_e]_b[_cons])))

** confidence interval for heritability
** using probit transformation and appropriate standard error
** (delta method used twice)

capture program drop _all
program define ciherit
   *ml display, first plus
   _coef_table, first plus
   noi _diparm lnsig_e lns1_1_1, label(heritability)                    ///
   func(exp(2*@2)/(exp(2*@1)+exp(2*@2)))                                ///
   deriv( -2*exp(2*@1)*exp(2*@2)/(exp(2*@1)+exp(2*@2))^2                ///
   -2*exp(4*@2)/(exp(2*@1)+exp(2*@2))^2+2*exp(2*@2)/(exp(2*@1)+exp(2*@2)))  ///
   level(95) ci(probit)
   disp in smcl in gr "{hline 13}" "{c BT}" "{hline 64}" _n
end

ciherit

*Repeat the same, but
*standardise heights
use adultheight.dta, clear
```

```
summ    heightp heightm
gen standp= (heightp- 173.3169)/ 8.093216
gen standm= (heightm- 161.1401)/6.490068
bysort sex: summ heighto
gen stando=(heighto-175.3364)/ 6.589212 if sex==1
replace stando=(heighto-162.3413)/ 6.077011   if sex==2

** reshape to long
gen y1=standm
gen y2=standp
gen y3=stando
gen family=_n
drop height* stand*
reshape long y, i(family) j(member)

** transform variables
*sex = 1 = male and 2 = female
replace sex=1 if member==2
replace sex=2 if member==1

gen M = member==1
gen P = member==2
gen O = member==3

gen var1 = M+O/2
gen var2 = P+O/2
gen var3 = O/sqrt(2)

*estimate heritability as above. Sex does not have an effect since adult height
was standardised by sex*
```

Tables 10.4 and 10.5: Tetrachoric correlation

```
clear
set mem 100m
set matsize 500
* the command rrrest needs to be downloaded after a keyword search

use hypertension.dta
* matpar: daughters parity;    gmpar : maternal parity
* binscls: manual social class of daughters husband
* gfbin2: manual social class of mother
* cmyrdel: centred age of daughter when she gives birth
* cgmyr: centred age of mother when she gives birth to daughter
* mhyp: pregnancy related hypertension in daughter
* gmhyp: pregnancy related hypertension in mother

*table 10.5
```

```
logistic  mhyp gmhyp gfbin2 cmyrdel cgmyr binscls gmpar gmpar matpar
*to get effects per 5 years of age:
lincom cmyrdel*5
lincom cgmyr*5


*table 10.4, compare coefficients with analysis in table 10.5
logit  mhyp gmhyp gfbin2 cmyrdel cgmyr binscls gmpar gmpar matpar
rrrest (gmhyp=  gmpar cgmyr gfbin2) ( mhyp= binscls cmyrdel matpar)

*test for equality of coefficients
test matpar=gmpar

*to get OR need to transform coefficients back onto exponential scale
```

Table 10.6

```
set mem 100m
set matsize 500
use aberdeengirls.dta

*zscore: foetal growth G2, mzscore: foetal growth G1
*mhtzsc: maternal height G1, gmhtzsc: grandmaternal height G0
*matpar: maternal parity G1, gmpar: grandmaternal parity G0
*binscls: paternal manual social class G1, gfbin2: grandpaternal social class G0

regress  zscore  mhtzsc cmyrdel binscls matpar
regress  mzscore  gmhtzsc  cgmyr gfbin2 gmpar
pwcorr mzscore zscore, sig

reg3  (mzscore   gmhtzsc   cgmyr gfbin2   gmpar) (zscore   mhtzsc   cmyrdel binscls
matpar)
testparm gmhtzsc mhtzsc, equal
testparm gfbin2 binscls, equal
testparm gmpar matpar, equal
```

Tables 10.7 and 10.8

```
set mem 100m
set matsize 500
use aberdeengirls.dta

*zscore: foetal growth G2, mzscore: foetal growth G1
*mhtzsc: maternal height G1, gmhtzsc: grandmaternal height G0
*matpar: maternal parity G1, gmpar: grandmaternal parity G0
*binscls: paternal manual social class G1, gfbin2: grandpaternal social class G0

**table 10.7
regress mzscore  gmhtzsc   cgmyr gfbin2   gmpar
regress mhtzsc  mzscore gmhtzsc gfbin2   gmpar
```

```
regress zscore mhtzsc  mzscore gmhtzsc gfbin2  gmpar cmyrdel binscls matpar

**table 10.8
reg3 (mzscore  gmhtzsc  cgmyr gfbin2  gmpar) ///
     (mhtzsc   mzscore gmhtzsc gfbin2  gmpar) ///
     (zscore mhtzsc mzscore gfbin2 cmyrdel  binscls matpar gmpar)


*grandmaternal height on offspring bwt: total=indirect, direct here set to zero
 nlcom [mzscore]_b[gmhtzsc]*[mhtzsc]_b[mzscore]*[zscore]_b[mhtzsc]+ ///
            [mzscore]_b[gmhtzsc]*[zscore]_b[mzscore]+ ///
            [mhtzsc]_b[gmhtzsc]*[zscore]_b[mhtzsc]

*grandmaternal height on maternal height: indirect
 nlcom [mzscore]_b[gmhtzsc]*[mhtzsc]_b[mzscore]

*grandmaternal height on maternal height: total
 nlcom [mzscore]_b[gmhtzsc]*[mhtzsc]_b[mzscore]+ ///
            [mhtzsc]_b[gmhtzsc]

*grandmaternal parity on offspring bwt: indirect
 nlcom [mzscore]_b[gmpar]*[mhtzsc]_b[mzscore]*[zscore]_b[mhtzsc]+ ///
            [mzscore]_b[gmpar]*[zscore]_b[mzscore]+ ///
            [mhtzsc]_b[gmpar]*[zscore]_b[mhtzsc]

*grandmaternal parity on offspring bwt: total
 nlcom [mzscore]_b[gmpar]*[mhtzsc]_b[mzscore]*[zscore]_b[mhtzsc]+ ///
            [mzscore]_b[gmpar]*[zscore]_b[mzscore]+ ///
            [mhtzsc]_b[gmpar]*[zscore]_b[mhtzsc]+ ///
            [zscore]_b[gmpar]

*grandmaternal parity on maternal height: indirect
 nlcom [mzscore]_b[gmpar]*[mhtzsc]_b[mzscore]

*grandmaternal parity on maternal height: total
 nlcom [mzscore]_b[gmpar]*[mhtzsc]_b[mzscore]+ ///
            [mhtzsc]_b[gmpar]

*grandpaternal manual social class on offspring bwt: indirect
 nlcom [mzscore]_b[gfbin2]*[mhtzsc]_b[mzscore]*[zscore]_b[mhtzsc]+ ///
            [mzscore]_b[gfbin2]*[zscore]_b[mzscore]+ ///
            [mhtzsc]_b[gfbin2]*[zscore]_b[mhtzsc]

*grandpaternal manual social class on offspring bwt: total
 nlcom [mzscore]_b[gfbin2]*[mhtzsc]_b[mzscore]*[zscore]_b[mhtzsc]+ ///
            [mzscore]_b[gfbin2]*[zscore]_b[mzscore]+ ///
            [mhtzsc]_b[gfbin2]*[zscore]_b[mhtzsc]+ ///
            [zscore]_b[gfbin2]
```

```
*grandpaternal manual social classon maternal height: indirect
 nlcom [mzscore]_b[gfbin2]*[mhtzsc]_b[mzscore]

*grandpaternal manual social class on maternal height: total
 nlcom [mzscore]_b[gfbin2]*[mhtzsc]_b[mzscore]+ ///
            [mhtzsc]_b[gfbin2]
            gmpar cmyrdel binscls matpar)
```

Figure 10.5

```
version 7.0
cap log close
clear
set mem 100m

use pateffect.dta
gen id=_n
regress mbwt fmht mmht
test fmht=mmht

egen meanheight= rowmean(fmht mmht)
gen diffheight= 0.5*(fmht-mmht)
regress mbwt meanheight diffheight

keep mbwt mean diff id
sort id
compress

save expat, replace

set more off
set seed 19562984

tempfile update sensitor
tempname pateff se isimul sens
postfile `sens' isimul pateff se using sensitor, replace

forvalues g=2.5 (2.5) 20 {
      display as text "gamma= " `g'
      use expat, replace

      forvalues i=1/100{
            qui cap drop miss
            display as text "simulation no.= " `i'
            qui sample `g'
            gen miss=1
            qui sort id
            qui save "`update'", replace
```

```
                qui use expat
                qui merge id using "`update'"
                qui replace meanheight=. if miss==1
                qui replace diffheight=. if miss==1
                qui cap drop _merge miss
                qui cap drop isimul pateff se
                qui regress mbwt meanheight diffheight
                gen pateff=_b[diffheight]
                gen se=_se[diffheight]
                gen isimul=`i'
                post `sens' (isimul) (pateff) (se)
        }
}
postclose `sens'

set more on
use sensitor, clear
gen gamma=int((_n-1)/100)
gen ciupper=pateff+1.96*se
gen cilower=pateff-1.96*se
tabstat pateff, by(gamma) s(mean)
tabstat cilower ciupper, by(gamma) s(min max)
```

Chapter 11

Random effects models for sibling and twin-based studies in life course epidemiology

Samuli Ripatti

Abstract

This chapter provides an introduction to statistical methods for twin and sibling studies using random effects models. The classic twin study begins with assessing the variance of a trait (called a phenotype by geneticists) in a large group, and attempts to estimate how much of this is due to genetic effects (heritability), how much appears to be due to shared environmental effects, and how much is due to unique environmental effects—events occurring to one twin but not another. Since heritability estimates are based on division of variances into between-pair and within-pair components, random effects models offer a uniform modelling framework for estimating these components of variance for a variety of traits measured on different scales. This chapter shows how three families of random effect models, random effects models for normally distributed traits, generalized linear mixed models for binary and count data, and frailty models for survival data may be used for modelling variances in longitudinal, or life course setting. The methods are illustrated using cognitive function and dementia onset data from The Swedish Adoption/Twin Study of Aging—a rich longitudinal dataset for aging. At the end of the chapter an appendix provides the R and Winbugs codes that are used in the analyses.

11.1 Introduction

Twin and family studies go back at least to the ancient physician Hippocrates (5th c. BCE), who attributed similar diseases in twins to shared material circumstances, and the stoic philosopher Posidonius (1st c. BCE), who attributed such similarities to shared astrological sex circumstances. The modern history of the twin study derives from Sir Francis Galton's pioneering use of twins to study the role of genes and environment on human development and behaviour. In his seminal 1875 paper 'The history of twins, as a criterion of the relative powers of nature and nurture'[1] he studied whether twins who were similar at birth diverged in dissimilar environments, and whether twins dissimilar at birth converged when reared in similar environments. He concluded that the evidence favoured nature rather than nurture.

From Chapter 4, we have seen that the power of twin designs arises from the fact that twins may be either monozygotic (MZ) developing from a single fertilized egg and therefore sharing all of their genes (with the exception of mitochondrial DNA)—or dizygotic (DZ) developing from two fertilized eggs and therefore sharing on average 50% of their genes, the same level of genetic similarity as found in non-twin full siblings. These known differences in genetic similarity, together with a testable assumption of equal environments for MZ and DZ twins[2] create the basis for the twin design for exploring the effects of genetic and environmental variance on a phenotype.[3]

11.1.1 Basic concepts in the twin study

Twin studies have long been recognized for their value in learning about the aetiology of disease. When studying associations between exposures of interest and traits, twin (and sibling) designs offer special opportunities for estimating the possible differential within-pair and between-pair effects. Carlin et al.[4] give an overview on these regression models and their interpretations. However, perhaps the greatest benefit of the twin design comes with the opportunity to model trait variances instead of mean effects and the basic logic of the twin study can be understood with very little mathematics beyond an understanding of correlation and the concept of variance.

The classic twin study begins with assessing the variance of a trait (called a phenotype by geneticists) in a large group, and attempts to estimate how much of this is due to genetic effects (heritability), how much appears to be due to shared environmental effects, and how much is due to unique environmental effects—events occurring to one twin but not the other.

In twin literature these three components are called A (additive genetics), C (common environment), and E (unique environment)—the so-called ACE Model. It is also possible to examine non-additive genetics effects, often denoted D for dominant effects. Given the ACE model, researchers can determine what proportion of variance in a trait is heritable, versus the proportions which are due to shared environment or unshared environment.

MZ twins have all their genes in common and if they were raised in a family share their early life environment. All differences between them in this framework can be attributed to unique or non-shared environment. The correlation r in a continuous trait we observe between MZ twins provides an estimate of A+C. Similarly, DZ twins have a common shared environment, and share 50% of their genes: so the correlation between DZ twins is a direct estimate of ½A + C, thus:

$$r^{MZ} = A + C$$
$$r^{DZ} = \tfrac{1}{2} A + C$$

The argument that MZ and DZ twins can be used to separate out genetic from environmental influences is based on the assumption that MZ and DZ twins experience the same degree of similarity in their environments, with respect to factors related to the trait of interest. Under this equal environment assumption, any excess similarity between MZ twins over that between DZ twins must be due to the greater proportion of genes shared by MZ twins rather than DZ twins. Under the equal environments assumption, the two equations above allow us to derive A, C and E:

$$A = 2(r^{MZ} - r^{DZ})$$
$$C = 2r^{DZ} - r^{MZ}$$
$$E = 1 - r^{MZ}$$

where r^{MZ} and r^{DZ} are simply the correlations of the trait in MZ and DZ twins respectively. Twice the difference between MZ and DZ twins gives us an estimate of A: the additive genetic effect.

C is simply the MZ correlation minus our estimate of A, and E is estimated directly by how much the MZ twin correlation deviates from 1.[5,6]

11.1.2 Extending this basic concept to the sibling study

In sibling data, the two siblings share on average half of their genes, thus being genetically comparable to DZ twins. The only difference is that siblings are not matched by age as DZ twins are. While similar comparisons of trait correlations are not available in sibling design, the intra-sibling correlation is a useful statistic for estimating the degree of *familial aggregation*—the effect of shared genes and early life environment—of the trait. The larger the correlation, the bigger is the effect of genes and shared early life environment in the variation of the trait.

11.2 Example of a twin study with over 20 years of follow-up: the Swedish Adoption/Twin Study of Aging

11.2.1 Design of the Swedish Twin Study

The methods in this chapter are illustrated using cognitive function and dementia onset data from The Swedish Adoption/Twin Study of Aging (SATSA)—a rich longitudinal dataset for the study of ageing. The Swedish Adoption/Twin Study of Aging (SATSA) was started in 1984 and is comprised of several longitudinal components. A comprehensive questionnaire was sent in the first component to all twins separated at an early age and reared apart and a control sample of twins reared together from the Swedish Twin Registry. The questionnaire included items concerning rearing, adult, and working environment, health status, health related behaviours (e.g. alcohol, tobacco, and dietary habits) as well as attitude and personality measures. The questionnaire phase is repeated every third year: Thus far more than 2,000 twins have responded to questionnaires sent in 1984, 1987, 1990, 1993, and 2004. In the second component a subsample of approximately 150 twin pairs reared apart and 150 twin pairs reared together have participated in four waves of in person testing including a health examination, structured interviews/tests of functional capacity, cognitive abilities, and memory. The first three waves were at three year intervals, the fourth was initiated in 1999, a fifth wave in 2002, and a sixth wave in 2005.

11.2.2 Longitudinal changes

Data from SATSA are analysed for the purpose of examining the relative importance of genetic and environmental factors for individual differences in aging related processes. Longitudinal changes as well as the relationships within and among domains (e.g. the importance of genetic effects for mediating the relationship between physical health and cognitive decline) for the elderly are of primary interest.

In our examples of random effects models we model individual longitudinal trajectories of scores for block design tests, one of the cognitive function tests that measures visual-spatial and motor skills. In this block design test the testee is required to take blocks that have all red sides, all white sides, and red and white sides and arrange them according to a given pattern. They are timed on this task compared to a normative sample.

Figures 11.1 and 11.2 show the trajectories on random subsets of 20 MZ and 20 DZ twin pairs. The two members of a pair are plotted with the same colours. The trajectories show considerable random fluctuation in the test scores, but also a trend towards lower scores as the twins grow older. Additionally, the trajectories for the two members of a pair seem to be a bit closer to each other in Figure 11.1 than in Figure 11.2, hinting at larger correlation between test scores for MZ pairs that for DZ pairs. Note also, that the individual trajectories have different lengths

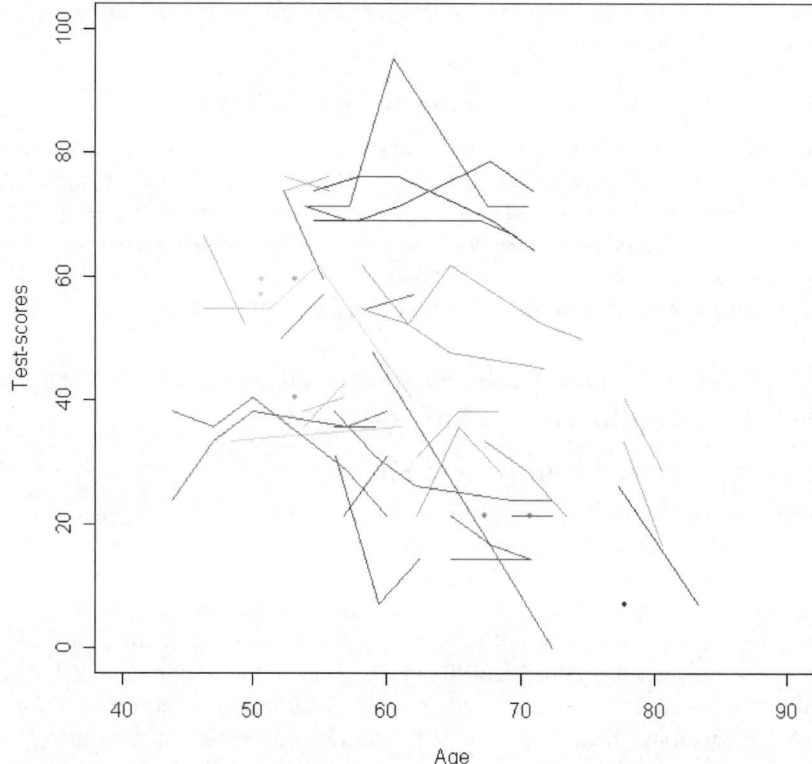

Fig. 11.1 Longitudinal trajectories of 20 randomly chosen MZ twins for block design test (see also colour plate 1).

reflecting the fact that some of the individuals drop out from the study. We'll return to different aspects of the scores in later sections.

11.3 On statistical software

The statistical analyses in this chapter can be done with various software packages. In our examples, we generally use R language and environment for statistical computing (http://www.r-project.org). There are several good textbooks and tutorials for R and many of them are listed in the R web pages. Here we assume a basic knowledge of the R functions. For Bayesian Markov Chain Monte Carlo estimation, we use WinBugs 1.4 (http://www.mrc-bsu.cam.ac.uk/bugs/winbugs/contents.shtml) which can also be accessed through R. Both software packages are flexible to operate and are freely available. Where applicable, we provide examples of the software code in an appendix at the end of this chapter.

11.4 Analysing cross-sectional twin data

11.4.1 Using random effects analysis of variance to infer within-pair associations

A simple way to estimate the within-pair correlation is to use one-way random effects analysis of variance (random ANOVA) to divide the variation into between pair and within pair components.

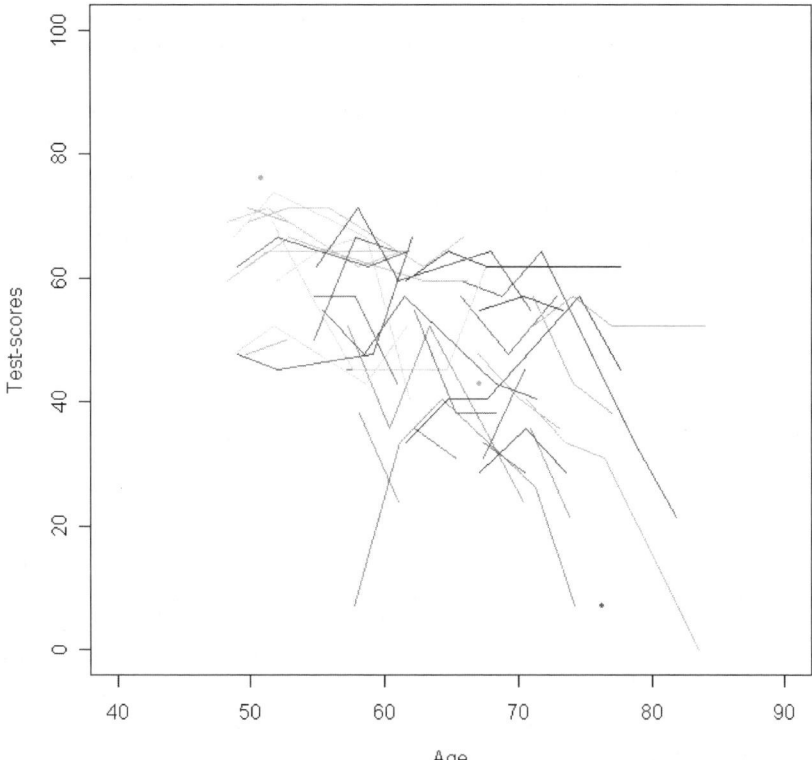

Fig. 11.2 Longitudinal trajectories of 20 randomly chosen DZ twins for block design test (see also colour plate 2).

If there is a genetic component to the trait variation, this can be seen by the MZ pairs having a larger proportion of their total variance between the pairs than in DZ pairs, and similarly MZ twins have a smaller proportion of their variance within pairs than DZ pairs.

The traditional fixed effects ANOVA for analysing sibling data were described in Chapter 3. Random effects ANOVA differs from the fixed effects ANOVA by assuming that the groups of interest, in our case the twin pairs, are a random sample of all the twin pairs in the population instead of a fixed set of 'groups'. This notion of random effects are introduced here and extended later on to longitudinal setting.

More formally, in random effects ANOVA the trait of interest Y is modelled as:

$$Y_{ij} = \mu + b_i + \varepsilon_{ij}, \tag{11.1}$$

where $i = 1, \ldots, n$ is an index for n pairs and $j = 1, 2$ for the two members in a pair, μ is the over-all average of trait Y, b_i is the random effect for pair i and ε_{ij} is the residual for individual j in pair i. In random effects ANOVA both the residuals and the random effects are assumed to follow a Normal distribution:

$$\varepsilon_{ij} \sim N(0, \sigma^2)$$
$$b_i \sim N(0, \sigma_b^2),$$

with σ^2 and σ_b^2 being the residual variance and the between-pair random effect variance, respectively. Note that with cross-sectional data with only one measurement per individual, it is not possible to differentiate the variance due to measurement error and an individual specific random fluctuation. However, with more structured models for longitudinal data described later in the chapter, both sources of variation may be estimated separately.

For family level data, i and j denote family and individual specific indices, respectively, with j possibly getting different numbers for different families, if the family sizes differ (for example, if this were applied to sibling data with differing numbers of siblings per family).

The variances of the two random components in the models can be used to calculate estimates for the intra-pair correlations. The correlation is simply the proportion of between-pair variance from the total variance:

$$r = \frac{\sigma_b^2}{(\sigma_b^2 + \sigma^2)}.$$

These intra-pair correlation estimates may further be used to divide the variance into heritability, shared environment, and non-shared environment.

The estimation of parameters for the random effect ANOVA can be done by maximizing the likelihood function of the data. However, it has been shown[7] that for unbiased variance estimates it is preferable to maximize a so called restricted maximum likelihood (REML). This maximization routine has been implemented in several statistical analysis packages, including PROC MIXED in SAS and lme-function in R. The R code for a cross-sectional random effects model is given in the appendix and we discuss here the interpretation of the model using the first wave of measurements in SATSA block test example.

The analysis shows that the standard deviation estimates (square roots of variances σ^2) are 15.4 and 9.9 for between and within pair variations, respectively (see appendix). These can be used to calculate the intra-pair correlations (estimated correlation for between MZ twins is 0.71).

11.4.1.1 Adding a covariate—adjusting for age

Both the fixed effects part and random effects part of Model 11.1 can easily be extended to incorporate covariate information. Here we extend the fixed effects part so that we can adjust for additional covariates measured for each individual, and in the next section we show how the random part can be extended to incorporate longitudinal information from each individual.

Model (11.1) can be rewritten as:

$$Y_{ij} = X_{ij}\beta + b_i + \varepsilon_{ij},$$
$$b_i \sim N(0, \sigma_b^2) \qquad (11.2)$$
$$\varepsilon_{ij} \sim N(0, \sigma^2)$$

where X_{ij} is a vector of covariates for individual j in pair i, and β is a vector of regression parameters. When the first item in X_{ij} is 1 for each individual, the first β is the intercept of the linear model. This extension allows for adding covariates that are either individual or twin pair specific. The level of variation in Y that the covariates explain is then reflected also in the variance estimates as can be seen in the appendix where statistical code and results for this example are shown.

R-code and output are shown in the appendix. The variance component estimates have changed a bit, particularly for between-pair variance which has dropped from a between pair standard deviation of 15.4 to 14.2. This follows from the fact that the two twins in a pair were called for testing at the same time, so the ages-at-testing vary more between pairs than within pairs. The change is also reflected in the intra pair correlation estimate which drops from 0.71 to 0.67.

The slope estimate −0.78 shows that on average one extra year of age corresponds to 0.78 drop in the block design test score.

11.5 Modelling repeated measures in twin data

In the previous section we showed how random effects ANOVA can be used to model cross-sectional twin data and extended the model to include covariates as additional fixed effects. In this section we extend the model into a full mixed effects linear model by allowing also the random effects to have more structure. This is needed when the data is longitudinal in the sense that it includes repeated measures taken from the same individual. Repeated measures introduces an additional layer of hierarchy to the model; now the measurements are correlated within twin pairs, but also the repeated measures taken for each individual may be more correlated with each other than with the measures of a co-twin. This is reflected also in the model below. Now, consider:

$$Y_{ij} = X_{ij}\beta + Z_{ij}b + \varepsilon_{ij},$$
$$b \sim N(0, D(\theta)) \qquad (11.3)$$
$$\varepsilon_{ij} \sim N(0, \sigma^2)$$

Here $b = (b_1, \ldots, b_q)$ is a vector of random effects and Z_{ij} is a design vector for individual ij. Random effects b are assumed to follow jointly a multivariate normal distribution with a variance/covariance matrix with parameters θ.

In our example there are up to five measurements of block test for each individual. In Figures 11.1 and 11.2 we see that the number of measurements vary from 1 to five for different individuals due to possible drop-out or failure to adequately complete the test. Also, the age range during which the measurements were taken varies between individuals since they were recruited at different ages. In the SATSA study, one of the primary goals has been to learn about the longitudinal effects of aging on cognitive function. A natural statistical modelling frame-work for studying aging is to fit a random growth curve to each individual as a function of age at the measurement, and to study how parameters in these growth curves vary and how correlated they are within twin pairs. Figures 11.3 and 11.4 show how the mean and the standard deviation of the scores develop over age.

In the appendix we show the R program code and output for the model with repeat data in SATSA MZ twins. In the random effects output (appendix example 11.2), we see that the between-pair standard deviation estimates are 42.1 and 0.57 for the intercept and slope, respectively in the MZ twins. Similarly, the within-pair standard deviation estimates are 23.9 and 0.39 for the random intercept and random slope, respectively. The estimates for intra-pair correlations are 0.76 and 0.68 respectively for intercepts and slopes, in the MZ twins.

The intra-pair correlation estimates for DZ twins are 0.45 and 0.51 respectively for intercept and slope (full analyses not shown). These estimates can be used together with MZ intra-pair correlations to estimate that the proportion of variance due to additive genetic effects is A = 2*(0.76 − 0.45) = 0.62 and 2*(0.68 − 0.51) = 0.34 for intercept and slopes, respectively. Similarly, the estimates for variance explained by shared environment is C = 2 × 0.45 − 0.76 = 0.14 and by unique environment is E = 1 − 0.76 = 0.24 for the intercepts and C = 2 × 0.51 − 0.68 = 0.34 and E = 1 − 0.68 = 0.32 for the slopes. Thus, additive genetic effects in this study are estimated to account for 62% of the variance in the average block test (cognitive function) score and 34% of the variance in its change with increasing age; shared environmental effects account for

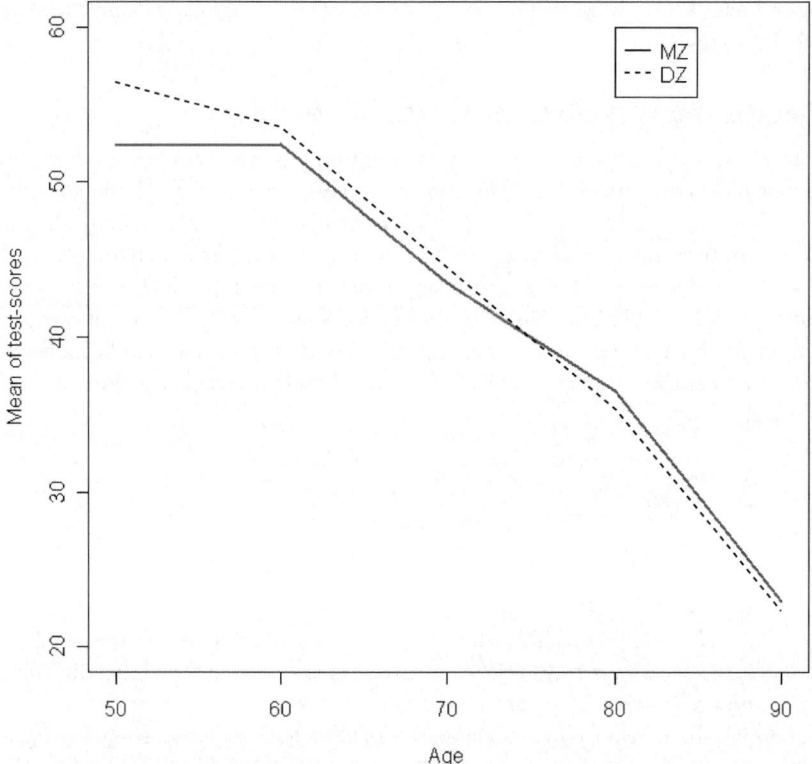

Fig. 11.3 Estimated means of the block design test scores over age (see also colour plate 3).

14% of the variance in the average score and 34% of the variance in change with age and unique environmental effects account for 24% of the variance in the average score and 32% of the variance in change with age.

11.6 Generalized linear mixed models (GLMM)

The generalized linear model (GLM) for independent individuals is specified through the probability distribution for the observations, and the link function relating the regression parameters to the means. Conditional on the means the observations are assumed to be statistically independent. The standard linear regression model is a GLM with normal distribution and identity link. The log-linear model for count data is a GLM with Poisson distribution and logarithmic link. The logistic regression model is a GLM with binomial distribution and logit link. These three special cases are useful standard GLMs with attractive theoretical properties.[8]

GLMs have also been extended to allow for random effects during the past two decades. Stiratelli, Laird and Ware[9] elegantly extend the Laird and Ware[10] mixed model for normally distributed repeated measures to the multivariate binary setting. Breslow and Clayton[11] give a thorough account of random effects generalized linear models, and call them generalized linear mixed models (GLMM).

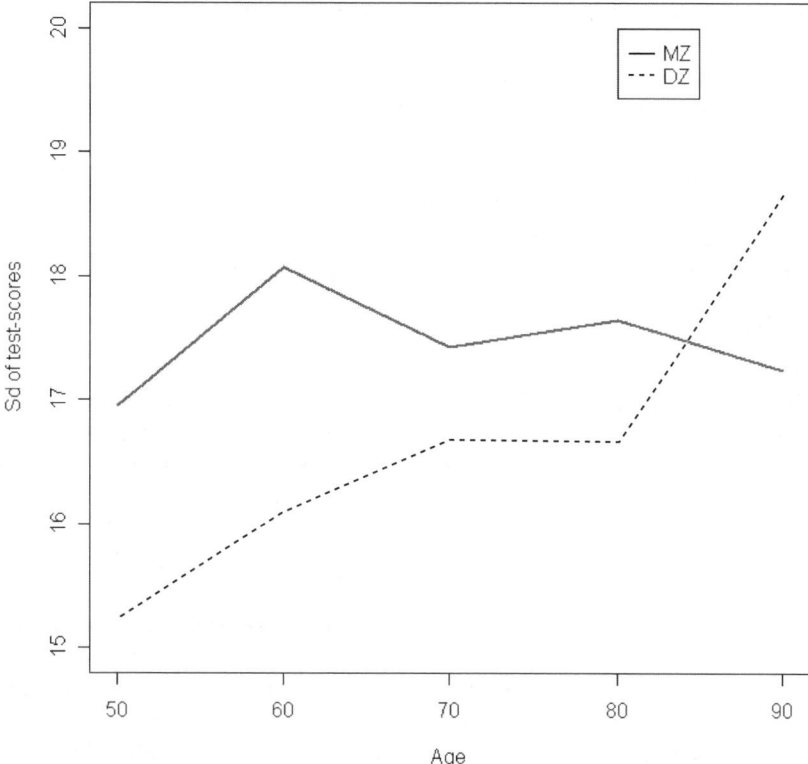

Fig. 11.4 Estimated average standard deviations of the block design test scores over age (see also colour plate 4).

In GLMM a transformation of the mean is modelled as a linear function of fixed parameters and normally distributed random effects. A link function connects the conditional mean and the linear predictor:

$$h(\mu_{ij}) = X_{ij}\beta + Z_{ij}b,$$
$$\mu_{ij} = E(Y_{ij} | b) \tag{11.4}$$
$$b \sim N(0, D(\theta))$$

and conditionally on random effects the outcome variable Y is assumed to follow an exponential family distribution, such as binomial (with typically a logit link) or Poisson distribution (with typically a logarithmic link).

While maximization of the likelihood is not feasible in GLMMs in the way it can be done in general linear mixed models, parameter estimation can be done using approximate likelihood methods[11] or using simulation-based likelihood and Bayesian methods. Approximate maximum likelihood methods based on penalized quasi-likelihood (PQL) are available in R library lme4 (cran.r-project.org).

To illustrate, how a GLMM model with repeated binary measurements can be fitted using R, we dichotomize the block design test score for the DZ twins. The statistical code and output are shown in example 11.3 in the appendix. The fixed effect estimate for slope is 0.218 (standard error = 0.022) corresponding to an odds ratio of 1.24 (exponentiate of 0.218) for the probability of the score being smaller than 45, per one year increase in age amongst the DZ twins. The variance component estimates lead to intra-pair correlations of 0.65 and 0.78 for intercept and slope, respectively. Similar analyses can be completed for the MZ twins and the results used in combination (as illustrated in Section 11.5 above) to estimate the contribution of additive genetic, shared environment, and unique environment to the variance in the average odds of the low block test (cognitive function score) and to the variance in change in the odds with increasing age.

11.7 Frailty models for age-at-onset data on twins

11.7.1 Why use frailty models?

In epidemiology, survival models have dominated the methodology for studying age at onset of a disease. This has largely been a result of the wide use of the Cox regression model,[12] where the risk for a disease is modelled as a function of time (commonly age) and measured covariate information. In quantitative genetic analyses of heritability of disease, the age at onset has received relatively little attention, and in the cases where it has been evaluated, survival models have rarely been applied. This is partly explained by the fact that genetic models have focused on variability in a latent continuous distribution of liability, whereas traditional survival methods have focused on the mean survival.

During the past decade, there has been progress in two kinds of latent variable models for age at onset analyses using twins. The first family of methods has expanded traditional structural equation models to survival data with threshold parameters connecting data on categorized age groups to an underlying latent normally distributed liability for disease. Twin models with multiple thresholds have been applied to age at onset responses.[13–16] The advantage of structural equation models lies in the simplicity of using the multivariate normal distribution for the liability to disease and the availability of software for these models. However, there are also problems and limitations with this approach. The age scale needs to be divided with arbitrary cut-off points and this classification causes loss of information in the data; left truncation and right censoring in the data are difficult to handle; the normality assumption of the liability is seldom justified for the age at onset distribution, which tends to have longer tails and an asymmetric shape. Additionally, there is no satisfactory way to take mortality into account in these models, which initially did not distinguish between death and disease onset outcomes.[14]

The problems with the multiple threshold mean models can be tackled with the second family of models, the semiparametric hazard based survival models. In the past few years, the traditional survival model methodology has been extended to include multivariate latent random effects or frailties,[16–19] which allow the inter-person variation in risks to be embedded in the model.

Frailty models have been extended into a multivariate random effect setting that can be used to partition the inter-person variation in age at onset of a chronic disease in twin studies, while fully taking into account the longitudinal aspects of the data including left truncation and right censoring. Their development has been parallel with generalized linear mixed models.[20]

11.7.2 Multivariate frailty model

For right-censored failure time data the random effects are referred to as frailties.[21] There is a rather extensive literature on so-called shared frailty models which are equivalent to random intercept models (Model 11.2) for normally distributed data with one level of random effects that are shared by members in the same cluster (in our case twin pair).[22]

A multivariate version of the Cox regression model is defined as a time dependent hazard for an event of interest:

$$\lambda_{ij}(t) = \lambda_0(t)\exp(X_{ij}\beta + Z_{ij}b),$$
$$b \sim N(0, D(\theta)) \tag{11.5}$$

where $\lambda_0(t)$ is a baseline hazard that is multiplied by the exponential function defining the relative risk for an individual j in pair i. The baseline hazard may also be given a parametric form, as we will do in the dementia example below. The relative risk is assumed to stay constant over the follow-up.

11.7.2.1 Modelling the onset of dementia in SATSA twins

We use these models to study heritability of dementia in the SATSA sample. Dementia is a late onset disorder, with prevalence increasing from 1.4% at age 65–69 to 15.8% at age 80–84[23] and beginning to level off at age 90–95.[24–25] In multiple threshold structural equation models for age of onset for Alzheimer's disease, Meyer and Breitner[14] report that genetic and shared environmental effects account for 37% and 35%, respectively, of the variance in liability. With a similar approach, Pedersen et al.[15] report that genetic and shared environmental effects account for 57% and 0% of the variance, respectively, for Alzheimer's disease. Although not previously reported, corresponding results for all dementia indicated that genetic effects accounted for 63% and shared environment for 24% of the variance.

The Study of Dementia in Swedish Twins,[26] used here for illustration, includes all members of the SATSA subsample who were born in 1935 or earlier and alive in 1987. The sample used in this example consists of 195 MZ pairs and 341 DZ pairs with both members screened for dementia at least once during the follow-up period (Table 11.1). Forty-four MZ and 68 DZ twins developed dementia and 72 MZ and 134 DZ twins died during the follow-up. Twenty MZ and 42 DZ twins both developed dementia and died during the follow-up. The overall dementia and mortality rates were similar for both types of twins. Kendall's τ,[18] a non-parametric descriptive measure for dependence within pairs, is larger for MZ twin pairs than for DZ twins indicating larger intra pair dependence for identical twins (see Table 11.1).

Table 11.1 Descriptive statistics of the sample of twins used in the analysis

	MZ	DZ
Number of individuals	390	682
Dementia:		
Number of dementia cases	44	68
Total person years	10803	19028
Rate of dementia	0.0041	0.0036
Kendall's τ(95% CI[1])	0.45(0.25,0.67)	0.20(0.033,0.36)
Death:		
Number of deaths	72	134
Total person years	3210	5642
Mortality rate	0.022	0.024

[1] Based on 100 bootstrap samples.

11.7.2.2 A frailty model for dementia

Because the age at onset of dementia is measured in whole years, we specify a discrete time multiplicative hazard model for twin pair i, $i = 1, \ldots, n$ ($n = 195$ and $n = 341$ for MZ and DZ, respectively) and individual j, $j = 1, 2$ at age k, $k = c, \ldots, K$ ($c = 37$, and $K = 93$ and $K = 95$ for MZ and DZ, respectively):

$$\lambda_{ijk} = \lambda_k \exp(b_i + b_{ij}) = \exp(\alpha_k + b_i + b_{ij}),$$
$$b \sim N(0, D(\theta)) \tag{11.6}$$

where b_i and b_{ij} are frailties or random effects specifying twin pair specific and individual specific log relative risks, respectively, and λ_k is the population specific average hazard of dementia at age k. The frailties are unobserved and random. The observed dementia times are assumed to be conditionally independent given the frailties.

11.7.3 Bayesian multivariate frailty models

We use this model to illustrate the possibilities for Bayesian modelling. Bayesian statistical methods are particularly useful when modelling data with hierarchical structures, such as in twin studies. With the developments in simulation-based Markov chain Monte Carlo methods for estimation and inference and development of generally available software, Bayesian methods have become computationally feasible.

For the hazard model, Clayton[27] shows how to sample from the non-parametric distribution for the conditional baseline hazard λ_k using a Gamma distribution as a prior distribution for the jump sizes in a discrete baseline hazard with one event in each time interval. Note that when a log-normal prior is assumed for the jumps, the resulting frailty model fits into the generalized linear mixed model framework with time modelled as a random effect.

The model is extended into a hierarchical Bayesian model by assigning prior distributions for the unobservables in the model. We assume that the two frailty components b_i and b_{ij} appear independently and follow Gaussian distributions with mean zero and variances σ^2_{pair} and σ^2_{ind}, respectively. The frailty variances σ^2_{pair} and σ^2_{ind} are assumed to be drawn independently from a flat Uniform (0,1000) hyper prior distribution. Because the data are quite sparse (44 MZ twins and 68 DZ twins developed dementia during the follow-up period) we smooth the baseline hazard using a second difference Gaussian prior distribution for the log-hazards α_k (see ref 11 for details) with variance $\sigma^2_\alpha/2$. The prior for σ^2_α is defined as an inverse Gamma (0.1,0.1) distribution. Markov chain Monte Carlo (MCMC) samples from the posterior distributions are drawn with Gibbs sampling[28] using WinBUGS software.[29]

Again, we define an intra pair correlation:

$$\rho = \frac{\sigma^2_{pair}}{\sigma^2_{pair} + \sigma^2_{ind}}$$

to measure the degree of association within twin pairs on the log-hazard scale. The variation in the baseline population hazard over age groups does not enter into this. MZ and DZ twins are contrasted by estimating this correlation separately for both types of twins. In accordance with standard twin models, these correlations can further be used to estimate the proportions of variance explained by genetic, and shared and non-shared environmental effects.[30]

For both models, Gibbs sampling was used with 20,000 samples drawn from the posterior distribution after a burn-in period of 1000 samples. Table 11.2 shows the medians and the

Table 11.2 Variance estimates (σ^2), intra pair correlations (ρ) and estimates for proportions of variance attributed to genes (A), shared environment (C) and non-shared environment (E) given by medians of the marginal posterior distributions with their 90% credible intervals for the simple frailty model

Parameter	MZ	DZ
σ^2_{pair}	3.97(1.69,8.25)	1.12(0.31,2.48)
σ^2_{ind}	0.50(0.012,2.68)	0.52(0.043,1.88)
σ^2_a	0.034(0.016,0.085)	0.028(0.014,0.070)
ρ	0.89(0.61,1.00)	0.69(0.27,0.96)
A	0.31(0,1)	
C	0.54(0,1)	
E	0.11(0.0036,0.39)	

90% credible intervals of the marginal posterior distributions for the parameters in the frailty model (11.6). The between pair variance estimate is substantially larger for MZ pairs (3.97 [1.69,8.25]) than for DZ pairs (1.12 [0.31,2.48]) and the individual specific variance is larger for DZ twins, although variation in the estimates is large (see Table 11.2). The posterior median of the smoothing parameter for the baseline hazard is almost the same for both types of twins. The differences in the intra pair correlations between MZ twins and the DZ twins reflect the differences in the variance components. The credible intervals for the intra pair correlations are much larger for the DZ twins showing that there is more information about the correlations in the MZ twins. This can also be seen in the plotted posterior distribution (solid line) in Figure 11.5. The flat prior distributions for the variance components lead to symmetric and slightly informative prior distributions (histograms in Figure 11.5) for intra pair correlations with mode at 0.5. The prior is conservative giving more distribution mass around the values of no genetic effect because a priori the intra pair correlations are assumed to be the same for MZs and DZs. Large credible intervals for the intra pair correlation in Table 11.2 are driven by the thick tails in the posterior distribution for the DZ twins. The WinBUGS code used to fit the model described above is shown in example 11.4 in the appendix.

11.8 Discussion: further extensions to the random effect models for twin and sib-pairs analyses

There are several ways that the random effect models for twins and sib-pairs presented here may be extended. It is obvious that the mean trajectories are rarely linear over different periods of life. The mixed model framework presented here uniformly allows for extension to the fixed and random effects to account for possible non-linear trend. The simplest extension is to add a quadratic term into the model to allow for curvilinear effects. With enough measurements per individual, this quadratic model may also be allowed to be subject specific and the variability in the quadratic function may then be studied.

Another extension to model non-linear effects could be to allow for bilinear effects with individual specific turning points in the model. This model would allow an individual to follow one trajectory until a turning point occurs and moves an individual to another trajectory. Indeed, evidence for such a behaviour has been presented for late age cognitive abilities with a turning point occurring close to death. These turning points may be related to measured

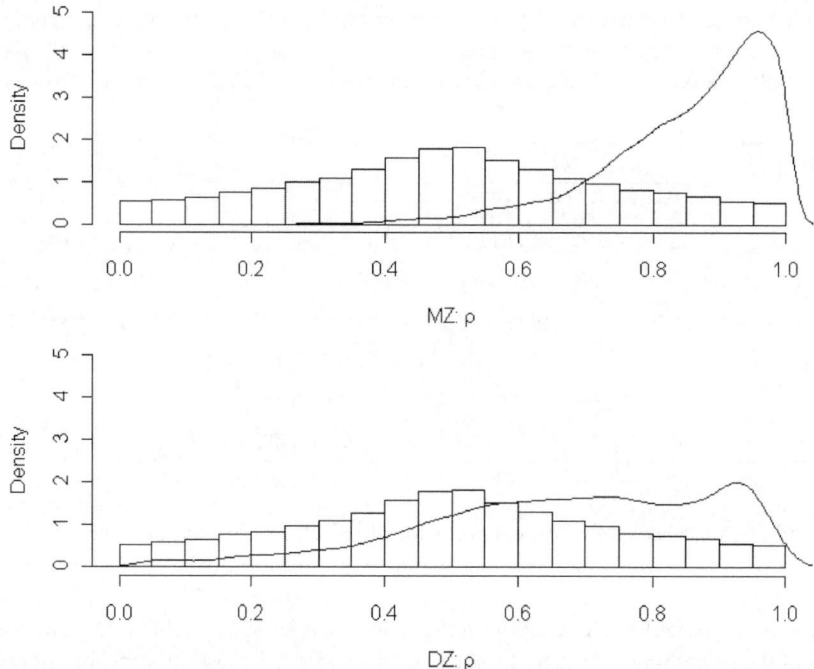

Fig. 11.5 Prior (histogram) and posterior (solid line) distributions for the intra pair correlations ρ, for MZ and DZ twins, based on the simple frailty model of dementia.

exposures (such as a divorce or an infarction) or they may be latent and estimated from the observed trajectories. Modelling jointly the risk of a turning point and the observed repeated measures leads to models incorporating both frailty methods and random effect models for repeated measurement.

Yet another extension to these time dynamic models is to incorporate more complex family structures. The variance/covariance matrix of the random effects can be extended to account for different levels of familial dependencies (see reference 31 for an example). However, the computational burden grows as the number of crossed (non-hierarchical) dependencies grows.

Finally, dealing with missing data is an important topic that has been ignored in this chapter. With longitudinal data, some level of drop-out will be inevitable and often this drop-out is selective in terms of traits of interest. When there exists extra information on causes of drop-out and strong predictors for dropping out (or any other causes of missing data), conditioning on these predictors in the analysis is advisable through multiple imputation and corresponding methods. In MCMC-based Bayesian estimation, multiple imputation can be naturally incorporated into the main analysis with missing data presenting another layer of unobservables along with the estimated parameters.

Acknowledgments

I would like to thank Juni Palmgren, Nancy Pedersen, and Margaret Gatz for our joint work on frailty models that was the basis for the frailty section, and Ida Lindqvist for preparing the figures for the chapter. The Swedish Twin Registry is thanked for their permission to use their wonderful longitudinal data on the chapter. The data used in the frailty example was collected with aid of

NIH Grants No. R01 AG008724 and R01 AG010175. The views expressed in this chapter are those of the author and not necessarily anyone named in the acknowledgements.

References

1. **Galton, F.** The history of twins, as a criterion of the relative powers of nature and nurture. *Fraser's Magazine* 1875; **12**: 566–76.
2. **Bouchard, T. and P. Propping.** *Twins as a Tool of Behavioral Genetics.* Chichester, John Wiley & Son Ltd, 1993.
3. **Neale, M. and L. Cardon.** *Methodology for Genetic Studies of Twins and Families.* Dordrecht, Netherlands, Kluwer Academic, 1992.
4. **Carlin, J., L. Gurrin, et al.** 'Regression models for twin studies: a critical review.' *International Journal of Epidemiology* 2005; **34**: 1089–99.
5. **Jinks, J. and D. Fulker.** Comparison of the biometrical genetical, MAVA, and classical approaches to the analysis of human behavior. *Psychol Bull* 1970; **73**(5): 311–49.
6. **Plomin, R., J. DeFries, et al.** *Behavioral Genetics.* New York, Freeman, 2001.
7. **Harville, D.** Maximum Likelihood approaches to variance component estimation and to related problems. *Journal of the American Statistical Association* 1977; **72**: 320–38.
8. **McCullagh, P. and J. Nelder.** *Generalized Linear Models.* London, Chapman and Hall, 1989.
9. **Stiratelli, R., N. Laird, et al.** Random effect models for serial observations with binary response. *Biometrics* 1984; **40**: 961–71.
10. **Laird, N. and J. Ware.** Random-effects models for longitudinal data. *Biometrics* 1982; **38**: 963–74.
11. **Breslow, N. and D. Clayton.** Approximate inference in generalized linear mixed models. *Journal of the American Statistical Association* 1993; **88**: 9–25.
12. **Cox, D.** Regression models and life tables. *Journal of the Royal Statistical Society Series B* 1972; **34**: 187–220.
13. **Pickles A, Neale M, et al.** A simple method for censored age-of-onset data subject to recall bias: Mother's reports of age of puberty in male twins. *Behavior Genetics* 1994; **24**: 457–69.
14. **Meyer, J. and J. Breitner.** Multiple threshold model for the onset of Alzheimer's disease in the NAS-NRC twin panel. *American Journal of Medical Genetics* 1998 **81**: 92–7.
15. **Pedersen, N., S. Posner, et al.** Multiple threshold models for genetic influences on age of onset for Alzheimer's disease: Findings in Swedish twins. *American Journal of Medical Genetics* 2001; **105**: 724–8.
16. **Pickles, A., R. Crouchley, et al.** Survival models for developmental genetic data: Age at onset of puberty and antisocial behaviour in twins. *Genetic Epidemiology* 1994; **11**: 155–70.
17. **Yashin, A. and A. Iachine.** Genetic analysis of durations: correlated frailty model applied to survival of Danish twins. *Genetic Epidemiology* 1995; **12**: 529–38.
18. **Hougaard, P.** Analysis of multivariate survival data. Heidelberg, Springer-Verlag, 2000.
19. **Ripatti, S. and J. Palmgren.** Estimation of multivariate frailty models using penalized partial likelihood. *Biometrics* 2000; **56**(4): 1016–22.
20. **Palmgren J. and S. Ripatti.** Fitting exponential family mixed models. *Statistical Modelling* 2002; **2**: 23–38.
21. **Vaupel, J., K. Manton, et al.** The impact of heterogeneity in individual frailty on the dynamics of mortality. *Demography* 1979; **16**: 439–54.
22. **Hougaard, P.** Modeling heterogeneity in survival data. *Journal of Applied Probability* 1991; **28**: 695–701.
23. **Ritchie, K., D. Kildea, et al.** The relationship between age and the prevalence of senile dementia: A meta-analysis of recent data. *International Journal of Epidemiology* 1992; **21**: 763–9.
24. **Fratiglioni, L., D. DeRonchi, et al.** Worldwide prevalence and incidence of dementia. *Drugs Aging* 1999; **15**: 365–76.
25. **Ritchie, K. and D. Kildea.** Is senile dementia 'age-related' or 'ageing-related'? Evidence from meta-analysis of dementia prevalence in the oldest old. *Lancet* 1995; **346**: 931–4.

26. **Gatz, M., N. Pedersen,** *et al.* Heritability for Alzheimer's disease: the study of dementia in Swedish twins. *Journals of Gerontology Series A: Biological Sciences and Medical Sciences* 1997; **52**: M117–M125.
27. **Clayton, D.** A Monte Carlo method for Bayesian inference in frailty models. *Biometrics* 1991; **47**: 467–85.
28. **Geman, S. and D. Geman.** Stochastic relaxation, Gibbs distributions, and the Bayesian restoration of images. *IEEE Transactions on Pattern Analysis and Machine Intelligence* 1984; **6**: 721–41.
29. **Lunn, D., A. Thomas,** *et al.* WinBUGS—a Bayesian modelling framework: concepts, structure, and extensibility. *Statistics and Computing* 1999; **10**: 325–37.
30. **Falconer, D.** *Introduction to Quantitative Genetics*. Edinburgh, Oliver & Boyd, 1960.
31. **Pankratz, V., M. de Andrade,** *et al.* Random-effects Cox proportional hazards model: general variance components methods for time-to-event data. *Genetic Epidemiology* 2005; **28**: 97–109.

Appendix: Statistical Codes used in analyses presented in Chapter 11

Example 11.1: Estimating random effects ANOVA using R

This example is described in Section 11.4.1 'Using random effects analysis of variance to infer within-pair associations', and is used initially for cross sectional data.

R has a special library for estimating linear and non-linear random effect models called nlme. Nlme is a collection of different functions for manipulating datasets, plotting them, modelling and testing them. The code below shows the first few lines of the data, how to transform it to a format suitable for lme-function and how to fit a random effects ANOVA to the MZ twins in the SATSA data. Once the grouped Data-function has been run, the syntax for lme is simple using the standard R model formula – lme automatically recognizes the data to be of hierarchical structure and treats pairs as random clusters.

```
> b.mz[1:6,]
  ID PAIR TEST1 AGE1
3  3    2  7.142857 81.10799
4  4    2 26.190476 81.10799
5  5    3 40.476190 78.80868
6  6    3 52.380952 77.65571
7  7    4  0.000000 56.77739
8  8    4 38.095238 56.77739
>
> tmp.mz <- groupedData(TEST1~1 | PAIR, data=b.mz)
> tmp.mz[1:6,]
Grouped Data: TEST1 ~ 1 | PAIR
  ID PAIR TEST1 AGE1
3  3    2  7.142857 81.10799
4  4    2 26.190476 81.10799
5  5    3 40.476190 78.80868
6  6    3 52.380952 77.65571
7  7    4  0.000000 56.77739
8  8    4 38.095238 56.77739
> f1 <- lme(TEST1~1, data=tmp.mz)
> f1
Linear mixed-effects model fit by REML
Data: tmp.mz
Log-restricted-likelihood: -895.1836
Fixed: TEST1 ~ 1
(Intercept)
42.41623
Random effects:
Formula: ~1 | PAIR
        (Intercept) Residual
StdDev:    15.37530 9.920616
Number of Observations: 216
```

```
Number of Groups: 108
>
> (15.38^2)/(15.38^2+9.92^2)
[1] 0.7062064
```

The groupedData-function adds meta information to the tmp.mz-object to tell that the data have a hierarchical structure with PAIR being a grouping variable. In the default output from the lme function we see that the standard deviation estimates (square roots of variances σ^2) are 15.4 and 9.9 for between and within pair variations, respectively. These can be used to calculate the intra-pair correlations (estimated correlation for MZ twins is 0.71) as is shown in the last lines of the output.

Example 11.1 continues: adding covariates

In lme, the fixed effects are added to the model by argument 'fixed' and a model formula outcome ~ fixed effect. Lme also automatically adds the intercept to the model. The intercept can be omitted from the mode by fixed=outcome~ -1 + effect. Below we show how adjusting for age at the time of testing changes the model estimates for SATSA data:

```
> f2 <- lme(TEST1~1, fixed=TEST1~AGE1, data=tmp.mz)
> f2
Linear mixed-effects model fit by REML
Data: tmp.mz
Log-restricted-likelihood: -888.1
Fixed: TEST1 ~ AGE1
(Intercept) AGE1
90.1605389 -0.7814371
Random effects:
Formula: TEST1 ~ 1 | PAIR
(Intercept) Residual
StdDev: 14.19431 9.894586
Number of Observations: 216
Number of Groups: 108
>
> 14.19^2/(14.19^2+9.89^2)
[1] 0.6730532
```

The variance component estimates have changed a bit, particularly for between-pair variance which has dropped from 15.4 to 14.2. This follows from the fact that the two twins in a pair were called for testing at the same time, so the ages-at-testing vary more between pairs than within pairs. The change is also reflected in the intra pair correlation estimate which drops from 0.71 to 0.67. The slope estimate −0.78 shows that on average one extra year of age corresponds to 0.78 drop in the block design test score.

Example 11.2: Modelling repeated measures in twin data using R

This example relates to the analyses described in Section 11.5 'Modelling Repeated Measures in Twin Data'

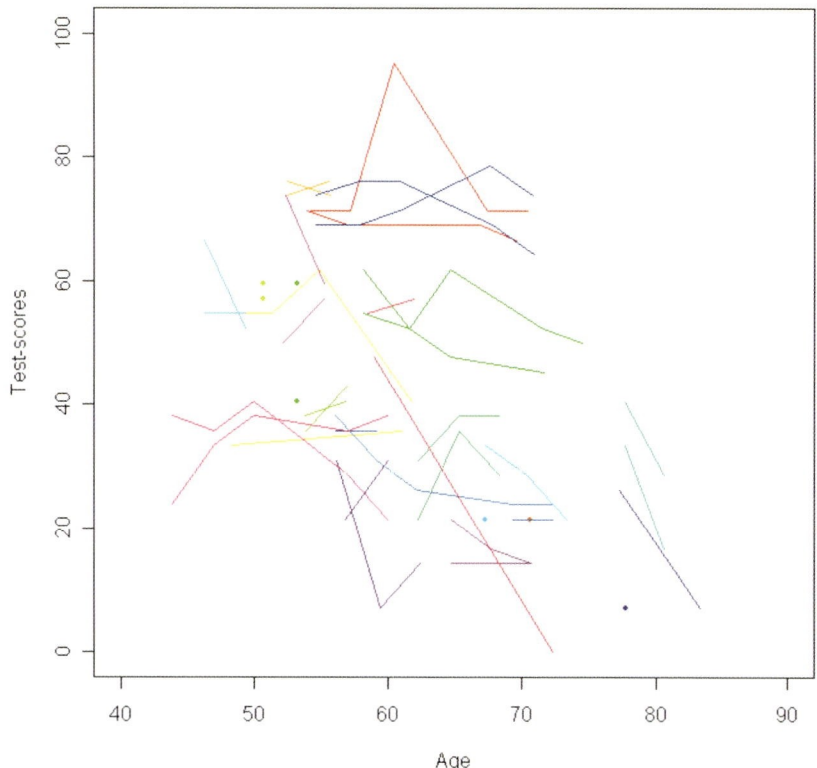

Plate 1 Longitudinal trajectories of 20 randomly chosen MZ twins for block design test.

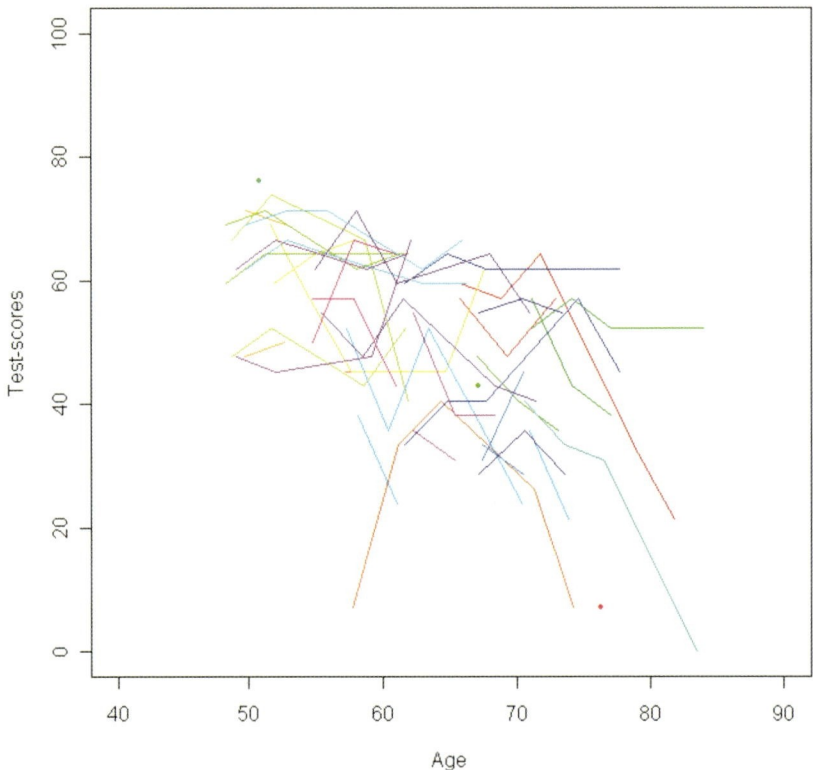

Plate 2 Longitudinal trajectories of 20 randomly chosen DZ twins for block design test.

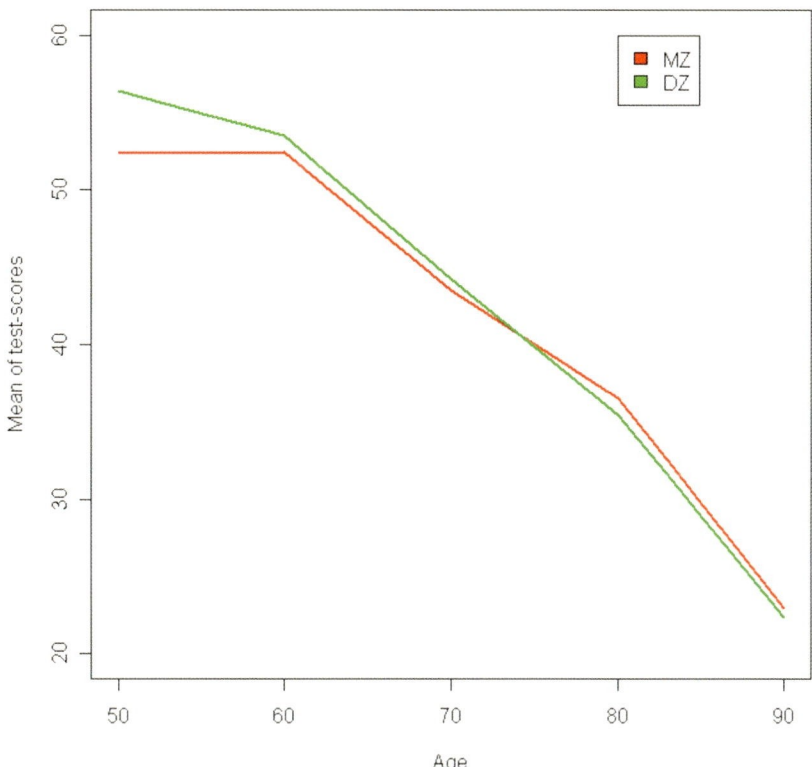

Plate 3 Estimated means of the block design test scores over age.

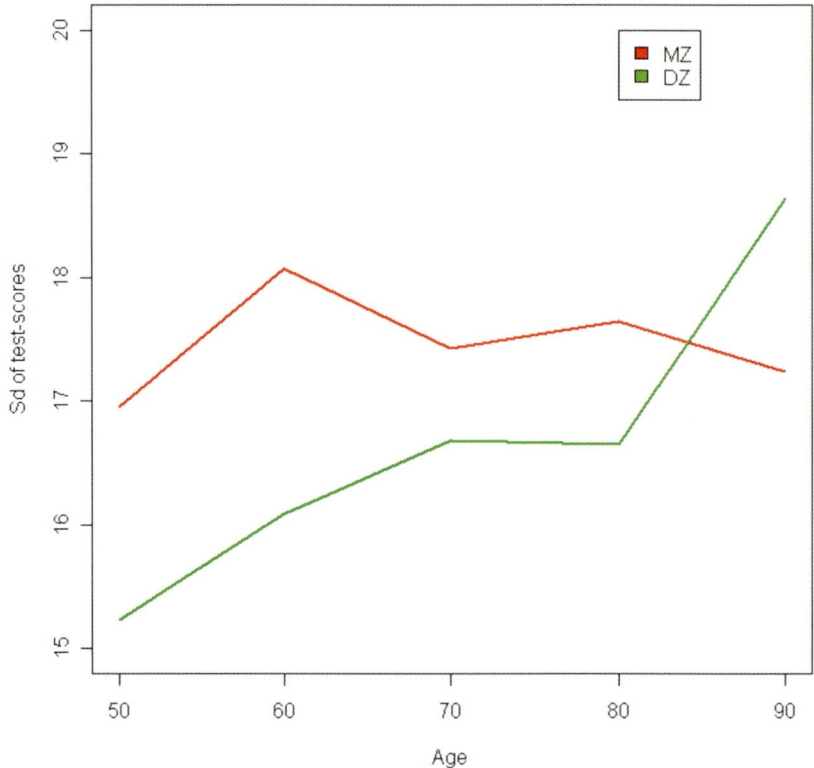

Plate 4 Estimated average standard deviations of the block design test scores over age.

In the example below, a random intercepts and slopes are fitted to the SATSA data for the MZ twins (as in example 11.1). We first transpose the data into a long format for the groupedData function:

```
> tmp.id <- rep(a.mz2$ID,5)
> tmp.pair < rep(a.mz2$PAIR,5)
> tmp.test <- c(a.mz2$TEST1,a.mz2$TEST2,a.mz2$TEST3,a.mz2$TEST4,a.mz2$TEST5)
> tmp.age <- c(a.mz2$AGE1,a.mz2$AGE2,a.mz2$AGE3,a.mz2$AGE4,a.mz2$AGE5)
> tmp.ipt <- rep(1:5,times=length(unique(a.mz2$ID)))
> tmp.mz2 <- groupedData(tmp.test~tmp.age | tmp.pair/tmp.id)
> tmp.mz2 <- tmp.mz2[!is.na(tmp.mz2$tmp.age) & !is.na(tmp.mz2$tmp.test),]
> tmp.mz2[1:12,]
Grouped Data: tmp.test ~ tmp.age | tmp.pair/tmp.id
   tmp.test  tmp.age tmp.pair tmp.id
1   7.142857 81.10799    2      3
2  26.190476 81.10799    2      4
3  40.476190 78.80868    3      5
4  52.380952 77.65571    3      6
5   0.000000 56.77739    4      7
6  38.095238 56.77739    4      8
7  64.285714 54.99178    5      9
8  59.523810 54.99452    5     10
9  78.571429 54.76918    6     11
10 83.333333 54.76918    6     12
11  7.142857 77.74726    7     13
12 26.190476 77.30479    7     14
```

We continue by fitting a random slope model to the five measurements for each individual with separate estimates for the pair level and for both individuals within a pair:

```
> f3 <- lme(tmp.test~tmp.age, data=tmp.mz2)
> f3
Linear mixed-effects model fit by REML
 Data: tmp.mz2
 Log-restricted-likelihood: -2784.263
 Fixed: tmp.test ~ tmp.age
(Intercept)     tmp.age
 88.193878   -0.721885
Random effects:
 Formula: ~tmp.age | tmp.pair
 Structure: General positive-definite
            StdDev     Corr
(Intercept) 42.0584568 (Intr)
tmp.age      0.5705153 -0.948
 Formula: ~tmp.age | tmp.id %in% tmp.pair
 Structure: General positive-definite
            StdDev     Corr
```

```
(Intercept) 23.9193533 (Intr)
tmp.age 0.3897896 -0.978
Residual 7.6341996
Number of Observations: 728
Number of Groups:
tmp.pair tmp.id %in% tmp.pair
108 216
> 42.0584568^2/(42.0584568^2+23.9193533^2)
[1] 0.7556073
> 0.5705153^2/(0.5705153^2+0.3897896^2)
[1] 0.6817587
```

In the random effects output, we see that the between-pair standard deviation estimates are 42.1 and 0.57 for the intercept and slope, respectively. Similarly, the within-pair standard deviation estimates are 23.9 and 0.39 for the intercept and slope, respectively. The last lines show the estimates for intra-pair correlations which are 0.76 and 0.68 for intercepts and slopes, respectively.

The intra-pair correlation estimates for DZ twins are 0.45 and 0.51 for intercept and slope, respectively. These estimates can be used together with MZ intra-pair correlations to estimate that the proportion of variance due to additive genetic effects is A = 2 (0.76 - 0.45) = 0.62 and 0.34 for intercept and slopes, respectively. Similarly, the estimates for variance explained by shared environment is C = 2 x 0.45 - 0.76 = 0.14 and by unique environment is E = 1- 0.76 = 0.24 for the intercepts and C = 2 x 0.51 – 0.68 = 0.34 and E = 1- 0.68 = 0.32 for the slopes.

Example 11.3: Generalized linear mixed model using R

To illustrate, how a GLMM model with repeated binary measurements can be fitted using R, we dichotomize the block design test score for the DZ twins. This example is described in Section 11.6 'Generalized linear mixed models'.

A new variable is created taking value 1 (TRUE in the output below) when test score is smaller than 45, and 0 (FALSE in the output) otherwise. Below we illustrate how a generalized linear mixed model for binary outcome, a logit link function and PQL estimation can be fitted using R:

```
> tmp.dz3 <- tmp.dz2
> tmp.dz3$bin <- tmp.dz2$tmp.test<45
> tmp.dz3$tmp.age <- tmp.dz3$tmp.age-65
> tmp.dz3[1:12,]
Grouped Data: tmp.test ~ tmp.age | tmp.pair/tmp.id
  tmp.test  tmp.age  tmp.pair tmp.id bin
1  7.142857 17.983563  1  1 TRUE
2 21.428571 17.983563  1  2 TRUE
3 78.571429 -9.600920  2  3 FALSE
4 38.095238 -9.598181  2  4 TRUE
5 47.619048 -8.650230  4  6 FALSE
6 45.238095 -8.997261  4  7 FALSE
7 42.857143 -9.344291  5  8 TRUE
8 47.619048 -8.202279  5  9 FALSE
9  7.142857 13.205019  6 10 TRUE
10 40.476190 13.205019  6 11 TRUE
```

```
11 21.428571 12.770327 7 12 TRUE
12 42.857143 12.770327 7 13 TRUE
>
> f3b2 <- lmer(bin~tmp.age +(tmp.age|tmp.id) + (tmp.age|tmp.pair),
family='binomial', data=tmp.dz3)
> f3b2
Generalized linear mixed model fit using Laplace
Formula: bin ~ tmp.age + (tmp.age | tmp.id) + (tmp.age | tmp.pair)
Data: tmp.dz3
Family: binomial(logit link)
AIC BIC logLik deviance
1307 1348 -645.3 1291
Random effects:
Groups Name Variance Std.Dev. Corr
tmp.id (Intercept) 7.225451 2.688020
tmp.age 0.022529 0.150098 -0.573
tmp.pair (Intercept) 3.910815 1.977578
tmp.age 0.006202 0.078753 0.366
number of obs: 1346, groups: tmp.id, 376; tmp.pair, 188
Estimated scale (compare to 1) 0.6480396
Fixed effects:
Estimate Std. Error z value Pr(>|z|)
(Intercept) 0.17053 0.23537 0.725 0.469
tmp.age 0.21806 0.02171 10.046 <2e-16 ***
--
Signif. codes: 0 '***' 0.001 '**' 0.01 '*' 0.05 '.' 0.1 ' ' 1
Correlation of Fixed Effects:
(Intr)
tmp.age -0.130
```

The model syntax for lmer is different from lme, the grouping variable for the random effect is given with a | symbol. (tmp.age | tmp.pair) means that the age variable is random (estimating the between-pairs variability in trend between). The fixed effect estimate for slope is 0.218 (se 0.022) corresponding to an odds ratio of 1.24 for the probability of the score being smaller than 45, per one year increase in age.

The variance component estimates lead to intra-pair correlations of 0.65 and 0.78 for intercept and slope, respectively.

Example 11.4 Bayesian Multivariate Frailty model using WinBUGS

This example shows the WinBUGS code used for the analyses described in Section 11.7.3 'Bayesian Multivariate Frailty Models'.

```
model
{
for (i in 1:N) {
    d[i] ~ dpois(mu[i])
mu[i] <- Y[i]*exp(alpha1[twid[i]]+
```

```
       alpha2[id[i]]+beta0+beta[age[i]])
                 }
       for (j in 1: Ntwid) {
                 alpha1[j] ~ dnorm(0, tau1)
                 }
       for (j in 1: Nid) {
                 alpha2[j] ~ dnorm(0, tau2)
                 }
       beta0 ~dnorm(0,0.00001)
       betamean[1] <- 2*beta[2] - beta[3]
       Nneighs[1] <- 1
       betamean[2] <- (2*beta[1] + 4*beta[3] - beta[4]) / 5
       Nneighs[2] <- 5
       for (k in 3: Nage - 2) {
                 betamean[k] <- (4*beta[k - 1] + 4*beta[k + 1] - beta[k -2] -
beta[k + 2]) / 6
                 Nneighs[k] <- 6
                 }
       betamean[Nage - 1] <- (2*beta[Nage] + 4*beta[Nage - 2] - beta[Nage - 3]) /
5
       Nneighs[Nage - 1] <- 5
       betamean[Nage] <- 2*beta[Nage - 1] - beta[Nage - 2]
       Nneighs[Nage] <- 1
       for (k in 1: Nage) {
                 betaprec[k] <- Nneighs[k] * tau3
                 }
       for (k in 1: Nage) {
                 beta[k] ~ dnorm(betamean[k], betaprec[k])
                 tau.like[k] <- Nneighs[k] * beta[k] * (beta[k] - betamean[k])
                 lambda[k] <- exp(beta0+beta[k])
                 }
       sigmasq1 ~ dunif(0,1000)
       sigmasq2 ~ dunif(0,1000)
       tau1 <- 1 / sigmasq1
       tau2 <- 1 / sigmasq2
       d1 <- 0.1 + sum(tau.like[]) / 2
       r1<- 0.1 + Nage / 2
       tau3 ~ dgamma(r1, d1)
       sigmasq3 <- 1 / tau3
       roo1 <- sigmasq1 / (sigmasq1 + sigmasq2 + sigmasq3)
       roo2 <- sigmasq1 / (sigmasq1 + sigmasq2)
}
```

Chapter 12

Discussant chapter—statistical considerations in family-based life course studies

Amanda Sacker

Abstract

This chapter summarizes some of the issues that have been described in the previous two chapters on statistical considerations in family studies. It aims to highlight some of the assumptions underlying the analytic methods and discuss how their use can impact the results. The statistical analyses outlined in this section share common features aimed at quantifying the association between genetic and environmental factors with phenotypic outcomes.
For some research, the focus is on heritability while for other work, the focus is on environmental issues while controlling for genetic influences. Modelling approaches for each are discussed, emphasizing potential problems and providing guidelines for careful interpretation. Examples from published empirical epidemiological work will be used to illustrate the breadth of analytical strategies adopted for family studies research.

12.1 Introduction

The fields of life course epidemiology and genetic epidemiology have grown rapidly over the last decade and it is timely to consider methods at the intersection of these two approaches. A review of models for intergenerational studies is provided by Nitsch and Mishra while models for twin data are reviewed by Ripatti. Both sets of authors build on simple statistical models to show the additional subtlety and complexity that is possible with longitudinal family data.

Ripatti has concentrated on the genetic contribution to variability in phenotypes. Nitsch and Mishra have demonstrated that while the aim of an intergenerational study can take the form of partitioning out the variance into its genetic and environmental components, another study might be more interested in controlling for the effect of genes when estimating environmental effects and vice versa. It is also possible to focus attention on covariate effects on the outcome and view the twin study as a unique method for adjusting for the confounding effect of genetic or environmental influences. In a useful review of regression models for twin studies,[1] Carlin *et al* present different parameterizations of a general regression model that allows for different covariate effects between and within twin pairs. Stata syntax is helpfully given for each parameterisation. These models can also be applied to other family relationships besides twins.

The discussion that follows takes two directions. The first is a critical review of some of the issues surrounding statistical approaches to family studies. Controversies about the assumptions underlying the statistical models and the interpretation of the results from the analyses are emphasized. I also try to draw attention to some limitations of the analytic models in common use in the field. The next section discusses heritability and its underlying assumptions; this is followed by a section on the limitations of the ACE model and a consideration of models that go beyond it; and a further section discusses the interpretation of shared and non shared variation in family studies.

The second part of this commentary then takes a more forward looking attitude and focuses on the advantages of life course models for family data. It gives examples of publications in the field, with the intention of interesting readers in further explorations into this exciting area of research. First, the advantages of a life course approach are discussed and then a discussion of latent variable models extends the introduction to this approach given by Nitsch and Mishra.

12.2 Heritability

Heritability is the proportion of phenotypic variation in a population that is attributable to genetic variation among individuals. The corollary of this definition is that the environmentability of a trait is the proportion of phenotypic variance attributable to environmental variance. It is important to bear in mind that these are abstract concepts that give no information about specific genes or environmental factors that influence phenotype expression. Moreover, they are population concepts that cannot be translated into attribution of individual characteristics to genes vs. environment. Heritability estimates depend on the variability of environmental influences in the population that is studied. This is important to bear in mind when translating findings on twin studies to the general population.

In this section, a narrow definition of heritability has been adopted whereby consideration is given to the proportion of phenotypic variance due to additive genetic variance only. However, it is worth considering the broader definition of heritability that encompasses all sources of genetic variation, including additive, dominant and epistatic[2] variance. The total phenotypic variance in the ACE model for example is taken to be the sum of gene and environmental components, but one should not forget the potential contribution of variance due to gene x environment interactions nor to gene environment covariation. While evolutionary biologists would argue that the contribution of epistatic variance, gene x environment interactions and gene environment covariation is small, psychiatric epidemiology and behaviour genetics tend to challenge this assumption.

There are other fundamental assumptions built into the models of heritability used in family studies that merit further examination. These are the equal environment assumption, the shared genes assumption and the assumption about heritability over the life course. Each is discussed in more detail below

12.2.1 The equal environment assumption

The traditional twin ACE model is predicated on the equal-environment assumption (EEA). That is, monozygotic (MZ) and dizygotic (DZ) twins are equally correlated in their exposure to environments of etiologic importance for the trait under study. In the chapter on intergenerational studies, an example is given where it is assumed that 'siblings have shared their environment since birth'. The validity of this EEA has been hotly debated from a theoretical and substantive view.[3,4] The validity of the EEA in sibling research seems at face value more dubious than in twin studies. It is violated when the correlation between environmental similarity and trait similarity is significantly greater than zero within zygosity or family groups.[5] Several methods have been outlined which attempt to detect violations of EEA.[5–7] Perhaps the methods of Derks *et al.* show the greatest promise: multivariate data is frequently available in case-control and cohort studies. While EEA seems to be a valid assumption for many traits, it is recommended that its validity is examined whenever possible.

12.2.2 The shared genes assumption

Family studies often use information on shared genes in their analyses. MZ twins share all of their genes but DZ twins and siblings share 50% of their genes *on average*, while half sibs have only 25% of their genes in common *on average*. Non-random mating will tend to inflate the similarity of genes within DZ pairs. The extent to which this violation of the shared genes assumption matters depends to a large extent on the phenotype under investigation. For example, assortive mating may be more important for research on intelligence than for research on neuroticism. It has been argued that the shared genes assumption, like the EEA, should not be seen as an assumption at all, but instead as a mechanism whose relevance can be tested using more complex study designs than the classical twin study design.[8] Longitudinal designs and models that include data from the extended family are two possible variations.

12.2.3 Heritability over the life course

Life course studies add an extra burden on the researcher to consider the theoretical assumptions related to gene action over the life course. Is it assumed that the same genes influence disease onset as disease progression? Are genetic influences assumed to be associated with linear increases in trait expression over the life span or does the shape of the gene-age trajectory differ for older and younger individuals?

Longitudinal family data conflates within subject phenotypic correlations over time and cross sectional within family phenotypic correlations, making analysis difficult.[9] It is often recommended that simple analyses are preferable to more complex ones[10] and the difficulty of analysing longitudinal family data may prevent many researchers from exploring its utility and benefits. The preponderance of research on age-related changes in the proportions of genetic and environmental influences has used cross-sectional designs,[11] but an understanding of the genetics of aging necessitates a life course perspective with longitudinal analyses.

12.3 Extensions and alternatives to the ACE model

In Section 12.2, a limitation of the ACE model was discussed. Specifically, its inability to take account of dominant genetic effects. Here, an alternative model that includes dominant variance is described, followed by a model to estimate both additive and dominant variance.

12.3.1 The ADE model

Under the assumption that shared environmental variance, C, is negligible, it is possible to estimate the proportions of variance of a phenotype attributable to additive and dominant genetic effects and unique environmental effects. MZ twins share all of their dominant genes, but DZ twins share 25% of dominant genes, *on average*. Analogous to the example in Chapter 11, the phenotypic variance can be partitioned into the three ADE components. More restricted versions of both the ACE and ADE model include the AE, CE and E models. The fit of the various models can be compared with fit statistics such as Akaike's Information Criterion (AIC)[12, 13] or the Bayesian Information Criterion (BIC)[14] which combine goodness-of-fit with degrees of freedom and do not require the models to be nested. The model with the lowest value of AIC or BIC is considered to have the best fit to the data.

12.3.2 The ACDE

In the full ACDE model, A, C, D, and E represent additive genetic factors, shared environmental factors, non additive dominant genetic factors, and non shared environmental factors, respectively. Using samples of MZ and DZ reared together twins, the model is under identified and it is not possible to estimate all four variances. However, if the sample is extended to include siblings, half-siblings, step-siblings, or reared apart twins, then the ACDE is identified. Table 12.1 summarizes the genetic and environmental concordance between these different family pairs.

Examples of both approaches outlined above are given in Jacobson and Rowe[15] and Ulrich et al.[16]

12.4 Shared vs. non-shared environment

Like the debates on the equal environment assumption, an equally vociferous debate has raged over shared and non shared environmental influences. Much of the debate has taken place between social scientists and behaviour geneticists. In both the previous chapters, the language used in the discussion of environmental effects has, on the whole, been carefully articulated but some additional comments on the shared vs. non shared environmental controversy might be useful here.

For behavioural geneticists, the definition of shared environment is a statistical one whereby the shared environment is simply all those factors that make family members similar on a phenotype.[17] In other words, an environmental factor would be assigned to the shared component of environmental variance with respect to a particular phenotype if and only if it had the effect of making family members similar to one another for that phenotype.[18] All other variance that does not covary between family members is subsumed under the non shared environmental variance.

By contrast, for social scientists, the definition of shared environment is usually a substantive one,[17] referring to aspects of the family home that the family members experience in common. This encompasses the physical and psychosocial conditions of the home but would not include

Table 12.1 Genetic and environmental concordance for different family pairs

	Genetic		Shared
	Additive	**Dominant**	**Environmental**
Reared together MZ twins	100%	100%	100%
Reared together DZ twins	50%	25%	100%
Reared together full siblings	50%	25%	100%
Reared together half siblings	25%	12.5%	100%
Reared together unrelated siblings	0%	0%	100%
Reared apart MZ twins	100%	100%	0%
Reared apart DZ twins	50%	25%	0%
Reared apart full siblings	50%	25%	0%
Reared apart half siblings	25%	12.5%	0%
Reared apart unrelated siblings	0%	0%	0%

aspects of the more distal environments like the neighbourhood or school. But consider DZ twins, who share friendships, attend the same school and use the same local amenities and a sibling pair, who have no friends in common and attend school in different locations. Clearly, from the social science viewpoint, the shared family environment for both sets of relatives is more similar than from the behavioural genetics viewpoint.

More importantly, from a behavioural genetics framework, the non shared environmental variance is that which is left over once genetic and shared environmental variance has been quantified. It is an amalgam of all the factors that make family members different from one another. Depending on the statistical design of the study, one of those factors will be measurement error. With a cross sectional design and a single measure of the phenotype in question, measurement reliability can have a large impact on the estimation of non shared environment. Life course studies with repeated measures offer one way to improve estimation of effect size because unreliability can be taken account of in the statistical model.

Another consideration is the interpretation of environmental influences beyond the substantive/statistical dichotomy. That is, that the definitions are population concepts. As such, they are uninformative about individual differences within the population. DZ twins share 50% of their genes, on average. This does not mean that 50% of the genes involved in a specific trait are shared by a particular twin pair. In a similar way, environmental variance is averaged over the whole population. If shared environmental variance in height is estimated to be 40% of the total variance in the population, this does not imply that 40% of your own height is caused by your family environment. In sensitive areas of research such as the epidemiology of criminality, for example, it is important that this distinction is transparent. A culture of victim blaming can result from misunderstanding the results of family genetic studies. These studies are also uninformative about differences between populations. For example, developmental delay in childhood has been shown to differ by ethnic group.[19] Inferences about the differences in genes and environment as an explanation for mean differences between ethnic groups cannot be made from estimates of genetic and environmental contributions to variation in developmental delay for ethnic subgroups.

12.5 Longitudinal models

In the previous section, some warnings about the interpretation of results from family studies in life course epidemiology were highlighted. In this section, two twin studies are described that exemplify the way that different results can be obtained for different study populations. Then studies are discussed that show some of the advantages of intergenerational family studies for hypothesis testing.

12.5 1 Twin studies on life time socio-economic position and health

Osler *et al.* carried out a study on 1,266 Danish twins in order to disentangle the influences of early genetic, prenatal, and rearing environmental factors from later environmental factors on adult health.[20] They examined a range of health related outcomes including height, BMI, grip strength, self-rated health, depression, cognition, and health behaviours. By examining MZ and DZ twins who were discordant for adult socio-economic position, they were able to explore the role of social causation for adult health, while controlling for genetic and childhood environmental factors. They reported that variability in most health outcomes was more strongly related to zygosity than to adult socio-economic position and therefore concluded that there was little evidence for social causation of adult health. The results did show that among DZ but not MZ female twins discordant on adult social class, the more socially advantaged female twin was more physically active.

In another study, Krieger et al. examined the same issue of life time socio-economic position and health in twins.[21] They had health and socio-demographic data on 308 female twin pairs in the US. In common with the Osler et al. study, they had measures of BMI, self-rated health and physical activity. In addition, measures of blood pressure, cholesterol, glucose, and waist-hip ratio were reported. Cardiovascular risk factors differed more among twins who were discordant on adult occupation class than concordant twin pairs. Within twin pairs discordant on occupational class, the working-class twin typically fared worse than the professional twin. Unlike the Osler et al. study, more socially advantaged DZ twins were no more physically active than their more disadvantaged co-twin. Poorer self-rated health was also more likely to be reported by the working class twin than the professional twin among the 51 MZ pairs discordant on class.

Why did one study conclude that health was associated with a non shared adult environmental variable and the other study make the opposing conclusion that health was not related to non shared adult socio-economic position? The question is really 'why should they be the same?'. One study was based in Denmark, a country with a strong social demographic welfare system while the other was based in the US, the proto-typical liberal welfare state.[22] Given that the two populations from which the conclusions are drawn are so different, it is unsurprising that the non-shared effects tell a different story. If estimates of genetic and shared variance were calculated, these would also yield inconsistent results.

12.5.2 Intergenerational studies on fetal development

The fetal over nutrition hypothesis proposes that greater maternal adiposity results in increased obesity in offspring. Lawlor et al. carried out a study on parent offspring trios to investigate this proposal.[23] They found evidence in favour of the hypothesis that maternal size during pregnancy has an effect on offspring BMI over and above that of shared familial mechanisms. The potential consequences of this finding are that children of obese female offspring will also have a tendency to obesity, continuing the obesity problem into subsequent generations. A later paper then went on to examine intergenerational increases in BMI with greater precision.[24] They compared measures of adult BMI in the parents and offspring *when they were the same age*. Maternal and paternal associations with their offspring's BMI were similar. Moreover, the substantially higher adult BMI for offspring than for parents could not be explained by measures of the fetal environment. In this study, the fetal over nutrition hypothesis was rejected as an explanation for inter generational increases in BMI. These studies exemplify the problem of sourcing data for inter generational studies. The generalizability of the results from the former study may have been hindered by the lack of comparable data between generations. Given that there are few data resources where individuals for two or more generations have reliable information from birth into adulthood, this issue is worth bearing in mind.

The fetal insulin hypothesis suggests that the same genetic polymorphisms lead to increased insulin resistance in adulthood and impaired growth in utero, and that these common genetic factors underlie the observed association between birth weight and the risk of cardiovascular disease in adulthood. A cross-sectional study found that maternal insulin resistance in older age was inversely related to the birth weight of their offspring,[25] thus supporting the fetal insulin hypothesis. A later inter-generational study of parental diabetes and offspring birth weight was able to explore this in more detail.[26] Diabetes in fathers and the birth weight of their offspring were inversely related. In contrast, diabetes in the mother increased the birth weight of offspring. However, there was some evidence for an interaction between maternal diabetes status and birth order, suggesting lower birth weight for offspring of mothers who were free of metabolic disturbances related to diabetes at the time of the child's birth. In this example, the fetal insulin hypothesis was supported by the evidence from both studies, but the latter study would have rejected the hypothesis if the analysis relied on main effects only. Additive genetic models that do not consider gene environment interactions may also be prone to type II errors.

12.6 Latent variable models

In Nitsch and Mishra's chapter, a subsection on path analysis describes how direct and indirect regression estimates can be estimated. Path analysis and more generally latent variable analysis have been used extensively for family studies in psychology and psychiatry but the methods are less well used in epidemiology. Many standard models can be analysed using either a latent variable or a multi level orientation. However, latent variable programs offer greater flexibility in specifying the model than most multi level software. It is also more intuitive to draw a diagram of the interdependencies of outcomes on all family members than to use dummy variables to denote family members in the context of multi level models. For more information on latent variable approaches to cross-sectional twin data, the reader is referred to Rijsdijk and Sham.[27] A particularly useful section on the implications of various assumptions, and methods to detect violations is provided. For the remaining part of this section, the focus will be on latent variable models for longitudinal twin and family data. Space considerations prevent a full discussion of the merits of the models. Instead, the following gives a hint to the potential of latent variable models for longitudinal family studies.

12.6.1 Latent variable models for longitudinal twin analysis

There are many ways to model ACE effects with longitudinal data. Svenberg *et al.* describe a Cholesky model of twins' self rated health over time.[28] The Cholesky model imposes a stratification structure on shared latent factors. For a phenotype measured on T occasions, there is a main factor that loads on all T, followed by another that only loads on the last T-1, and so forth, until the T-th factor that loads only on the last measure. This model assumes that there is one main factor of global importance, followed by a succession of orthogonal factors of decreasing commonality to the phenotype. In a longitudinal genetic analysis of HDL cholesterol in twins,[29] a variation of the Cholesky model is shown, which models differential gene expression during development by specifying general and specific genetic effects, general and specific shared environmental effects and specific non shared environmental effects.

A different approach is taken by McArdle and Hamagami.[30] They combine a cross sectional ACE biometric model with a latent growth curve model to specify a latent growth model for biometric data in twins. This paper then details some sophisticated latent difference score models of dynamic change for twins' biometric data. Although these latter models are not recommended for the novice in latent variable modelling, they show how complex theories can be translated into statistical models.

12.6.2 Latent variable models for longitudinal intergenerational analysis

Happily, latent variable models for intergenerational family data are simpler to understand. Despite this, there are limited applications in the literature. Wickrama and colleagues provide an example of modelling the differential contribution of mothers and fathers to intergenerational transmission of health related behaviours.[31] An example of testing mediating hypotheses on the intergenerational transmission of depression is shown in Hammen *et al.*[32] Meanwhile, a path model of aggressive behaviour in three generations is outlined by Conger *et al.*[33] As the cohort studies described by Nitsch and Mishra mature, intergenerational latent variable models may also come of age.

12.7 Conclusions

A wide diversity of statistical models can be considered for longitudinal family studies. Some of the implicit assumptions and limitations of these models have been articulated more explicitly here. Guided by the seven deadly sins of dyadic data analysis,[10] seven deadly sins of life course family models are summarized:

- Treating the individual instead of the family as the unit of analysis.
- Confusing substantive and statistical definitions of the environment.
- Translating population effects into individual predictions.
- Ignoring potential complexity of genetic inheritance without testing the suitability of the additive model.
- Assuming family members share equal environmental determinants.
- Presuming the direction of influence from one family member to another without reciprocal influences.
- Ignoring measurement error.

References

1. **Carlin JB, Gurrin LC, Sterne JAC, Morley R, Dwyer T.** Regression models for twin studies: a critical review. *International Journal of Epidemiology* 2001; **34**(5): 1089–99.
2. **Cordell HJ.** Epistasis: what it means, what it doesn't mean, and statistical methods to detect it in humans. *Hum Mol Genet* 2002; **11**: 2463–8.
3. **Joseph J.** Twin Studies in Psychiatry and Psychology: Science or Pseudoscience? *Psychiatric Quarterly* 2002; **73**(1): 71–82.
4. **Faraone SV, Biederman J.** Nature, nurture, and attention deficit hyperactivity disorder. *Developmental Review* 2000; **20**: 568–81.
5. **Derks EM, Dolan CV, Boomsma DI.** A Test of the Equal Environment Assumption (EEA) in Multivariate Twin Studies. *Twin Research and Human Genetics* 2006; **9**(3): 403–11.
6. **Hettema J, Neale M, Kendler K.** Physical similarity and the equal-environment assumption in twin studies of psychiatric disorders. *Behavior Genetics* 1995; **25**(4): 327–35.
7. **Kendler K, Neale M, Kessler R, Heath A, Eaves L.** A test of the equal-environment assumption in twin studies of psychiatric illness. *Behavior Genetics* 1993; **23**(1): 21–7.
8. **Boomsma D, Busjahn A, Peltonen L.** Classical twin studies and beyond. *Nature Reviews Genetics* 2002; **3**: 872–82.
9. **Burton PR, Scurrah KJ, Tobin MD, Palmer LJ.** Covariance components models for longitudinal family data. *International Journal of Epidemiology* 2005; **34**(5): 1063–77.
10. **Kenny D, Kashy D, Cook W.** *Dyadic Data Analysis.* The Guildford Press, New York, 2006.
11. **Shanahan MJ, Hofer SM, Shanahan L.** Biological Models of Behavior and the Life Course. In: Mortimer JT, Shanahan MJ, eds. *Handbook of the Life Course.* Plenum, New York, 2003.
12. **Akaike H.** Factor analysis and AIC. *Psychometrika* 1987; **52**: 317–32.
13. **Bozdogan H.** Model section and Akaike's information criteria (AIC): The general theory and its analytical extensions. *Psychometrika* 1987; **52**: 345–70.
14. **Raftery AE.** Bayesian Model Selection in Structural Equation Models. In: Bollen KA, Long JS, eds. *Testing Structural Equation Models.* Sage, Newbury Park. pp. 163–80, 1993.
15. **Jacobson KC, Rowe DC.** Genetic and shared environmental influences on adolescent BMI: interactions with race and sex. *Behavior Genetics* 1998; **28**(4): 265–78.
16. **Ulrich V, Gervil M, Kyvik KO, Olesen J, Russell MB.** The inheritance of migraine with aura estimated by means of structural equation modelling. *J Med Genet* 1999; **36**(3): 225–7.

17 Carey G. *Human Genetics for the Social Sciences* Sage Publications Ltd, London, 2003.
18 **Plaisance KS.** Behavioral Genetics and the Environment: The Generation and Exportation of Scientific Claims [Doctoral Dissertation]. University of Minnesota, 2006.
19 **Kelly Y, Sacker A, Schoon I, Nazroo J.** Ethnic variations in achievement of developmental milestones by 9 months of age: the Millennium Cohort Study. *Developmental Medicine and Child Neurology* 2006; **48**: 825–30.
20 **Osler M, McGue M, Christensen K.** Socioeconomic position and twins' health: a life-course analysis of 1266 pairs of middle-aged Danish twins. *Int J Epidemiol*, 2007; dyl266.
21 **Krieger N, Chen JT, Coull BA, Selby JV.** Lifetime socioeconomic position and twins' health: an analysis of 308 pairs of United States women twins. *PLoS Medicine* 2005; **2**(7): e162.
22 **Esping-Andersen G.** *The Three Worlds of Welfare Capitalism*. Polity Press, Cambridge, 1990.
23 **Lawlor DA, Davey Smith G, O'Callaghan M, Alati R, Mamun AA, Williams GM,** *et al.* Epidemiologic evidence for the fetal overnutrition hypothesis: findings from the Mater-University Study of Pregnancy and Its Outcomes. *Am J Epidemiol* 2006;,kwk030.
24 **Kivimaki M, Lawlor DA, Davey Smith G, Elovainio M, Jokela M, Keltikangas-Jarvinen L,** *et al.* Substantial intergenerational increases in body mass index are not explained by the fetal overnutrition hypothesis: the Cardiovascular Risk in Young Finns Study. *Am J Clin Nutr* 2007; **86**(5): 1509–14.
25 **Lawlor DA, Davey Smith G, Ebrahim S.** Birth weight of offspring and insulin resistance in late adulthood: cross sectional survey. *BMJ* 2002; **325**(7360): 359–
26 **Hypponen E, Davey Smith G, Power C.** Parental diabetes and birth weight of offspring: intergenerational cohort study. *BMJ* 2003; **326**(7379): 19–20.
27 **Rijsdijk FV, Sham PC.** Analytic approaches to twin data using structural equation models. *Briefings in Bioinformatics* 2002; **3**(2): 119–33.
28 **Svedberg P, Gatz M, Lichtenstein P, Sandin S, Pedersen NL.** Self-rated health in a longitudinal perspective: a 9-year follow-up twin study. *J Gerontol B Psychol Sci Soc Sci* 2005; **60**(6): S331–S340.
29 **Nance W, Bodurtha J, Eaves L, Hewitt J, Maes H, Segrest J,** *et al.* Models for the longitudinal genetic analysis of same-age twins: application to HDL cholesterol. *Twin Research and Human Genetics* 1998; **1**: 3–8.
30 **McArdle JJ, Hamagami F.** Structural equation models for evaluating dynamic concepts within longitudinal twin analyses *Behavior Genetics* 2003; **33**(2): 137–59.
31 **Wickrama KAS, Conger RD, Wallace LE, Elder GH, Jr.** The intergenerational transmission of health-risk behaviors: adolescent lifestyles and gender moderating effects. *Journal of Health and Social Behavior* 1999; **40**(3): 258–72.
32 **Hammen C, Shih JH, Brennan PA.** Intergenerational Transmission of Depression: Test of an Interpersonal Stress Model in a Community Sample. *Journal of Consulting and Clinical Psychology*, 2004; **72**(3): 511–522.
33 **Conger RD, Neppl T, Kim KJ, Scaramella L.** Angry and aggressive behavior across three generations: a prospective, longitudinal study of parents and children. *Journal of Abnormal Child Psychology* 2003; **31**(2): 143–60.

Part IV

Some illustrative examples of the use of family-based studies in life course epidemiology

Chapter 13

Family-based studies applied to the influence of early life factors on cardiovascular disease

Debbie A Lawlor and David A Leon

Abstract

There is good evidence that associations exist between, fetal and other early life factors, and subsequent risk of cardiovascular disease (CVD) that can be replicated in a range of settings. These associations provide the evidential basis for the *developmental origin of CVD* in humans, which posits that susceptibility to CVD in later life is importantly influenced by the nature of the *in utero*, infant, and childhood environment. However, much of this evidence is from cohort studies of unrelated individuals, and it has been argued that these associations may be explained by confounding by genetic variation or uncontrolled aspects of the environment. Family-based studies have been increasingly used to try and differentiate between these competing explanations. In the area of the developmental origins of CVD the limited number of twin studies, to date, has generally suffered from having insufficient statistical power. However, the largest single twin study has found persuasive evidence that the inverse association of birth weight with raised blood pressure in young adult men is unlikely to be explained by socioeconomic or genetic confounding. Studies in sibships, have also suggested that fixed familial factors (including socioeconomic position and maternal genotype) do not explain the associations of birth weight with CVD events or variations in blood pressure. Intergenerational studies in which offspring birth weight has been related to disease in parents provide further support for an intrauterine developmental origin of the association between birth weight and CVD. These studies demonstrate the potential of family-based studies in throwing light on the developmental origins of CVD. However, there is a need to move beyond the examination of birth weight with CVD to using family-based studies for exploring mechanisms underlying other life course exposures of relevance to CVD.

13.1 Introduction

CVD accounts for the majority of deaths in high income countries and is an increasing cause of morbidity and mortality in low and middle income countries.[1] Coronary heart disease (CHD) and stroke, the main manifestations of CVD, are rare until middle age and more than half of the deaths due to these causes occur over the age of 70 years. Until recently, most of our knowledge concerning aetiological risk factors focused on factors acting in adult life such as diet, smoking, physical activity, hypertension and adult obesity.[2] There is indeed good evidence that these major adult risk factors explain much of the geographical and secular variations in CVD events, and it has been suggested that there is no need to seek further aetiological risk factors for CVD.[3, 4] Moreover, there are a range of drugs now available that are highly effective in secondary prevention (that work by reducing adult risk factors such as elevated blood pressure and total or low density lipoprotein cholesterol) which, together with reductions in smoking, have contributed to the sharp decline in CVD mortality in high income countries.[5–8] It has also been proposed that combinations of these agents, in the so-called 'polypill' may provide an important approach to primary prevention if they were taken widely by people in middle age or older regardless of diagnosed CVD.[9] However, even strong advocates of these pragmatic perspectives would no doubt agree that ultimately it would be most desirable to reduce the risk of developing CVD in the first instance, not least through reducing the population prevalence of raised blood pressure, adverse lipid profiles and other physiological risk factors without the need for population-wide pill prescription. To achieve this requires a better understanding of the pre-adult determinants of CVD and its risk factors.

It has been known for decades that the pathophysiological process of atherosclerosis, which ultimately leads to CHD and ischaemic strokes, begins in childhood and young adulthood.[10–12] Cardiovascular risk factors, such as high blood pressure, obesity, dyslipidaemia, and insulin resistance are present in childhood, associated with atherosclerosis and endothelial dysfunction, and track into adulthood.[13–16] A growing body of research has highlighted the potential role of pre-adult influences that may operate through various different life course models on CVD risk factors and end points (summarized in previous life course book chapters[17–20]).

Within this body of research, family-based studies have been increasingly used to explore the nature of associations (whether they are causal or explained by bias or confounding) and possible mechanisms underlying the associations of pre-adult risk factors with later disease outcomes. Previous chapters in this book have outlined the theoretical underpinning and statistical approaches to these studies. This chapter will summarize evidence from family-based studies that have been used to explore the life course epidemiology of CVD, in particular the nature of the association between *in utero* environment and fetal growth and later disease risk. Our focus on this specific area is justified by the fact that the interpretation of these statistical associations remains a particularly controversial one that has generated more research than that of life course influences acting later in infancy or childhood.

This chapter starts with a brief summary of these controversies and proposed mechanisms surrounding the inverse association of birth weight with CVD and then goes on to detail the contribution of family-based studies to answering these questions. Towards the end we briefly describe the limited number of family-based studies that have looked at other aspects of the life course epidemiology of CVD and end with a discussion of future research potential.

13.2 The inverse association of birth size with cardiovascular disease and risk factors

A large number of studies have demonstrated inverse associations (sometimes 'reverse-J' shaped) between birth size (most commonly birth weight) and CVD endpoints,[21] and risk factors, including blood pressure,[20] fasting glucose,[19] insulin,[19] total cholesterol and triglycerides,[22, 23] and positive associations with high density lipoprotein cholesterol (HDL-c).[23] Conversely, birth weight is positively associated with body mass index,[24] and with both total fat mass and lean mass assessed by DXA scan in children.[25] The strength of the associations of lower birth weight with adverse CVD events and risk factors is generally smaller, often considerably so, than those between risk factors, for example body mass index and waist circumference, measured in adult life and these outcomes.

There are a number of different interpretations of the inverse associations of birth weight with CVD risk:

- Impaired intrauterine nutrition/growth alone or in combination with various post-natal nutrition/growth trajectories programmes later CVD risk,[23, 26–28] possibly through epigenetic mechanisms.[29]

- The associations are largely, or entirely, due to the effects of genetic variants that have pleiotropic effects influencing both fetal growth and later insulin resistance and hence CVD risk.[30]

- The associations are largely, or entirely, due to confounding (by for example socioeconomic position or shared familial behaviours such as smoking, low levels of physical activity and high fat diets), statistical artefact and/or publication bias.[31, 32]

Family-based studies have the potential to help differentiate between some of these competing interpretations, although they cannot in themselves contribute to resolving the role of statistical artefact and publication bias.

13.2.1 Twin studies of birth weight and cardiovascular disease risk

From relatively early on in the debate about the early origins of CVD as formulated by Barker[26] and others, it has been recognized that twins provide a potentially powerful way to deepen and indeed test the developmental origins hypothesis.[33] There are two respects in which twins can be informative. The first is entirely specific to the developmental origins field and the role of impaired fetal growth. Twins, compared to singletons, experience intrauterine growth retardation and have on average birth weights that are 900g lower than those of singletons. Thus, there is the question as to whether twins *per se* have an elevated risk of CVD and levels of associated risk factors. The second is the more general application of twin data to separating out non-genetic (environmental) and genetic effects (see Chapters 4, 11 and 12 for details of the theoretical underpinning and statistical methods of this application of twin studies).

If the fetal growth impairment experienced by twins occurs through similar processes to that experienced by growth impaired singletons, one would expect twins to be at greater risk of CVD. The salience of comparing twins with singletons (or the general population which is largely singletons) is reinforced by the fact that there is evidence that twins tend to exhibit upward growth centile crossing when compared to singletons, a phenomenon sometimes referred to as 'catch-up growth'. This can be inferred from the observation that while twins at birth weigh considerably less than singletons and are shorter in length, by adult life the twin deficit in height relative to singletons is almost entirely eliminated and that in weight largely so.[34] Though there may be some weak association between higher socioeconomic position and occurrence of dizygotic twins (DZ), the likelihood of having a monozygotic (MZ) twin pregnancy is not influenced by socioeconomic position or maternal cigarette smoking. Thus any association between multiplicity status (being a twin versus a singleton) is unlikely to be strongly confounded by social class or smoking. It is therefore striking that there is almost no evidence that twins *per se* have an excess risk of CVD. In one study of 8,174 female and 6,612 male twins (both MZ and DZ combined) CHD mortality was no greater than that in the general population, suggesting that the intrauterine growth, and subsequent catch-up growth, experienced by twins was not associated with increased CHD risk.[35] These results were confirmed in a second study of nearly 20,000 twins in which all-cause and CVD mortality were found to be similar among MZ twins, DZ twins and the general population.[36] In addition, twins do not appear to have higher blood pressure than singletons in general[37] or their non-twin siblings,[38] and being a twin is not importantly associated with other CVD risk factors.[39]

There are a number of potential explanations for this apparent inconsistency in the evidence. The most obvious is that the assumption that the form of fetal growth impairment and later catch-up growth experienced by twins is similar to that which underlies singleton fetal growth impairment (and catch up) is wrong. The point in gestation when the *in utero* growth of twins starts to diverge below that of singletons is unclear, although it seems that it is evident at 30 weeks.[40] Singleton fetal growth impairment also seems to begin in the third trimester (i.e from ~ 26 weeks). However, there is a need for further research that (a) contrasts *in utero* growth patterns in twins, singletons with fetal growth impairment, and singletons with no growth impairment and (b) identifies the underlying mechanisms that control these *in utero* growth patterns. Such research would require serial ultrasound scans throughout pregnancy, conducted using standard protocols, in all three groups, but we believe that investment in such research is valuable. This is an important issue to clarify and its resolution may throw light on the distinctive nature of the pathophysiological processes involved in growth retardation of singletons that is associated with later increased risk of CVD.

We now turn to considering the more traditional use of twin studies (see Chapters 4, 11 and 12) to separate genetic from environmental effects underlying the association of early life factors with CVD risk. Published twin studies vary in the analytic strategy they adopt, in part depending upon the question being addressed. However, in the context of trying to understand the underlying mechanisms (genetic versus non-genetic) for the association of birth weight with CVD a logical progression would be as follows. One would start by either treating all of the twins as individuals (with statistical methods that produce robust standard errors, taking account of the fact that twins in a pair are not independent) and simply assess the association between birth weight and CVD in the twin population, or by more formally assessing the association of average birth weight for each twin-pair with average CVD risk for each twin pair (*between* twin study). If an inverse association between birth weight and CVD is found between twins this suggests that twins *per se* do not differ from the general populations in which this association has been demonstrated. Next, a *within* twin pair analysis is undertaken that would be equivalent to matching on factors that are identical within twin pairs. If there is no association within monzygotic (MZ) pairs between birth weight and CVD (i.e. MZ twins with disease compared to their co-twins without disease do not differ from each other with respect to birth weight) but the association is seen in dizygotic (DZ) twins, this suggests that factors which are identical between MZ twins (but not DZ twins) explain the association. Since MZ twins are genetically identical (with the exception of the mitochondrial DNA), a mechanism involving pleiotropic effects by non-mitochondrial fetal genetic variants would be an obvious explanation for the birth weight-CVD association. However, approximately two-thirds of MZ twins share a placenta (i.e. they are monozygotic monochorionic pairs—as described in more detail in Chapter 4), therefore the lack of an association specifically within MZ twins may also be consistent with non-genetic placental factors for which most MZ twins are also matched.[41] If there is no association within either MZ or DZ twins (i.e. when the analysis is undertaken with matching on factors that are identical within either MZ of DZ twin pairs), but there is a between pairs association then this must be explained by fixed maternal factors that are identical for both MZ and DZ twins. These factors would include familial socioeconomic circumstances and maternal birth characteristics and growth across her life, maternal environmental exposures up to the time of the twin pregnancy, and other fixed maternal characteristics such as her genotype, smoking, diet, and alcohol consumption and age during the twins pregnancy. If the within twin pair associations for both MZ and DZ pairs are similar to the between twin association, this suggests that fetal nutrition (which varies within both twin types and also between singletons) or any other factor that is not identical within twin pairs explains the association.

Twin studies that have adopted some or all of the strategy outlined above have been used to explore the association of birth weight (and less commonly other perinatal exposures such as maternal body mass index during pregnancy and maternal age[42]) with blood pressure,[43, 44] dyslipidaemia,[45] glucose intolerance,[46] insulin resistance,[42] diabetes,[47, 48] indicators of adiposity and body composition,[49, 50] and CHD events.[51, 52] Results from the small number of studies with CHD endpoints are largely inconclusive because of inadequate statistical power to detect differences in associations between MZ and DZ twins. There are more studies of blood pressure (treated as a continuous variable) than any binary CVD or risk factor outcome. A systematic review and meta-analysis of twin studies examining the association of birth weight with blood pressure failed to provide conclusive evidence for a stronger role for either genetic or environmental factors.[43] This was attributed to small sample sizes and between study variation in the way in which zygosity was defined and blood pressure measured. However, this meta-analysis excluded a subsequently published study based on the Swedish Twin Registry that is the largest of its kind.[44] Rather than analysing mean blood pressure, a binary outcome of hypertension was used. This was ascertained on the basis of self-reports of diagnosed hypertension combined with taking anti-hypertensive medication on a daily basis. Birth weight was abstracted from original birth records. From the 16,000 twin pairs available for analysis, 594 DZ and 250 MZ pairs were identified that were discordant for hypertension, and who were baptised at birth thus minimizing the likelihood of incorrectly assigning birth weights to each member of the pair, an important source of bias noted in previous studies.[37] Within MZ pairs a 500g lower birth weight was associated with an odds ratio of hypertension of 1.74 (95% CI 1.13, 2.70), and within DZ pairs of 1.34 (95% CI 1.07, 1.69). The equivalent association in the whole cohort was 1.42 (95%CI: 1.25, 1.61). This study, therefore, provides the strongest evidence to date that the inverse association of birth weight with hypertension is independent of genetic and environmental factors shared by twins including maternal and fetal genotype (except fetal mitochondrial DNA), physiology in pregnancy, socio-economic factors and gestation. It thus supports the contention that this inverse association is indeed caused by some aspect of fetal nutrition or *in utero* development represented by birth weight and that differs between both MZ and DZ pairs. The use of self-report of hypertension and treatment may have resulted in outcome measurement error, but this is likely to be non-differential with respect to recorded birth weight and would be expected to lead to an underestimation of any association. Furthermore any bias due to non-differential measurement error in the outcome should not differ by twin status and therefore could not explain the similarity in associations within DZ and MZ twins and in the whole-population analysis.

To our knowledge, only two within twin analysis have looked at the association of birth weight with CHD events,[51, 52] and none have looked at the association with stroke risk. The same research group undertook the two CHD studies on two independent samples of Swedish twins. In the first study, there was no association between birth weight, birth length, ponderal index or head circumference and acute myocardial infarction within 118 same sex twin pairs (MZ and DZ combined), though low birth weight was associated with increased myocardial infarction between twins in the whole cohort, suggesting that fixed maternal factors such as familial socioeconomic position, maternal education, her growth and development in *utero* and early life and maternal genotype explained the association.[51] In the second study there was an association between low self-reported birth weight and increased risk of angina between 4,594 same sex twins and also within 55 pairs of same sex DZ twins who were selected to be discordant for self-reported angina.[52] However, within 37 MZ twin pairs, discordant for angina, there was no association with birth weight. Self-reported birth weight was validated in a sub-group of the study and found to be accurate.[52] These findings suggest that non-mitochondrial fetal genetic factors or other factors that are uniquely shared within MZ twin pairs could explain the low birth weight-CHD association. However, further studies based on larger numbers of twin pairs are necessary to be certain that these results are not due to chance. As noted in Chapter 4, these studies are an illustration of the need for very large sample sizes to fully exploit the potential of within and between twin study analyses in this area, something that in practice may not be feasible.

13.2.2 Sibling studies of birth weight and cardiovascular disease risk

Analysis of sibling singleton pairs or larger groups can also be informative about the nature of the associations between early life factors and CVD risk as discussed in more general terms in Chapter 3. Unlike MZ twins, singleton siblings born to the same mother and father only share 50% of their genotype. Moreover, unlike MZ and DZ twin pairs, singleton sibling groups do not share the same intrauterine environment and are likely to have different gestational ages. In addition, a number of maternal factors that vary between consecutive pregnancies, for example maternal age, are necessarily different for siblings but identical for twins. However, singleton siblings do share fixed maternal characteristics that include their mother's own *in utero* and post-natal development, pre-adult nutritional status, attained height, pelvic size, socioeconomic position, and educational level. Thus, sibling studies provide a useful method for distinguishing between fixed maternal/family characteristics and those factors that vary between full-siblings in explaining the associations between perinatal exposures and later outcomes. The overall analytical approach is similar to that described above for between and within twin study analyses, but as noted above for siblings the characters that are 'fixed' and therefore controlled for are not as extensive as for twins.

To our knowledge only three studies have employed this design to explore the association of birth weight with CVD outcomes. The outcome examined in all three of these Swedish studies was blood pressure,[53–55] and their key findings were in broad agreement: in childhood,[53] and young adult life,[54, 55] there was an inverse association between birth weight and mean systolic blood pressure within sibships having accounted for length of gestation. In the largest of these studies an inverse associations of birth weight and gestational age with systolic blood pressure were found both within and between sibships without adjustment for concurrent height, weight or BMI.[55] The authors of this study concluded that the inverse associations of birth weight and gestational age with later blood pressure were not explained by confounding due to family socioeconomic position, maternal skeletal size or factors from across the earlier part of a mother's life course. Instead the most likely alternative explanations for these associations involved differences between pregnancies (to the same mother) in maternal metabolic or vascular health during pregnancy and/or differences in placental implantation. Differences in maternal metabolic or vascular capacity between pregnancies might be related to her behaviours such as smoking, diet and physical activity. However, in common with many life course studies (see Chapter 6) none of the sibling studies that examined the birth weight-CVD association had information on these behaviours or on measurements of maternal vascular and metabolic health in order to be able to test these hypotheses.

Since full siblings on average do share 50% of their genotype, genetic variants related to both fetal growth and later blood pressure could also explain this association. However, adjustment for father's blood pressure (that had been measured at the same mean age as the participant's blood pressure was measured) did not alter the within or between sibship associations of birth weight and blood pressure, despite the father-son blood pressures being positively correlated.

The authors suggested that, in so far as the positive correlation between father's and son's blood pressure when both are measured at the same age is related to genetic factors, the lack of impact of adjustment for father's blood pressure on the associations suggests that they are unlikely to be caused by fetal genetic factors.[55] It is interesting to compare findings from this large sibling study to those from the largest twin study to date[44] (described earlier in this chapter). On the basis of similar associations within and between siblings, the authors of the sibling study concluded that maternal vascular or metabolic health during pregnancy or differences in placental implantation between pregnancy may explain the association of birth weight with later higher blood pressure. However, in the twins study the similarity of the birth weight-hypertension association within DZ and MZ twins to that seen in the general (singleton) population, would argue against maternal metabolic and cardiovascular health during pregnancy explaining the association, since this will be the same for both twins. Furthermore, as noted earlier the fact that two-thirds of MZ twins share a placenta means that these twin results also argue against differences in placentation as an explanation. As noted in section 13.2.1 the extent to which twins may differ in important ways with respect to intrauterine growth from singletons may limit how generalizable twin studies of birth weight associations are to the general population. Furthermore, whilst both the twin study described above is large and well-conducted, further studies are required to replicate its findings.

13.2.3 Intergenerational studies of offspring birth weight and parental cardiovascular disease risk

A third family-based design has been developed specifically to detect evidence that common genetic factors underlie the inverse associations observed between fetal birth weight and later CVD risk. Unlike twin and sibship designs, this approach utilizes information across two consecutive generations, investigating the association of offspring birth weight with CVD risk factors and events in their parents (see Chapter 2 for more detailed description of the theoretical underpinning of these studies). If the birth weight-CVD association seen in individuals is at least partly explained by genetic influences derived from both maternal and paternal genetic variants one would expect that offspring birth weight would be inversely associated with CVD in both mothers and fathers. As explained in more detail in Chapter 2, in this context detecting an association of offspring birth weight with fathers' CVD risk is of particular importance, because such an association would be consistent with the transmission of genes, at least once socioeconomic factors were accounted for. In contrast, many factors that could influence maternal CVD risk (for example, maternal diet and smoking) could also influence the intrauterine environment, and thus birth weight of her offspring.

A recent meta-analysis of all published studies of the association of offspring birthweight with parental CVD endpoints found that amongst mothers the pooled confounder adjusted hazard ratio of CVD mortality for a one standard deviation increase in offspring birthweight was 0.75 (95%CI: 0.67, 0.84) and among fathers the equivalent association was 0.93 (95%CI: 0.91, 0.95), with statistical evidence of a difference between these two effects $p < 0.001$[56] (see Figure 2.5; Chapter 2).

As discussed in Chapter 2, in more detail, the generally stronger associations with maternal CVD can be explained by a number of different mechanisms[57] all of which could be operating simultaneously:

1. 'Fetal programming', whereby fetal undernutrition in the mother programmes her increased cardiovascular disease and also leads to lower birth weight offspring due to a smaller pelvic size.

2. Direct effects of maternal health-related behaviours, such as smoking, heavy alcohol consumption, and poor diet, both on offspring birth weight and on maternal cardiovascular disease risk.
3. Maternal imprinting (i.e. the phenotype resulting from a particular gene locus is differentially modified by the sex of the parent contributing that particular allele).
4. Other epigenetic effects (i.e. a change in the outcome of a gene that is controlled by non-genetic factors so that the phenotype resulting from a particular gene is modified by environmental exposures).
5. Paternal misclassification, as some fathers in these studies will not be the biological parents and this would be expected to dilute the paternal association, assuming this is largely driven by genetic variants related to both birth size and insulin resistance and hence CVD.
6. It is also plausible that the weak association in fathers is fully explained by residual confounding.
7. Finally, it is possible that some of the offspring birth weight-maternal cardiovascular disease association reflects lower offspring birth weight due to pregnancy related health-compromising factors in some mothers (i.e. reverse causality). In this case the expectation would be that the elevated cardiovascular mortality risk would be greater for periods closer in time to the index pregnancy and, as with other cases of health-related selection, this effect would reduce over time. For coronary heart disease mortality this was found in analyses of one of the largest studies to date and this time-related effect explains some of the heterogeneity between studies relating offspring birth weight to maternal cardiovascular disease risk (Figure 2.5a; Chapter 2).[56]

The implausibly high levels of non-paternity (30%) that would be required to explain the magnitude of difference in maternal-paternal associations for cardiovascular disease endpoints and the non-specificity of the association in fathers, with similar magnitude associations for other outcomes that could be due to confounding,[56] have led to the suggestions that these intergenerational studies support a maternal (most likely specific intrauterine) explanation for the inverse association of birth weight with CVD risk seen in the general population.[56]

This intergenerational design has also been used with the same rationale to explore the associations of size at birth with insulin resistance[58–60] and type 2 diabetes.[59, 61–65] These have reported contradictory results, with inverse[58, 61, 62], positive,[63, 65] and null[64] associations of offspring birth weight with insulin resistance/type 2 diabetes reported in mothers and inverse[59, 61–63, 65] or null[60, 64] associations reported in fathers.

Two important issues may explain these contradictions. First, type 2 diabetes is frequently asymptomatic, with up to 50% of individuals with this condition remaining undiagnosed.[66] When outcome in parents has relied solely on self-report or medical record doctor diagnosis of type 2 diabetes, as it has in most of these studies, non-differential misclassification may have biased findings towards the null. This bias should be similar for both mothers and fathers since there is no evidence that the prevalence of undiagnosed diabetes varies by gender. Furthermore, this would not affect studies of insulin resistance or hyperglycaemia determined by fasting blood samples, which have also reported contradictory results.

The second issue is likely to be more important for intergenerational studies relating offspring birth weight to parental insulin resistance or diabetes. Gestational diabetes is associated with increased risk of type 2 diabetes in the mother in later life and also with greater offspring birth weight.[67, 68] The effects of maternal hyperglycaemia on fetal growth and adiposity are not limited to women with diagnosed diabetes during pregnancy. Among non-diabetic mothers there is a linear or 'j' shaped association between fasting and post-challenge glucose concentrations during pregnancy and greater birth size and other adverse perinatal outcomes.[69–71] Thus, in mothers a positive association of offspring birth weight and her risk of later type 2 diabetes and insulin resistance would be expected because of the established effect of maternal glycaemia on offspring birth weight.[60, 63, 65] Any effect of other mechanisms (intrauterine programming or genes with pleiotropic effects resulting in lower birth weight and insulin resistance) might be somewhat masked in these intergenerational studies. This line of reasoning in itself suggests that the intergenerational design may not be as helpful for studying insulin resistance/glucose intolerance/diabetes as it is for CVD itself.[60, 63, 65]

One of the studies relating offspring birth weight to parental diabetes used a novel approach by exploring the intergenerational association of birth weight with parental diabetes within twin pairs.[65] In essence this examined whether the twin whose offspring had the lower birth weight for gestational age was the most likely to be diagnosed with diabetes. The size of effects from these analyses were very similar to those observed in the unpaired analysis, with fathers showing an inverse association and mothers a positive association with offspring birth weight within twin pairs. This suggests that the inverse association in fathers, and the positive association in mothers (in this study), is not generated primarily by factors that are shared by twins—as these are precisely accounted for by the within twin-pair analysis. Regrettably, this study was too small to undertake this sort of analysis stratified by zygosity. This would have provided a key test of the fetal insulin hypothesis. Further studies of this sort would be worth undertaking, although there are few contexts in which large intergenerational datasets of twins could be assembled.

13.2.4 Summary of evidence from family-based studies of the association of birth size with CVD

Overall the studies described above suggest that the inverse association of birth size with adverse CVD outcomes seen in the general population are independent of fixed familial characteristics such as socioeconomic position and maternal development, growth, and behaviours up to the point of her first pregnancy (that are likely to be similar for siblings). With the exception of raised blood pressure in young adult males, the work to date cannot exclude a purely fetal genetic mechanism. However, with respect to CVD outcomes the intergenerational studies are more strongly supportive of intrauterine mechanisms for this association. Comparing offspring-parental associations for insulin resistance/type 2 diabetes outcomes are complicated by the effect of maternal glycaemia on her offspring adiposity and without large studies that have information on maternal glycaemia during pregnancy such studies are limited in the contribution they can potentially make to understanding the mechanisms linking lower birth weight to increase type 2 diabetes risk. Finally, whilst theoretically a robust study design for distinguishing fetal genetic from intrauterine mechanisms, likely differences in patterns of fetal growth between twins and non-twins, potential biases in the allocation of birth weight to each twin within a pair, and the very large sample sizes that are required for these studies to distinguish effects within MZ twins from those within DZ twins (particularly for binary outcomes) with adequate precision, limit the extensive use of twin studies in practice.

13.3 Parental exposures and offspring CVD outcomes

The focus of research on the early origins of CVD have largely focused on birth weight as a risk factor to date. However, recent interest has shifted to modifiable maternal behaviours during pregnancy. In this section we describe some family based study designs – comparing maternal and paternal behaviour associations – that have been applied to try and understand whether maternal behaviours affect offspring CVD risk factors via intrauterine mechanisms. Chapter 2 describes the theoretical underpinning of this approach in more detail.

13.3.1 Maternal behaviours during pregnancy and offspring cardiovascular risk factors

There is evidence that maternal smoking during pregnancy influences offspring obesity[72-75] and suggestions that maternal diet during pregnancy influences offspring blood pressure.[76, 77] However, such associations might be explained by confounding factors that influence maternal behaviour and her offspring's health. For example, mothers who smoke during pregnancy might also engage in other risky health behaviours, such as low levels of physical activity and a high fat diet. It is plausible that behaviours in parents and offspring will be positively associated with each other. Thus, maternal smoking in pregnancy might be associated with offspring obesity via shared maternal-offspring adverse behaviours rather than a specific intrauterine mechanism. One approach to this issue is to compare the strength of associations between an exposure among mothers and offspring outcomes and the same exposure among fathers and the offspring outcomes (see Chapter 2 for a detailed explanation of the assumptions behind this approach).

Using this approach results from the Avon Longitudinal Study of Parents and their Children (ALSPAC) suggest that the relationship between maternal smoking during pregnancy and greater adiposity in offspring is not due to intrauterine mechanisms but is most likely due to confounding by shared familial socioeconomic and behavioural characteristics. In ALSPAC, both maternal and her partner's smoking during the time of the mother's pregnancy were associated with greater BMI in their offspring at age 7.[78] Furthermore, when a more direct measure of adiposity—DXA scan determined fat mass—was used as the outcome similar findings were observed.[78] A more recent study in a large cohort of Bavarian children confirms the near identical association of maternal smoking during pregnancy and offspring obesity at age 5.8 years (odds ratio 2.3; 95%CI: 1.3, 2.7) to that for paternal smoking (at the time of the mother's pregnancy) and offspring obesity at age 5.8 years (odds ratio 2.0; 95%CI: 1.8, 3.1).[79] Similar findings were also observed in ALSPAC with respect to parental smoking and offspring blood pressure, again suggesting that the previously reported association of maternal smoking during pregnancy with offspring blood pressure is not explained by intrauterine mechanisms.[80]

As discussed in Chapter 2 some have suggested that the association between father's smoking and offspring body mass index reflects epigenetic influences, and that such male-line intergenerational responses have important health implications.[81] However, it seems unlikely that two different mechanisms could explain the maternal smoking-offspring body mass index association (the suggested mechanism being that exposing the developing fetus to nicotine adversely affects development of hypothalamic function and through this mechanism impacts upon appetite control over the life course and hence increases the risk of future obesity[82, 83]) and the paternal smoking-offspring body mass index association (the suggested mechanism being a male-line epigenetic effect[81]) and produce the same magnitude of association for each.[84] A more likely explanation is that the same mechanism explains both associations; confounding by socioeconomic position and other behaviours (diet and physical activity) that are related to smoking and shared by all family members is likely.

To our knowledge there are no published studies to date that have compared the associations of maternal diet during pregnancy with offspring CVD related outcomes to similar associations of paternal diet around the time of his partner's pregnancy. Such a study could provide a robust means of testing the causal association of maternal diet with offspring outcomes, but few studies have the resources and the practical capabilities of collecting accurate paternal diet, as well as maternal diet, during pregnancy (Chapter 6).

13.3.2 The developmental overnutrition hypothesis

The developmental over nutrition hypothesis suggests that greater exposure to maternal hyperglycaemia and obesity during pregnancy results in increased offspring adiposity in later life.[24, 85] If greater maternal adiposity during pregnancy does programme offspring to greater obesity this would result in the obesity epidemic progressing across generations irrespective of environmental or genetic changes.[86] This possibility is also referred to as the intergenerational acceleration hypothesis with proponents suggesting that such a phenomenon may have a sound basis in mammalian biology.[87]

This hypothesis can be investigated by comparing maternal-offspring body mass index associations with paternal-offspring body mass index associations. A similar magnitude of effect of maternal and paternal adiposity on offspring measures of adiposity would suggest that the associations were driven by factors that are just as likely to be passed from father to offspring as they were from mother to offspring (i.e. this would not support the developmental over nutrition hypothesis). As discussed in Chapter 2 evidence to date suggests that a specific maternal effect of greater adiposity during pregnancy on her offspring adiposity in later life is at most weak and unlikely to have been a major driver of the obesity epidemic seen in recent years.[88–91]

13.3.3 Effects of in utero exposure to diabetes in pregnancy—the Pima Indian Studies

Some of the study designs described in this chapter, although excellent in conception, have failed to produce clear and definitive results because of limited power or poor measurement of exposures or outcome. Before finishing this selective review of the utility of family designs for resolving issues to do with the early origins of CVD it is essential to mention a small set of family studies that have made important progress by providing good evidence that *in utero* exposure to maternal diabetes increases the later risk of diabetes in the offspring—itself an important risk factor for CVD.

The Pima Indians have been studied extensively because of their very high rates and early age at onset of type 2 diabetes. In the first of a pair of elegant studies it was demonstrated that fasting hyperinsulinemia occurred at an earlier age in the offspring of women who had abnormal glucose tolerance during pregnancy, and these offspring were more obese and had higher rates of abnormal glucose tolerance than those whose mothers who did not have abnormal glucose tolerance in pregnancy.[92] However, this could potentially be explained by confounding with genetic predisposition for earlier onset of disturbances of insulin mediated glucose metabolism. This possibility was excluded in a second study which used a discordant sib-pair design.[93] For this, sib-pairs were identified who were discordant for diabetes at a particular age. Of these a further subset were ones in which the mother was diagnosed with diabetes herself between the pregnancies of her discordant children. The analysis showed that it was more likely that the diabetic sib was born after the mother had been diagnosed with diabetes than before. A parallel analysis looking at the timing of paternal diagnosis of diabetes failed to find any association of birth order with pattern of discordance in the offspring.[93] This provided good evidence that exposure to diabetes *in utero* increases the risk of diabetes later in life, a conclusion that was anticipated many years earlier by Freinkel in his important but often overlooked theory of fuel mediated teratogenesis.[94, 95]

13.4 Conclusions and implications for further research

This selective review of the use of family-based designs to throw light on the association of early life factors with later risk of CVD illustrates the potential of these special approaches to break the impasse that arises from the endless replication of associations in studies whose design does nothing to critically test the hypotheses of interest. While these designs are not a panacea, and as described above (and in more detail in previous chapters in this book) have problems of their own, their judicious use can move our understanding forward. The main obstacle to exploiting these designs further stands not in their own shortcomings, but in the difficulty of identifying populations in which the requisite data is collected on families and in which there are sufficient numbers to estimate effects with precision (problems that are highlighted in Chapter 6, as well as other previous chapters in this book). Fortunately, the full range of potentially useful populations, particularly those in the Nordic countries with extensive record linkage possibilities, has not yet been exhausted. Further progress in this area is therefore likely, particularly through careful combining of results or individual level data in meta- or pooled analyses.

References

1 **Lopez AD, Murray CC.** The global burden of disease, 1990–2020. *Nat Med* 1998; **4**: 1241–3.
2 **Marmot M, Elliott P.** *Coronary Heart Disease Epidemiology, from Aetiology to Public Health*. Oxford University Press, Oxford, 1992.
3 **Magnus P, Beaglehole R.** The real contribution of the major risk factors to the coronary epidemics, time to end the 'only-50%' myth. *Arch Intern Med* 2001; **161**: 2657–60.
4 **Beaglehole R, Magnus P.** The search for new risk factors for coronary heart disease, occupational therapy for epidemiologists? *Int J Epidemiol* 2002; **31**: 1117–22.
5 **Law MR, Wald NJ, Rudnicka AR.** Quantifying effect of statins on low density lipoprotein cholesterol, ischaemic heart disease, and stroke, systematic review and meta-analysis. *BMJ* 2003; **326**: 1423.
6 **Antithrombotic Trialist' Collaboration.** Collaborative meta-analysis of randomised trials of antiplatelet therapy for prevention of death, myocardial infarction, and stroke in high risk patients. *BMJ* 2002; **324**: 71–86.
7 **Unal B, Critchley JA, Capewell S.** Explaining the decline in coronary heart disease mortality in England and Wales between 1981 and 2000. *Circulation* 2004; **109**: 1101–7.
8 **Unal B, Critchley JA, Fidan D, Capewell S.** Life-years gained from modern cardiological treatments and population risk factor changes in England and Wales, 1981–2000. *Am J Public Health* 2005; **95**: 103–8. disease by more than 80%. *BMJ* 326: 1419.
9 **Wald NJ, Law MR.** A strategy to reduce cardiovascular disease by more than 80%. *BMJ* 2003; **326**: 1419.
10 **Enos MW, Holmes LCR, Beyer CJ.** Coronary disease among United States soldiers killed in action in Korea. *JAMA* 1953; **152**: 1090–3.
11 **McNamara JJ, Molot MA, Stremple JF, Cutting RT.** Coronary artery disease in combat casualties in Vietnam. *JAMA* 1971; **216**: 1185–7.
12 **Strong JP, Malcom GT, McMahan CA, Tracy RE, Newman WP, Herderick EE** *et al.* Prevalence and extent of atherosclerosis in adolescents and young adults. Implications for prevention from the pathobiological determinants of Atherosclerosis in Youth Study. *JAMA* 1999; **281**: 727–35.
13 **McCarthy HD, Ellis SM, Cole TJ.** Central overweight and obesity in British youth aged 11–16 years, cross sectional surveys of waist circumference. *BMJ* 2003; **326**: 624.
14 **Freedman DS, Dietz WH, Srinivasan SR, Berenson GS.** The relation of overweight to cardiovascular risk factors among children and adolescents, The Bogalusa Heart Study. *Pediatrics* 1999; **103**: 1175–82.
15 **Tounian P, Aggoun Y, Dubern B, Varille V, Guy-Grand B, Sidi D** *et al.* Presence of increased stiffness of the common carotid artery and endothelial dysfunction in severely obese children, a prospective study. *Lancet* 2001; **358**:1400–4.
16 **Fagot-Campagna A, Pettitt DJ, Engelgau MM, Burrows NR, Geiss LS, Valdez R** *et al.* Type 2 diabetes among North American children and adolescents, an epidemiologic review and a public health perspective. *J Pediatr* 2000; **136**: 664–72.
17 **Lawlor DA, Ebrahim S, Davey Smith G.** coronary heart disease and stroke. In, Kuh D, Hardy R, eds. *A Life Course Approach to Women's Health*. Oxford University Press, Oxford, pp 86-120, 2002.

18 Lawlor DA, Ben-Shlomo Y, Leon DA. Pre-adult influences on cardiovascular disease. In, Kuh D, Ben-Shlomo Y, eds. *A Life Course Approach to Chronic Disease Epidemiology. Second ed.* Oxford University Press, Oxford, pp 41–76, 2004.

19 Forouhi N, Hall E, McKeigue P. A life course approach to diabetes. In, Kuh D, Ben-Shlomo Y, eds. *A Life Course Approach to Chronic Disease Epidemiology. Second ed.* Oxford University Press, Oxford, pp 165–88, 2004.

20 Whincup PH, Cook DG, Geleijnse JM. A life course approach to blood pressure. In, Kuh D, Ben-Shlomo Y, eds. *A Life Course Approach to Chronic Disease Epidemiology. Second ed.* Oxford University Press, Oxford, pp 218–39, 2004.

21 Huxley R, Owen CG, Whincup PH, Cook DG, Rich-Edwards J, Davey Smith G *et al.* Is birth weight a risk factor for ischemic heart disease in later life? *Am J Clin Nutr* 2007; **85**: 1244–50.

22 Owen CG, Whincup PH, Odoki K, Gilg JA, Cook DG. Birth weight and blood cholesterol level, a study in adolescents and systematic review. *Pediatrics* 2003; **111**:1081–9.

23 Gluckman PD, Hanson MA. The developmental origins of the metabolic syndrome. *Trends Endocrinol Metab* 2004; **15**: 183–7.

24 Gillman MW. A life course approach to obesity. In, Kuh D, Ben-Shlomo Y, eds. *A Life Course Approach to Chronic Disease Epidemiology.* 2nd ed. Oxford University Press, Oxford, pp 189–217, 2004.

25 Rogers IS, Ness AR, Steer CD, Wells JC, Emmett PM, Reilly JR *et al.* Associations of size at birth and dual-energy X-ray absorptiometry measures of lean and fat mass at 9 to 10 y of age. *Am J Clin Nutr* 2006; **84**: 739–47.

26 Barker DJ. Fetal programming of coronary heart disease. *Trends Endocrinol Metab* 2002; **13**: 364–8.

27 Bateson P, Barker D, Clutton-Brock T, Deb D, D'Udine B, Foley RA *et al.* Developmental plasticity and human health. *Nature* 2004; **430**: 419–21.

28 Lucas A, Fewtrell MS, Cole TJ. Fetal origins of adult disease-the hypothesis revisited. *BMJ* 1999; **319**: 245–9.

29 Waterland RA, Michels KB. Epigenetic Epidemiology of the Developmental Origins Hypothesis. *Ann Rev Nutr* 2007; **27**: 363–88.

30 Hattersley AT, Tooke JE. The fetal insulin hypothesis, an alternative explanation of the association of low birthweight with diabetes and vascular disease. *Lancet* 1999; **353**: 1789–92.

31 Tu YK, West R, Ellison GT, Gilthorpe MS. Why evidence for the fetal origins of adult disease might be a statistical artifact, the 'reversal paradox' for the relation between birth weight and blood pressure in later life. *Am J Epidemiol* 2005; **161**: 27–32.

32 Huxley R, Neil A, Collins R. Unravelling the 'fetal origins' hypothesis, is there really an inverse association between birth weight and future blood pressure? *Lancet* 2002; **360**: 659–65.

33 Paneth N, Susser M. Early origin of coronary heart disease (the 'Barker hypothesis'). *BMJ* 1995; **310**: 411–12.

34 Pietilainen KH, Kaprio J, Rissanen A, Winter T, Rimpela A, Viken RJ *et al.* Distribution and heritability of BMI in Finnish adolescents aged 16y and 17y, a study of 4884 twins and 2509 singletons. *Int J Obes Relat Metab Disord* 1999; **23**:107–55.

35 Vagero D, Leon D. Ischaemic heart disease and low birth weight, a test of the fetal- origins hypothesis from the Swedish Twin Registry. *Lancet* 1994; **343**: 260–3.

36 Christensen K, Wienke A, Skytthe A, Holm NV, Vaupel JW, Yashin AI. Cardiovascular mortality in twins and the fetal origins hypothesis. *Twin Res* 2001; **4**: 344–9.

37 Johansson-Kark M, Rasmussen F, De Stavola B, Leon DA. Fetal growth and systolic blood pressure in young adulthood, the Swedish Young Male Twins Study. *Paediatr Perinat Epidemiol* 2002; **16**: 200–9.

38 Williams S, Poulton R. Twins and maternal smoking, ordeals for the fetal origins hypothesis? A cohort study. *BMJ* 1999; **318**: 897–900.

39 Phillips DI, Davies MJ, Robinson JS. Fetal growth and the fetal origins hypothesis in twins—problems and perspectives. *Twin Res* 2001; **4**: 327–31.

40 Taylor GM, Owen P, Mires GJ. Foetal growth velocities in twin pregnancies. *Twin Res* 1998; **1**: 9–14.

41 Phillips DI. Twin studies in medical research, can they tell us whether diseases are genetically determined? *Lancet* 1993; **341**: 1008–9.

42 Loos RJF, Phillips DIW, Fagard R, Beunen G, Derom C, Mathieu C, *et al.* The influence of maternal BMI and age in twin pregnancies on insulin resistance in the offspring. *Diabetes Care* 2002; **25**: 2191–6.

43 McNeill G, Tuya C, Smith WC. The role of genetic and environmental factors in the association between birthweight and blood pressure, evidence from meta-analysis of twin studies. *Int J Epidemiol* 2004; **33**: 995–1001.

44 Bergvall N, Iliadou A, Johansson S, de FU, Kramer MS, Pawitan Y *et al.* Genetic and shared environmental factors do not confound the association between birth weight and hypertension, a study among Swedish twins. *Circulation* 2007; **115**: 2931–8.

45 Ijzerman RG, Stehouwer CD, Van Weissenbruch MM, De Geus EJ, Boomsma DI. Evidence for genetic factors explaining the association between birth weight and low-density lipoprotein cholesterol and possible intrauterine factors influencing the association between birth weight and high-density lipoprotein cholesterol, analysis in twins. *J Clin Endocrinol Metab* 2001; **86**: 5479–84.

46 Baird J, Osmond C, MacGregor A, Snieder H, Hales CN, Phillips DI. Testing the fetal origins hypothesis in twins, the Birmingham twin study. *Diabetologia* 2001; **44**: 33–9.

47 Iliadou A, Cnattingius S, Lichtenstein P. Low birth weigth and type-II diabetes, A study on 11 226 Swedish twins. *Int J Epidemiol* 2004; **33**: 948–53.

48 Poulsen P, Vaag AA, Kyvik KO, Moller Jensen D, Beck-Nielsen H. Low birth weight is associated with NIDDM in discordant monozygotic and dizygotic twin pairs. *Diabetologia* 1997; **40**: 439–46.

49 Loos RJF, Beunen G, Fagard R, Derom C, Vlietinck R. Birth weight and body composition in young adult men—a prospective twin study. *International Journal of Obesity* 2001; **25**: 1537–45.

50 Loos RJ, Beunen G, Fagard R, Derom C, Vlietinck R. Birth weight and body composition in young women: a prospective twin study. *Am J Clin Nutr* 2002; **75**: 676–82.

51 Hubinette A, Cnattingius S, Ekbom A, de Faire U, Kramer M, Lichtenstein P. Birthweight, early environment, and genetics: a study of twins discordant for acute myocardial infarction. *Lancet* 2001; **357**: 1997–2001.

52 Hubinette A, Cnattingius S, Johasson ALV, Henriksson C, Lichtenstein P. Birth weight and risk of angina pectoris: analysis in Swedish twins. *European Journal of Epidemiology* 2003; **18**: 539–44.

53 Leon DA, Koupil I, Mann V, Tuvemo T, Lindmark G, Mohsen R *et al.* Fetal, developmental and parental influences on childhood systolic blood pressure in 600 sib pairs: The Uppsala Family Study. *Circulation* 2005; **112**: 3478–85.

54 Bergvall N, Iliadou A, Tuvemo T, Cnattingius S. Birth characteristics and risk of high systolic blood pressure in early adulthood, socioeconomic factors and familial effects. *Epidemiology* 2005; **16**: 635–40.

55 Lawlor DA, Hubinette A, Tynelius P, Leon DA, Davey Smith G, Rasmussen F. Associations of gestational age and intrauterine growth with systolic blood pressure in a family-based study of 386,485 men in 331,089 families. *Circulation* 2007; **115**: 562–8.

56 Davey Smith G, Hyppönen E, Power C, Lawlor DA. Offspring birth weight and parental mortality, prospective observational study and meta-analysis. *Am J Epidemiol* 2007; **166**: 160–9.

57 Davey Smith G. Genetic risk factors in mothers and offspring. *Lancet* 2001; **358**: 1268.

58 Lawlor DA, Davey Smith G, Ebrahim S. Birth weight of offspring and insulin resistance in late adulthood, cross sectional survey using data from the British Women's Heart and Health Study. *BMJ* 2002; **325**: 359–62.

59 Wannamethee SG, Lawlor DA, Whincup PH, Walker M, Ebrahim S, Davey Smith G. Birthweight of offspring and paternal insulin resistance and diabetes in late adulthood, cross-sectional survey. *Diabetologia* 2004; **47**:12–18.

60 Knight B, Shields BM, Hill A, Powell RJ, Round A, Hamilton W *et al.* Offspring birthweight is not associated with paternal insulin resistance. *Diabetologia* 2006; **49**: 2675–8.

61 Davey Smith G, Sterne JA, Tynelius P, Rasmussen F. Birth characteristics of offspring and parental diabetes, evidence for the fetal insulin hypothesis. *J Epidemiol Community Health* 2004; **58**: 126–8.

62 Hypponen E, Davey Smith G, Power C. Parental diabetes and birth weight of offspring, inter-generational cohort study. *BMJ* 2003; **326**:19–20.

63 Lindsay RS, Dabelea D, Roumain J, Hanson RL, Bennett PH, Knowler WC. Type 2 diabetes and low birth weight. The role of paternal inheritance in the association of low birth weight and diabetes. *Diabetes* 2000; **49**: 445–9.

64 Adams J, Pearce MS, White M, Unwin NC, Parker L. No consistent association between birthweight and parental risk of diabetes and cardiovascular disease. *Diabet Med* 2005; **22**: 950–3.

65 Bergvall N, Lindam A, Pawitan Y, Lichtenstein P, Cnattingius S, Iliadou A. Importance of familial factors in associations between offspring birth weight and parental risk of type-2 diabetes. *Int J Epidemiol* 2008; **37**: 185–92.

66 Thomas MC, Walker MK, Emberson JR, Thomson AG, Lawlor DA, Ebrahim S et al. Prevalence of undiagnosed Type 2 Diabetes and Impaired Fasting Glucose in an older British population. *Diabetic Medicine* 2005; **22**: 789–93.

67 Jovanovic L, Pettitt DJ. Gestational diabetes mellitus. *JAMA* 2001; **286**: 2516–18.

68 Kjos SL, Buchanan TA. Gestational diabetes mellitus. *N Engl J Med* 1999; **341**: 1749–56.

69 Scholl TO, Sowers M, Chen X, Lenders C. Maternal glucose concentration influences fetal growth, gestation, and pregnancy complications. *Am J Epidemiol* 2001; **154**: 514–20.

70 Sermer M, Naylor CD, Gare DJ, Kenshole AB, Ritchie JW, Farine D et al. Impact of increasing carbohydrate intolerance on maternal-fetal outcomes in 3637 women without gestational diabetes. The Toronto Tri- Hospital Gestational Diabetes Project. *Am J Obstet Gynecol* 1995; **173**: 146–56.

71 Farmer G, Russell G, Hamilton-Nicol DR, Ogenbede HO, Ross IS, Pearson DW et al. The influence of maternal glucose metabolism on fetal growth, development and morbidity in 917 singleton pregnancies in nondiabetic women. *Diabetologia* 1988; **31**: 134–41.

72 Power C, Jefferis BJ. Fetal environment and subsequent obesity, a study of maternal smoking. *Int J Epidemiol* 2002; **31**: 413–19.

73 Toschke AM, Montgomery SM, Pfeiffer U, von KR. Early intrauterine exposure to tobacco-inhaled products and obesity. *Am J Epidemiol* 2003; **158**: 1068–74.

74 von KR, Toschke AM, Koletzko B, Slikker W, Jr. Maternal smoking during pregnancy and childhood obesity. *Am J Epidemiol* 2002; **156**: 954–61.

75 Mamun AA, Lawlor DA, Alati R, O'Callaghan MJ, Williams GM, Najman JM. Does maternal smoking during pregnancy have a direct effect on future offspring obesity? Evidence from a prospective birth cohort study. *Am J Epidemiol* 2006; **164**: 317–25.

76 Campbell DM, Hall MH, Barker DJ, Cross J, Shiell AW, Godfrey KM. Diet in pregnancy and the offspring's blood pressure 40 years later. *Br J Obstet Gynaecol* 1996; **103**: 273–80.

77 Shiell AW, Campbell-Brown M, Haselden S, Robinson S, Godfrey KM, Barker DJ. High-meat, low-carbohydrate diet in pregnancy, relation to adult blood pressure in the offspring. *Hypertension* 2001; **38**: 1282–8.

78 Leary SD, Davey Smith G, Rogers IS, Reilly JJ, Wells JC, Ness AR. Smoking during pregnancy and offspring fat and lean mass in childhood. *Obesity* 2006; **14**: 2284–93.

79 von Kries R, Bolte G, Baghi L, Toschke AM, for the GME Study Group. Parental smoking and childhood obesity—is maternal smoking in pregnancy the critical exposure? *Int J Epidemiol* 2008; **37**: 210–16.

80 Brion MJ, Leary SD, Davey Smith G, Ness AR. Similar associations of parental prenatal smoking suggest child blood pressure is not influenced by intrauterine effects. *Hypertension* 2007; **49**: 1422–8.

81 Pembrey ME, Bygren LO, Kaati G, Edvinsson S, Northstone K, Sjostrom M et al. Sex-specific, male-line transgenerational responses in humans. *Eur J Hum Genet* 2006; **14**: 159–66.

82 Kane JK, Parker SL, Matta SG, Fu Y, Sharp BM, Li MD. Nicotine up-regulates expression of orexin and its receptors in rat brain. *Endocrinology* 2000; **141**: 3623–9.

83 Slotkin TA. Fetal nicotine or cocaine exposure, which one is worse? *J Pharmacol Exp Ther* 1998; **285**: 931–45.

84 **Mackay DJ.** Model comparison and Occams Razor. In Mackay DJ, edr. *Information Theory, Inference and Learning Algorhythms*. Cambridge University Press, Cambridge, 2003.

85 **Pettitt DJ, Knowler WC.** Diabetes and obesity in the Pima Indians, A cross-generational vicious cycle. *The Journal of Obesity and Weight Regulation* 1988; **7**: 61–75.

86 **Ebbeling CB, Pawlak DB, Ludwig DS.** Childhood obesity, public-health crisis, common sense cure. *Lancet* 2002; **360**: 473–82.

87 **Taylor PD, Poston L.** Developmental programming of obesity in mammals. *Exp Physiol* 2007; **92**: 287–98.

88 **Lawlor DA, Davey Smith G, O'Callaghan M, Alati R, Mamun AA, Williams GM** *et al.* Epidemiologic evidence for the fetal overnutrition hypothesis, findings from the mater-university study of pregnancy and its outcomes. *Am J Epidemiol* 2007; **165**: 418–24.

89 **Davey Smith G, Steer C, Leary S, Ness A.** Is there an intra-uterine influence on obesity? Evidence from parent-child associations in the Avon Longitudinal Study of Parents and Children (ALSPAC). *Arch Dse Child* 2007; **92**: 876–80.

90 **Kivimäki M, Lawlor DA, Davey Smith G, Elovainio M, Jokela M, Keltikangas-Järvinen L** *et al.* Substantial inter-generational increases in body mass index are not explained by the fetal overnutrition hypothesis, The Cardiovascular Risk in Young Finns. *Am J Clin Nutr* 2007; **86**: 1509–14.

91 **Lawlor DA, Timpson N, Harbord RM, Leary S, Ness A, McCarthy MI** *et al.* Exploring the developmental overnutrition hypothesis using parental-offspring associations and the *FTO* gene as an instrumental variable for maternal adiposity. The Avon Longitudinal Study of Parents and Children (ALSPAC). *PLoS Medicine* 2008; **5**: e33. doi:101371/journal.pmed0050033.

92 **Pettitt DJ, Bennett PH, Saad MF, Charles MA, Nelson RG, Knowler WC.** Abnormal glucose tolerance during pregnancy in Pima Indian women. Long-term effects on offspring. *Diabetes* 1991; **40**: 126–30.

93 **Dabelea D, Hanson RL, Lindsay RS, Pettitt DJ, Imperatore G, Gabir MM** *et al.* Intrauterine exposure to diabetes conveys risks for type 2 diabetes and obesity, a study of discordant sibships. *Diabetes* 2000; **49**: 2208–11.

94 **Freinkel N, Metzger BE.** Pregnancy as a tissue culture experience, the critical implications of maternal metabolism for fetal development. In Ciba Foundation, editor. Pregnancy Metabolism, Diabetes and the Fetus (Ciba Foundation Symposium No. 63). Excerpta Medica, Amsterdam The Netherlands, pp. 3–23, 1979.

95 **Freinkel N.** Of pregnancy and progeny. *Diabetes* 1980; **29**: 1023–35.

Chapter 14

How family-based studies have added to the understanding of life course epidemiology of mental health

Stephani L Hatch and Gita D Mishra

Abstract

This chapter reviews some of the key family-based studies that have identified links between various illnesses and behaviours in parents and siblings with psychiatric disorders in study members. It also describes how sibling and twin studies are beginning to produce results that quantify the relative contribution of genetic and environmental effects. We conclude with recommendations from the perspective of life course epidemiology to move beyond the established associations and to increase our understanding of the underlying mechanisms involved in psychiatric disorders. Specifically, we describe the range of characteristics in terms of study design, and type and scope of data that should be incorporated in future large population based studies.

14.1 Introduction

Up to 30% of the world's population suffer from mental disorders every year, with more than two-thirds receiving inadequate or no treatment, even in countries with the best health resources.[1] It is estimated that 14% of the total global burden of disease is attributable to mental disorder.[2] Mental or neuropsychiatric disorders cover many conditions, including the various types of depression, psychoses, and alcohol- and substance-use disorders. They are believed to contribute more to morbidity among the non-communicable diseases than heart disease, stroke, and cancer.[2] But a lack of appreciation and understanding of the links between mental disorders and other health conditions means that their full impact is likely to be far higher.

Mental health is a complex area of research due to the variety of mental disorders, difficulties in their measurement, and the multifarious mix of factors from genetic to social and environmental influences that potentially influence their onset and severity. Nevertheless over several decades, family-based studies derived from treatment and primary care settings, as well as community-based and population-based studies, have contributed significantly to advancing our understanding of the course, consequences, and comorbidities of mental disorders. In previous chapters, family-based studies have largely been interpreted as those studies that either describe familial clustering of a disease or health related outcome or those studies that have exploited within and between familial association to develop better mechanistic understanding of disease (for example, partitioning genetic from shared and individual environmental determinants).

But in mental health, family-based studies have often been focussed on exploring directly the effect of relationships between different family members (parents-offspring, wife-husband, siblings) on mental disorder, such as the impact of parental behaviour or discord on offspring mental health.

As discussed in Chapters 2 to 4, within the three broad categories of intergenerational, sibling, and twin studies, there are numerous sub-types of family-based studies. Also there is often an overlap between intergenerational studies and sibling studies, especially in mental health when the analysis focuses on the relationship of disorders between first degree relatives. Twin and sibling samples permit the exploration of genetic and environmental factors, particularly in the consideration of shared environments that play an important part in transmission (see Chapters 4 and 11 for further information on the theoretical underpinning and statistical methods in twin studies).

In mental health research recruitment for family-based studies has often relied upon the use of probands, that is drawing the sample from those individuals with the disorder under investigation.[3–5] Family members of the proband are then examined to determine the degree that they have the same disorder. In addition to identifying the extent of intergenerational influences, they permit insights on the key characteristics of psychiatric disorders, such as the age of onset, their course and episodic nature, and the occurrence of any comorbidity. The main disadvantage of these studies is their lack of representativeness with respect to the general population due to their sampling method. They also often rely on retrospective reporting (e.g. identifying the timing of onset for siblings and parents of probands), but they may still obtain prospective data, for example incident risk in offspring who at the time of establishment of the cohort through probands are clearly younger than the expected age of disease onset. Family-based studies in mental health epidemiology have also been drawn from clinic settings or the relevant community at risk for specific disorders. Again these are unlikely to be representative of the general population.

In contrast, longitudinal population based studies, such as national birth cohort studies, by definition aim to be representative of the general population of a similar age. As in other fields of research (for instance Chapter 13), with prospective data they can detect wide ranging influences on mental health by allowing for testing of hypothesized pathways from early life experience to adult mental health. Typically, this involves pathways related to material and social resources (e.g., social class from family of origin) and parental behaviour, while controlling for important potential confounders reflecting both family and educational domains.[6–10]

The established methodology for assessing psychiatric disorders is via validated symptom-based measures or instruments. Measurement strategies generally focus on identifying symptoms, either via self-completed questionnaires or through interview surveys. Small studies, e.g. clinic based samples, tend to utilize clinicians for these assessments, but larger community studies usually rely on trained interviewers to capture mental health status. In clinical terms, current diagnostic criteria to determine the absence or presence of a disorder are normally based on the Diagnostic and Statistical Manual of Mental Disorders, fourth edition, (DSM-IV)[11] or a coding according to the International Classification of Diseases (ICD-10).[12] Other measures have been developed specifically for clinical diagnostic assessments, such as the revised Clinical Interview Schedule (CIS-R)[13] and the World Health Organisation's Composite International Diagnostic Interview (CIDI).[14] Many larger studies, however, utilize simple measures of traits such as the Center for Epidemiologic Studies Depression Scale (CES-D)[15] and the General Health Questionnaire (GHQ).[16]

About half of all mental disorders begin before the age of 14 years (http://www.who.int/features/factfiles/mental_health/mental_health_facts/en/index.html), with research also suggesting that genetic and early childhood psychosocial risk factors are important to understanding the timing of the onset of mental disorders at different life stages.[17–22] To underline this role in both the development and mechanisms of psychopathology, the chapter focuses on the key family-based studies over the last decade that have examined early life exposures. We particularly describe research that identifies prenatal and early childhood exposures that influence some of the most common child and adolescent mental disorders, such as depression, anxiety, antisocial disorders, and substance use.

The chapter reviews results from some of the key intergenerational studies, followed by sibling and twin studies that have contributed to a more detailed understanding of mental disorders over the last decade, although this list is by no means exhaustive. We have concentrated on highly prevalent psychiatric disorders such as depression or substance-use disorder. Recent studies presenting findings on the impact of environmental and genetic factors on common mental disorders, as well as the how the interplay between the two may influence psychopathology findings are also discussed.[23] We conclude by offering suggestions to enable family-based studies to contribute more effectively to understanding psychiatric epidemiology from a life course perspective.

14.2 Intergenerational studies

Intergenerational studies have largely been used to explore how parental characteristics (e.g. their experience of mental health, their behaviours and parenting skills, their socioeconomic background) influence the risk of mental ill-health in their offspring. For instance, a number of studies have confirmed a two- to threefold increased risk for major depressive disorder and anxiety disorder among children and adolescents with at least one depressed parent in comparison to those without depressed parents.[19, 24–29] Although the increased risk of poor mental health outcomes among the offspring of parents with psychological distress is well established, the mechanisms for intrafamilial transmission are often not well understood.[3, 30–38]

14.2.1 Mental health of parents and offspring

In a family-based study comprised of a proband sample (n = 125) of depressed parents undergoing treatment and controls (n = 95), Weissman and colleagues followed offspring into adulthood over 20-years.[19] This study not only indicated the high probability of transmission, but also included findings related to the degree of risk passed through the generations. Nearly half of all children with both a depressed grandparent and parent were found to have some form of psychopathology (i.e., depressive disorder, any anxiety, disruptive disorder, or substance disorder), in comparison to remaining 11% with one depressed grandparent, 17% with one depressed parent, and 23% in families where neither grandparent or parent were depressed (not excluding other forms of pscychopathology).[5] It was also found that children (average age 10 years) with both a grandparent and parent with major depressive disorder have the highest risks for anxiety and an increased likelihood for prepubertal onset of anxiety.[5]

Although these types of studies provide insights on some important associations, a key critique is of their small sample size and use of samples drawn from subjects under treatment rather than being representative of the general population. The Dunedin Multidisciplinary Health and Development Study in New Zealand (Dunedin Longitudinal Study), is a birth cohort of 1,037 subjects. Results indicate that those with either major depressive disorder or anxiety disorder were more likely to have mothers with greater internalizing symptoms, in comparison to healthy counterparts.[39] Those participants with major depressive disorder tended to have a more complex family history of depression. In another longitudinal study, the National Survey of Health and Development (NSHD; also known as the 1946 British Birth Cohort) with over 5,000 participants parental mental health was associated with mental health among females in early adulthood[19] and maternal neuroticism during childhood was also linked with the adult mental health of male offspring.[10]

The Early Development Stages of Psychopathology (EDSP) is another longitudinal study that investigated substance-use and other mental disorders in a representative population sample of more than 3,000 individuals in Germany. It assessed the impact of major depression in parents on the course of depression in offspring by collecting intergenerational data on the age of onset, course, and severity of the disorder.[27] Findings from this study confirmed earlier results that major depression among parents was associated with increased offspring risk for depression (odds ratio [OR] for one parent with disorder, 2.7; 95% confidence interval [CI], 2.1–3.5; and OR for two parents with disorder, 3.0; 95% CI, 2.2–4.1).[27]

While such results point to the role of genetic and various shared environmental factors, they also indicate the possibility for these effects to operate in both directions, for instance psychopathology in offspring leading to depression in their parents.[3, 40–42] Further complications arise since mental disorders may not occur singularly but as a group of comorbid disorders. In findings that were consistent with earlier results from other studies, research from a nationally representative sample of children in the US suggested that the offspring of parents with depression were approximately twice as likely to have multiple mental health problems as children of parents without depression.[38, 43]

The presence of comorbid disorders also extends to other psychiatric disorders early in the life course.[44] The Michigan Longitudinal Study (MLS) followed three cohorts of children from families with alcoholic parents and children from matched families without an alcoholic parent (see Zucker *et al.*[45] for additional details). Evidence from the study indicated an increased risk for externalizing symptoms that persisted into adolescence where parents had comorbidity of antisocial or depressive disorders with alcoholism.[46] In a small proband study, the child and adolescent male offspring of a parent, particularly a mother, with comorbidity of substance-use and depressive disorder were found to have increased risk for conduct disorder, in comparison to sons of controls without any disorder.[47] The findings from this study are consistent with other studies that report an increased risk for externalizing symptoms for children who parents have comorbid antisocial and alcoholic disorders versus those parents with alcohol disorder only or controls.[48–49]

14.2.2 Early life exposures and mental health

Current literature on developmental psychopathology suggests that the course and correlates of disorders is a function of age of onset.[17] The findings differentiating childhood, adolescent, and adult onset of major depressive disorder indicate that each time period may represent distinct subtypes of disorder, with some suggestion that genetic and early childhood psychosocial risk factors are both key in understanding these differences.[18–22]

Numerous studies have consistently linked postnatal depression with emotional and behavioural problems in offspring during childhood.[50] The Avon Longitudinal Study of Parents and Children (ALSPAC) followed over 13,000 women from pregnancy and addressed the timing of exposures for childhood mental health by examining maternal psychological distress from both the antenatal and postnatal periods. Research found that antenatal anxiety in late pregnancy and postnatal depression are separate risks for behaviour or emotional problems in children at 4 years, after controlling for a range of confounding factors from maternal age to alcohol use.[51–52] In other findings, even very low levels of alcohol consumption in early pregnancy were associated with offspring mental health problems from early to middle childhood, controlling for alcohol use before pregnancy, maternal alcohol use during childhood, and postnatal maternal depression.[53]

Birth cohort studies can provide prospective data on the social and economic status of the parents, often based on the social class of the father as measured by his occupation. The National Collaborative Perinatal Project (NCPP), a large scale population based study, found that lower childhood social class based on father's occupation was associated with increased reporting of depressive symptoms at age 18–39 years for men and women, as measured by the Diagnostic Interview Schedule[54] and after controlling for family history of mental illness.[55] Using the same instrument, results from the Dunedin Longitudinal Study linked lower socioeconomic status to major depressive disorder as well as its occurrence with the comorbidity of generalized anxiety disorder in adulthood.[41] The National Child Development Study (NCDS, 1958 British birth cohort), revealed a similar relationship for depression as measured by the Clinical Interview Schedule[56] at 45 years of age.[57]

In contrast, analysis of 1970 British Birth Cohort Study, found no evidence for a link between lower childhood social class and depression and anxiety at 26 years, as measured by the Malaise Inventory.[58][6] Similarly when using the Present State Exam[59] for assessment, no relationship was found between the adult mental health at 36 years and childhood social class or the educational qualifications of parents.[9] Other indicators of childhood social environment, however, such as living in council housing and experiencing overcrowding in the home, were identified as linked with poorer adult mental health.[9]

An explanation for these disparate findings may lie in research that compared results from different instruments. In a subsequent analysis of the 1970 British Birth Cohort Study, it was found that when using the GHQ-12 and controlling for the same set of potential confounders, lower childhood social class was associated with symptoms of depression and anxiety at 30 years, whereas this was not the case when using measures from the Malaise Inventory that was administered at the same age.[7] In addition, this finding is replicated in a recent analysis of birth cohort data followed from the same time period. Hence, one of the methodological challenges in establishing the role of various factors on mental disorder lies in understanding the strengths and weaknesses of the instruments being used that may vary according to age and type of disorder.

Early life exposures may also have highly specific consequences on adult mental health. For instance, childhood experiences reflective of the maternal relationship may be important in understanding the occurrence of postnatal depression in the adult offspring. Women in the NSHD who recalled receiving a low level of maternal care or experienced maternal separation for more 3.5 days in early childhood were found to be at increased risk for postnatal depression, compared to other women.[60] This remained the case after adjusting for their current psychological status and adult relationship with their mother. Such findings are significant, since childbearing years are the high risk period for major depression in women.[61] But the mechanism of this link remains unclear, for instance childbirth may just act as trigger and lead to anxiety in mothers and recall of unhappy memories from their own childhood. More prospective information is needed to better understand potential long term effects of mother-child relationships on postnatal depression.

14.2.3 Parental behaviour

The literature of developmental psychopathology has long identified parental behaviour as an important risk factor for mental ill health in offspring,[62] but determining the direction of this relationship remains problematic. While many family-based studies of mental health have tended to focus on maternal practices during early childhood, they have often omitted information on paternal behaviours or influence. Their methodological strength, however, lies in the use of multiple family informants and corroborating evidence from medical and family service records.[19,51,63]

Differentiating the roll of each factor is complex since parental behaviours of interest and mental disorders often do not occur separately. The Children in the Community Study, a longitudinal study in New York State, assessed 782 families during the childhood and adolescence of the offspring. Consistent with earlier findings on the relationship between parental psychopathology and maladaptive parental behaviour,[30, 65] results from the study indicated that maternal major depressive disorder was associated with problematic maternal behaviour in the home during the child rearing years.[64] This indicates that maladaptive parental behaviour may be an important mediator in the association between parental and offspring psychopathology.[65] From data spanning four time points and involving numerous measures of parental behaviours, it was also found that in comparison to parents with episodic psychiatric disorders, those with persistent psychiatric disorders were more likely to have offspring with psychiatric disorders in adulthood.[65]

Regarding paternal influence, results from the 1958 British birth cohort found no evidence for influence on adolescent and adult mental health of the paternal involvement in childhood (e.g., outings with the father, father managing the child, reading to the child and interest in the child's education).[8] However, the information on paternal behaviour was based on reports from the mother, and should be treated with some caution. It points to the more general need for longitudinal studies to take a far more comprehensive approach to monitoring parental behaviour.

Intergenerational studies can also elucidate the impact of parenting behaviours in terms of the emotional unavailability of parents and marital or family discord,[66] particularly divorce—although the evidence is mixed.[67] For women in the 1946 British Birth Cohort, it was found that that divorce or separation of parents has had adverse effect on their mental health in early adulthood and for those women who themselves were divorced/separated in mid-adulthood.[9–10] Among male cohort members, temporary parental separation and paternal death before age 18 (and especially if this occurred between the ages 5–11 years) was shown to be associated with increased reporting of symptoms of anxiety and depression.[10] However, more recent evidence suggests that symptoms of depression and anxiety in offspring may be present prior to the divorce event, and some studies have since refocused analysis to concentrate on the negative effects of parental discord and other problems in the home on children's emotional and behavioural problems.[67]

The health behaviours of parents, such as alcohol consumption (as described in Section 14.2.1), have been investigated extensively in relationship to poor offspring mental health. The majority of the evidence consistently links heavy and moderate alcohol consumption by parents with poor behavioural and emotional outcomes for children and adolescents.[68–70] Parental care and bonding are other factors that can affect mental health in offspring. In an Australian cohort of school students it was found that low maternal and paternal care held independent associations for depression in adolescence, as measured by CIDI and CIS-R.[71] In a subsample of women and their daughters from a longitudinal study, the findings suggest that parental bonding (via the self-reported Parental Bonding Instrument[72]) was associated across generations and independent of depression, temperament, and socioeconomic status.[73] In the longitudinal 20 year follow-up of this study, for offspring of depressed parents, no relationship was found between family discord (e.g., parent-child discord, low family cohesion, affectionless control, and parental divorce) and depression and anxiety in the offspring.[74] However, for offspring of parents without depression, affectionless parental control (as identified by the same instrument) was associated with a nearly fivefold increased risk of major depressive disorder during adolescence (OR, 4.8, p=0.05) and a 14-fold increase risk of substance-use disorder (OR, 14.3, p=0.01) in adulthood.[74]

14.2.4 Summary of intergenerational studies

Intergenerational studies have formed a major part of the epidemiological research on offspring mental health, specifically in terms of investigating the influence of parental characteristics, from their mental health and comorbidities to their socioeconomic background and parenting skills, on the risk of mental disorders in offspring from childhood to later adult life. Few studies have looked over more generations, beyond parental affects, and explored how grandparental characteristics influence offspring mental health.

The family studies described above are by no means exhaustive, but they have illustrated the complex web of factors that affect mental health in families: relationships between either the same or different types of metal disorder across generations; the direction of these relationships, in the influence of children on their parents; the role of shared environments, such as socioeconomic conditions; differences due to timing of exposures; and disparities in the timing of onset for mental health. Furthermore, we identified the critical role of the instruments used to assess mental health across the life course and required, and taking a comprehensive approach to gathering prospective data, such as on both maternal and paternal behaviours. Large multi-generational longitudinal studies, with repeat measurements of behaviours and 'outcomes' on all generations, are needed to untangle the different possibilities, but few such studies currently exist.

14.3 Sibling and twin studies

As discussed in earlier chapters (Chapters 3, 4, and 11), sibling and twin studies have particular advantages for researchers investigating the relative contribution of genetic and environmental effects. In terms of mental health, a key part of the research has been to investigate the length and direct interaction between sibling relationships and studies have therefore focused on the complex developmental processes within sibling relationships that lead to poor mental health outcomes.[75] In attempting to conceptualise sibling relationships over the life course, it is important for researchers to understand how the quality of these relationships tends to change as siblings develop.

14.3.1 Family type and the quality of sibling relationships

A number of studies have indicated a strong link between negative sibling relationships (e.g., conflict and aggression) and poor mental health in childhood and adolescence.[76, 77] However, the direction of the associations are difficult to determine, given that the presence of conduct problems and other externalising behaviours in one sibling is itself likely to result in a negative sibling relationship, as well as vice versa.[78] In a longitudinal sibling sample drawn from the community, adolescents with severe antisocial behaviour reported more negative relationships with their siblings, in comparison to controls.[78] But to create a more comprehensive picture of how relationships within the family may influence the mental health of family members, recent family-based studies have assessing parental and sibling behaviours and family characteristics through multiple informants.

In this respect, two important sibling studies are the Avon Brother and Sisters Study (ABSS), a substudy of ALSPAC on 192 families, that has concentrated on the importance of family type (e.g., stepfamilies, single mother families) and the Non-shared Environment in Adolescent Development (NEAD) sibling study of 720 families (two-parent families with a pair of adolescent siblings—including twins—of the same gender and no more than four years apart in age). Both have been able to investigate the joint influences of sibling and parent-child, relationships on externalising behaviours (e.g., antisocial) in adolescents from non-stepfamilies and stepfather families.[79]

These studies utilize data from full, half, and adopted siblings to further elucidate the influence of family types and relationship dynamics for both parent-child and sibling dyads from early childhood through adolescence. Their findings have often contradicted other earlier studies. For example, a number of other studies, with poorer study designs, have found that sibling relationships are more likely to be negative in stepfamilies,[77, 80–82] but this was not detected in the ABSS.[83] However in ABSS it was found that negativity (conflict and aggression) was more likely in sibling relationships in single-mother families in comparison to other family types. The ABSS study is one of the few to have included assessments of positive sibling relationships, and finds that they appear to moderate the association between childhood adversity and internalizing symptoms (but not externalizing symptoms), regardless of the quality of the mother-child relationship.[84]

In the NEAD study, negative or hostile sibling relationships were linked with externalizing behaviours in boys in stepfamilies and similarly, but with greater impact, in non-stepfamilies.[85] For girls in this study, hostile sibling relationships were associated with adolescent externalising behaviours, but only in non-stepfamilies. There is also evidence of higher correlations between negative sibling relationships and higher level of adjustment problems in two-parent families.[83] However the main contribution from this study has been as a sibling-twin study, as is discussed in a later section.

14.3.2 Twins studies and depression

As described in Chapter 4, the advantages of twin studies lies in their ability to go beyond purely descriptive statistics and identify various genetic and environmental influences and their interactions. A meta-analysis of five methodologically rigorous twin studies, with a combined sample of more than 21,000 individuals, supported earlier evidence that depression is in part an inherited trait, and the influence of heritability persists into later life.[86] The aggregate of estimate of heritability of major depression was estimated to be 37% (95% CI of 31%–42%).[86] This result was recently replicated using data from a large representative sample of more than 15,000 twin pairs from the national Swedish Twin Registry (38%). It should be noted, particularly for research on mental disorders, that differences in heritability can be sensitive to how narrowly or broadly a disorder is defined in each study. Furthermore, as heritability is a relative measure of genetic contribution to the variation in a trait or disease outcome (relative to total genetic and environmental contribution), it may be sensitive to differences in the prevalence of non-genetic (environmental) risk factors between populations and variations in environmental factors over time.

The Swedish study also confirmed findings of other twin studies[87, 88] that sex differences exist in genetic risk factors for major depression, specifically that the heritability of having a liability to major depression is greater in women than in men (42% versus 29%). However they did not find any evidence to support the suggestion that shared environmental risk factors (such as parental rearing practises or social class) were important in the development of major depression either in the males or females. A limitation of this study is that major depression was only assessed at one time point.

As was discussed earlier, understanding the timing of onset of disorders has been a key part of mental health research. It is well established from epidemiological studies that there is a marked rise in the prevalence of depression between the ages of 13 to 15 years. Over a three year period, a longitudinal study from the UK surveyed 1,820 twin and sibling pairs aged 12–19 years at three time points. It was found that depressive symptoms at all time points were moderately heritable with substantial non-shared environmental contributions. The detailed findings suggested changes in both genetic and environmental factors occurred across development. A population based life course study may help explain if developmentally sensitive genetic factors are 'switched on' at critical periods leading to some of the biological and pubertal changes—as well as cognitive maturation—that occur during adolescence, and that these in turn greatly effect the rates of depression.

14.4 Using cohort studies to investigate gene-environment interaction

In the last decade or so there has been a re-emergence of interest in gene-environment interplay.[89] This could be thought of as a situation where the risk from an environmental exposure varies according to genotype or where the genotype effect varies according to environment. In 2003, using data from Dunedin Longitudinal Study, Caspi and colleagues set out to investigate the observation that stressful experiences lead to depression in some people, but not in others.[90] They found that a functional polymorphism in the promoter region of the serotonin transporter (5-HTT) gene was found to moderate the influence of stressful life events on depression.

As this result has important implications for the investigation of how the gene-environment interaction affects health, it has inspired a flurry of replication studies.[91] The majority identified interaction effects in a similar direction to the original study, although for two this was observed only among women.[92, 93] However in one of the larger studies, with over 4,000 participants, no evidence of an interaction was found between genotype and adverse experiences in childhood or adulthood on the risk of depression.[94] Another recent study also failed to replicate the earlier interaction.[95] These mixed results could be due to differences in the type of environmental stress measures used, random variation between samples or an effect of publication bias (it may be more likely that those with a 'positive' replication are submitted and accepted for publication). Nonetheless, the consistency of findings from most of these studies suggests that the effects of stressful events might indeed be mediated by 5-HTT gene.

14.5 Conclusions and future directions

This chapter has largely concentrated on descriptive results from family-based studies that link various disorders and behaviours in parents and siblings with mental health outcomes in the study member. This reflects how in mental health research, such studies are used to explore family relationships, and their changing quality and quantity, in terms of their effects on mental disorders. We have also seen how sibling and twin studies are beginning used to produce results that quantify the relative contribution of genetic and environmental effects. So from the perspective of life course epidemiology, to move beyond the established associations and increase our understanding of the underlying mechanisms involved in mental health, more longitudinal prospective studies need to be undertaken with large population based samples.

Specifically, we suggest a number of addition features that these life course studies should embody. First, to further our understanding of the factors that influence the onset, course, and comorbidity patterns of psychiatric disorders, there is a need for more multigenerational prospective study designs. It is also necessary have assessments of psychiatric disorders closely spaced to capture patterns of episode recurrence. This will allow a better characterization of their trajectories and the identification of both familial and individual level factors across the life course that may shape initial differences in these trajectories and their decline. Repeated measures across generations, including grandparents, also may afford researchers an opportunity to attempt to untangle possible bi-directional associations of familial transmission of mental disorders.

Second, more attention to the characterisation of families types and their disparate composition would add important contextual information to the understanding of environmental factors.

Analysis undertaken by studies, such as ALSPAC, suggests that family typologies may be useful for inferences about the family environment. In life course epidemiology, they may assist with understanding the mental health consequences resulting from changing family formation over time. Creating typologies at the family level could also aid in identifying the long-term processes of psychiatric symptoms within groups characterised by disadvantaged social status (e.g., low socioeconomic status, ethnic minorities), particularly in multicultural contexts.

Finally, to improving the scope and the quality of the data collected in family-based studies, researchers should consider nesting sub-samples of family members within birth cohort studies and other longitudinal population-based studies. For example, interviewing the spouses and partners, offspring and continuing to include parents of cohort members. Particularly, there should be more paternal information, instead of gleaning information from maternal assessments. This type of familial inclusion also provides useful external corroborating information. Furthermore assessments should cover multiple domains (e.g., home, school, work) that may be important to understanding environmental exposures experienced by all family members.

In summary, we have seen that family-based studies have identified numerous intergenerational associations linking a wide range of mental disorders. It has also been evident that sibling and twin studies provide useful insights to unravel the various mechanisms that may explain these relationships. Specifically, future research should focus on the extent that (a) genetic transmission causes vulnerability to mental disorder in parents, offspring, and siblings; (b) environmental influence of parental mental disorder leading to offspring mental disorder; or the alternate direction that offspring mental disorder leads to parental mental disorder; and (c) both the shared and the non-shared familial environmental factors increase vulnerability for psychiatric disorder in parents, offspring, and siblings. Thus, combining family-based study designs with the life course perspective has the potential to reframe and further our understanding of many of the key findings in psychiatric epidemiology in a manner that allows for better understanding of aetiology, context, long term processes, and the consequences of the familial transmission of psychiatric disorders.

References

1 Thornicroft G. Most people with mental illness are not treated. *Lancet* 2007; **370**: 807–8.
2 Prince M, Patel V, Saxena S, Maj M, Maselko J, Phillips MR, *et al*. No health without mental health. *Lancet* 2007; **370**: 859–77
3 Warner V, Weissman MM, Mufson L, Wickramaratne PJ. Grandparents, parents, and grandchildren at high risk for depression: A three-generation study. *Journal of the American Academy of Child & Adolescent Psychiatry* 1999; **38**: 289–96.
4 Harrington R, Rutter M, Weissman M, Fudge H, Groothues C, Bredenkamp D, *et al*. Psychiatric disorders in the relatives of depressed probands. I. Comparison of prepubertal, adolescent and early adult onset cases. *Journal of Affective Disorders* 1997; **42**: 9–22.
5 Mondimore FM, Zandi PP, MacKinnon DF, McInnis MG, Miller EB, Schweizer B, *et al*. A comparison of the familiality of chronic depression in recurrent early-onset depression pedigrees using different definitions of chronicity. *Journal of Affective Disorders* 2007; **100**: 171–7.
6 Cheung YB. Early origins and adult correlates of psychosomatic distress. *Social Science & Medicine* 2002; **55**: 937–48.
7 Flouri E. Psychological outcomes in midadulthood associated with mother's child- rearing attitudes in early childhood: Evidence from the 1970 British birth cohort. *European Child & Adolescent Psychiatry* 2004; **13**: 35–41.
8 Flouri E, Buchanan A. The role of father involvement in children's later mental health. *Journal of Adolescence* 2003; 26, 63–78.

9. **Rodgers B.** Adult affective disorder and early environment. *British Journal of Psychiatry* 1990; **157**: 539–50.
10. **Rodgers B.** Pathways between parental divorce and adult depression. *Journal of Child Psychology and Psychiatry* 1994; **55**: 1289–1308.
11. **American Psychiatric Association.** *Diagnostic Statistical Manual of Mental Disorders*, 4th edn. American Psychiatric Association, Washington, DC, 1994.
12. World Health Organisation. *Composite international diagnostic interview (CIDI, Version 1.0)* World Health Organisation, Geneva, 1990.
13. **Lewis G, Pelosi AJ, Araya R, Dunn G.** Measuring psychiatric disorder in the community: A standardized assessment for use by lay interviewers. *Psychological Medicine* 1992; **22**: 465–86.
14. **Prince M, Stewart R, Ford T, Hotopf M.** *Practical psychiatric epidemiology.* Oxford University Press, London, 2004.
15. **Radloff LS.** The CES-D scale: A self report depression scale for research in the general population. *Applied Psychological Measurement* 1977; **1**: 385–401.
16. **Goldberg G, Williams P.** *A user's guide to the general health questionnaire.* NFER-Nelson, Windsor, Berkshire, 1988.
17. **Rutter M, Kim-Cohen J, Maughan B.** Continuities and discontinuities in psychopathology between childhood and adult life. *Journal of Child Psychology and Psychiatry* 2006; **47**: 276–95.
18. **Harrington RC, Fudge H, Rutter M, Pickles A, Hill J.** Adult outcomes of childhood and adolescent depression:1. Psychiatric status. *Archives of General Psychiatry* 1990; **47**: 465–73.
19. **Weissman MM, Wickramaratne P, Nomura Y, Warner V, Pilowsky D, Verdeli H.** Offspring of Depressed Parents: 20 Years Later. *American Journal of Psychiatry* 2006; 163: 1001–8.
20. **Harrington R, Rutter M, Fombonne E.** Developmental pathways in depression: Multiple meanings, antecedents, and endpoint. *Development and Psychopathology* 1996; **8**: 601–16.
21. **Jaffee SR, Moffitt TE, Caspi A, Fombonne E, Poulton R, Martin J.** Differences in early childhood risk factors for juvenile-onset and adult-onset depression. *Archives of General Psychiatry* 2002; **59**: 215–22.
22. **Kessler RC, Magee WJ.** Childhood adversities and adult depression: basic patterns of association in a US national survey. *Psychological Medicine* 1993; **23**: 679–90.
23. **Rutter M, Silberg J, O'Connor T, Simonoff E.** Genetics and child psychiatry. *Journal of Child Psychology and Psychiatry* 1999; **40**: 19–55.
24. **Kendler KS, Davis CG, Kessler RC.** The familial aggregation of common psychiatric and substance use disorders in the National Comorbidity Survey: a family history study. *British Journal of Psychiatry* 1997; **170**: 541–48.
25. **Klein DN, Lewinsohn PM, Seeley JR, Rohde P.** A family study of major depressive disorder in a community sample of adolescents. *Archives of General Psychiatry* 2001; **58**:13–20.
26. **Kovacs M, Devlin B, Pollock M, Richards C, Mukerji P.** A controlled family history study of childhood-onset depressive disorder. *Archives of General Psychiatry* 1997; **54**: 613–23.
27. **Lieb R, Isensee B, Hofler M, Pfister H, Wittchen HU.** Parental major depression and the risk of depression and other mental disorders in offspring: A prospective-longitudinal community study. *Archives of General Psychiatry* 2002; **59**: 365–74.
28. **Olfson M, Marcus SC, Druss B, Pincus HA, Weissman MM.** Parental depression, child mental health problems, and health care utilization. *Medical Care* 2003; **41**: 716-21.
29. **Williamson DE, Birmaher B, Axelson DA, Ryan ND, Dahl RE.** First episode of depression in children at low and high familial risk for depression. *Journal of the American Academy of Child & Adolescent Psychiatry* 2004; **43**: 291–97.
30. **Downey G, Coyne JC.** Children of depressed parents: an integrative review. *Psychological Bulletin* 1990; **108**: 50-76.
31. **Merikangas KR, Prusoff BA, Weissman MM.** Parental concordance for affective disorders: psychopathology in offspring. *Journal of Affective Disorder* 1988; **15**: 279–90.

32 Orvaschel H, Walsh-Allis G, Ye W. Psychopathology in children of parents with recurrent depression. *Journal of Abnormal Child Psychology* 1988; **16**: 17–28.

33 Weissman MM, Gammon D, John K, Merikangas KR. Children of depressed parents. *Archives of General Psychiatry* 1987; **44**: 847–53.

34 Fendrich M, Warner V, Weissman MM. Family risk factors, parental depression, and psychopathology in offspring. *Developmental Psychology* 1990; **26**: 40–50.

35 Weissman MM, Fendrich M, Warner V, Wickramaratne PJ. Incidence of psychiatric disorders in offspring at high and low risk for depression. *Journal of the American Academy of Child & Adolescent Psychiatry* 1992; **31**: 640–48.

36 Warner V, Mufson I, Weissman MM. Offspring at high and low risk for depression and anxiety: mechanisms of psychiatric disorder. *Journal of the American Academy of Child & Adolescent Psychiatry* 1995; **33**: 1256–64.

37 Weissman MM, Warner V, Wickramaratne P, Moreau D, Olfson M. Offspring of depressed parents: 10 years later. *Archives of General Psychiatry* 1997; **54**: 932–40.

38 Hammen C, Burge D, Burney E, Cheri A. Longitudinal study of diagnoses in children of women with unipolar and bipolar affective disorder. *Archives of General Psychiatry* 1990; **47**: 1112–17.

39 Moffitt TE, Avshalom C, Harrington H, Milne BJ, Melchoir M, Goldberg D, et al. Generalized anxiety disorder and depression: childhood risk factors in a birth cohort followed to age 32. *Psychological Medicine* 2007; **37**: 441–52.

40 Mitchell J, McCauley E, Burke P, Calderon R, Schloredt K. Psychopathology in parents of depressed children and adolescents. *Journal of the American Academy of Child & Adolescent Psychiatry* 1989; **28**: 352–57.

41 Todd R, Geller B, Neuman R, Fox LW, Hickok J. Increased prevalence of alcoholism in relatives of depressed and bipolar children. *Journal of the American Academy of Child & Adolescent Psychiatry* 1996; **35**: 716–24.

42 Neuman R, Geller B, Rice JP, Todd R. Increased prevalence and earlier onset of mood disorders among relatives of prepubertal versus adult probands. *Journal of the American Academy of Child & Adolescent Psychiatry* 1997; **36**: 466–73.

43 Beardslee WR, Versage EM, Cladstone TR. Children of affectively ill parents: a review of the past 10 years. *Journal of the American Academy of Child & Adolescent Psychiatry* 1988; 31: 1134–41.

44 Angold A, Costello EJ, Erkanli A. Comorbidity. *Journal of Child Psychology and Psychiatry* 1999; **40**: 57–87.

45 Zucker RA, Fitzgerald HE, Refior SK, Puttler LI, Pallas DM, Ellis DA. The clinical and social ecology of childhood for children of alcoholics: Description of a study and implications for a differentiated social policy. In: Fitzgerald HE, Lester BM, Zuckerman BS, eds. *Children of Addiction: Research, health and policy issues* New York: Garland Press. pp. 174–222, 2000.

46 Hussong AM, Wirth RJ, Edwards MC, Curran PJ, Chassin LA, Zucker RA. Externalizing symptoms among children of alcoholic parents: Entry points for an antisocial pathway to alcoholism. *Journal of Abnormal Psychology* 2007; **116**: 529–42.

47 Nunes EV, Weissman MM, Goldstein RB, McAvay G, Seracini AM, Verdell H, et al. Psychopathology in children of parents with opiate dependence and/or major depression. *Journal of the American Academy of Child & Adolescent Psychiatry* 1998; **37**: 1142–51.

48 Puttler LI, Zucker RA, Fitzgerald HE, Bingham CR. Behavioral outcomes among children of alcoholics during the early and middle childhood years: Familial subtype variations. *Alcoholism: Clinical and Experimental Research* 1998; **22**: 1962–72.

49 Wong M, Zucker R, Puttler L, Fitzgerald H. Heterogeneity of risk aggregation for alcohol problems between early and middle childhood: Nesting structure variations. *Development and Psychopathology* 1999; **11**: 727–44.

50 Goodman SH, Gotlib IH. Risk for psychopathology in the children of depressed mothers: a developmental model for understanding mechanisms of transmission. *Psychological Review* 1999; **106**: 458–90.

51 O'Connor TG, Heron J, Golding J, Beveridge M, Glover V. Maternal antenatal anxiety and children's behavioural/emotional problems at 4 years. Report from the Avon Longitudinal Study of Parents and Children. *British Journal of Psychiatry* 2002; **180**; 502–8.

52 O'Connor TG, Heron J, Glover V. Alspac Study Team. Antenatal anxiety predicts child behavioral/emotional problems independently of postnatal depression. *Journal of the American Academy of Child & Adolescent Psychiatry* 2002; **41**: 1470–77.

53 Sayal K, Heron J, Golding J, Emond A. Prenatal alcohol exposure and gender differences in childhood mental health problems: A longitudinal population-based study. *Pediatrics* 2007; **119**: e426–e34.

54 Robins LN, Helzer JE, Croughan J, Ratcliff KS. National Institute of Mental Health Diagnostic Interview Schedule. Its history, characteristics, and validity. *Archives of General Psychiatry* 1981; **38**: 381–99.

55 Gilman SE, Kawachi I, Fitzmaurice GM, Buka SL. Socioeconomic status in childhood and the lifetime risk of major depression. *International Journal of Epidemiology* 2002; **31**: 359–67.

56 Lewis G, Pelosi AJ, Araya R, Dunn G. Measuring psychiatric disorder in the community: a standardized assessment for use by lay interviewers. *Psychological Medicine* 1992; **22**: 465–86.

57 Power C, Atherton K, Strachan DP, Shepherd P, Fuller E, Davis A, et al. Life-course influences on health in British adults: Effects of socio-economic position in childhood and adulthood. *International Journal of Epidemiology* 2007; **36**: 532–39.

58 Rutter M, Tizard J, Whitmore K. *Education, Health and Behaviour*. Longmans, London, 1970.

59 Wing JK, Cooper JE, Sartorious N. *Present State Examination*. Cambridge University Press, London, 1974.

60 McLaren L, Kuh D, Hardy R, Mishra G. Postnatal depression and the original mother-child relationship: A prospective cohort study. *Journal of Affective Disorder* 2007; **100**: 211–19.

61 Weissman MM, Jensen P. What research suggests for depressed women with children. *Journal of Clinical Psychiatry* 2002; **63**: 641–47.

62 Kendler KS. Parenting: a genetic-epidemiologic perspective. *American Journal of Psychiatry* 1996; **153**; 11–20.

63 Pine D, Cohen P, Gurley D, Brook J, Ma Y. The risk for early-adulthood anxiety and depressive disorders in adolescents with anxiety and depressive disorders. *Archives of General Psychiatry* 1998; **55**: 56–64.

64 Johnson JG, Cohen, P, Kasen S, Brook JS. Maternal psychiatric disorders, parenting, and maternal behavior in the home during the child rearing years. *Journal of Child and Family Studies* 2006; **15**: 97–114.

65 Johnson JG, Cohen P, Kasen S, Smailes E, Brook JS. Association of maladaptive parental behaviour with psychiatric disorder among parents and their offspring. *Archives of General Psychiatry* 2001; **58**: 453–60.

66 Avison WR. The impact of mental illness on the family. In: Aneshensel C, Phelan J, editors. *Handbook of the Sociology of Mental Health*. Kluwer Academic/Plenum Publishers, New York, pp.495–518, 1999.

67 Kelly JB. Children's adjustment in conflicted marriage and divorce: A decade review of the research. *Journal of the American Academy of Child and Adolescent Psychiatry* 2000; **39**: 963–73.

68 Hill SY, Lowers L, Locke-Wellman J, Shen SA. Maternal smoking and drinking during pregnancy and the risk for child and adolescent psychiatric disorders. *Journal of Studies on Alcohol* 2000; **61**: 661–68.

69 Knop J, Penick EC, Jensen P, Nickel EJ, Gabrielli WF, Mednick SA, et al. Risk factors that predicted problem drinking in Danish men at age thirty. *Journal of Studies on Alcohol* 2003; **64**: 745–55.

70 Merikangas KR, Dierker LC, Szatmari P. Psychopathology among offspring of parents with substance abuse and/or anxiety disorders: a high-risk study. *Journal of Child Psychology and Psychiatry* 1998; **39**: 711–20.

71 Patton GC, Coffey C, Posterino M, Carlin JB, Wolfe R. Parental 'affectionless control' in adolescent depressive disorder. *Social Psychiatry and Psychiatric Epidemiology* 2001; **36**: 475–80.

72 Parker G, Tupling H, Brown LB. A parental bonding instrument. *British Journal of Medical Psychology* 1979; **52**: 1–10.

73. Miller L, Kramer R, Warner V, Wickramaratne P Weissman M. Intergenerational transmission of parental bonding among women. *Journal of the American Academy of Child & Adolescent Psychiatry* 1997; **36**: 1134–39.

74. Pilowsky DJ, Wickramaratne P, Nomura Y, Weissman MM. Family discord, parental depression, and psychopathology in offspring: 20-year follow-up. *Journal of the American Academy of Child & Adolescent Psychiatry* 2006; **45**: 452–60.

75. Brody GH. Sibling relationship quality: its causes and consequences. *Annual Review of Psychology* 1998; **49**: 1–24.

76. Bank L, Patterson GR, Reid JB. Negative interaction patterns as predictors of later adjustment problems in adolescent and young adult males. In: G Brody, editor. *Sibling Relationships: The Causes and Consequences*. Ablex, New Jersey. pp. 197–229, 1996.

77. Hetherington EM, Clingempeel WG. Coping with marital transitions: A family system perspective. *Monographs of the Society for Research in Child Development* 1992; **57**: 2–3.

78. Slomkowski C, Cohen P, Brook J. The sibling relationships of adolescents with antisocial and comorbid mental disorders: an epidemiological investigation. *Criminal Behaviour and Mental Health* 1997; **7**: 353–68.

79. Reiss D, Hetherington EM, Plomin R, Howe GW, Simmens SJ, Henderson SH, *et al*. Genetic questions for environmental studies. Differential parenting and psychopathology in adolescence. *Archives of General Psychiatry* 1995; **52**: 925–36.

80. Hetherington EM, Stanley-Hagan M. The adjustment of children with divorced parents: A risk and resiliency perspective. *Journal of Child Psychology and Psychiatry* 1999; **40**: 129–40.

81. Hetherington EM, Henderson SH, Reiss D, Anderson ER, Bridges M, Chan R, *et al*. Adolescent siblings in stepfamilies: Family functioning and adolescent adjustment. *Monographs of the Society for Research in Child Development* 1999; **64**:

82. MacKinnon CE. Sibling interactions in married and divorced families: Influence of ordinal position, socioeconomic status, and play context. *Journal of Divorce* 1989; **12**: 221–34.

83. Deater-Deckard K, Dunn J, Lussier G. Sibling relationships and social-emotional adjustment in different family contexts. *Social Development* 2002; **11**: 571–90.

84. Gass K, Jenkins J, Dunn J. Are sibling relationships protective? A longitudinal study. *Journal of Child Psychology and Psychiatry* 2007; **48**: 167–75.

85. Kim JE, Hetherington EM, Reiss D. Associations among family relationships, antisocial peers, and adolescents' externalizing behaviors: gender and family type differences. *Child Development* 1999; **70**: 1209–30.

86. Sullivan PF, Neale MC, Kendler KS. Genetic epidemiology of major depression: review and meta-analysis, *American Journal of Psychiatry* 2000; **157**: 1552–62.

87. Bierut LJ, Heath AC, Bucholz KK, Dinwiddie SH, Madden PA, Statham DJ, *et al*. Major depressive disorder in a community-based twin sample: are there different genetic and environmental contributions for men and women? *Archives of General Psychiatry* 1999; **56**: 557–63.

88. Kendler KS, Gardner CO, Neale MC, Prescott CA. Genetic risk factors for major depression in men and women: similar or different heritabilities and same or partly distinct genes? *Psychological Medicine* 2001; **31**: 605–16.

89. Moffitt TE, Caspi A, Rutter M. Strategy for investigating interactions between measured genes and measured environments. *Archives of General Psychiatry* 2005; **62**: 473–81.

90. Caspi A, Sugden K, Moffitt TE, Taylor A, Craig IW, Harrington H, *et al*. Influence of life stress on depression: moderation by a polymorphism in the 5-HTT gene. *Science* 2003; **301**: 386–89.

91. Zammit S, Owen MJ. Stressful life events, 5-HTT genotype and risk of depression, *British Journal of Psychiatry* 2006; **188**: 199–201.

92. Eley TC, Sugden K, Corsico A, Gregory AM, Sham P, McGuffin P, *et al*. Gene-environment interaction analysis of serotonin system markers with adolescent depression, *Molecular Psychiatry* 2004; **9**: 908–15.

93 **Grabe HJ, Lange M, Wolff B, Volzke H, Lucht M, Freyberger HJ, et al.** Mental and physical distress is modulated by a polymorphism in the 5-HT transporter gene interacting with social stressors and chronic disease burden. *Molecular Psychiatry* 2005; **10**: 220–24.

94 **Surtees PG, Wainwright NW, Willis-Owen SA, Luben R, Day NE, Flint J.** Social adversity, the serotonin transporter (5-HTTLPR) polymorphism and major depressive disorder. *Biological Psychiatry* 2006; **59**: 224–29.

95 **Gillespie NA, Whitfield JB, Williams B, Heath AC, Martin NG.** The relationship between stressful life events, the serotonin transporter (5-HTTLPR) genotype and major depression. *Psychological Medicine* 2005; **35**: 101–11.

Chapter 15

How family-based studies have added to understanding the life course epidemiology of reproductive health

Susan MB Morton and Janet Rich Edwards

Abstract

Reproductive events throughout a woman's life course tend to be both a product of the cumulative exposures a woman has been subject to before that event, as well as a marker for her likely future health. While genetic contributions influence fertility, development, growth and reproduction of the next generation, all of these critical events in life are subject to external, environmental influences. This is true for individual women and within families of individuals. Perhaps given the shared genes and environments within and across generations in a family it is therefore not surprising that family studies consistently demonstrate a higher degree of consistency in reproductive outcomes at all points in the life course for those who share a family connection, than for individuals who do not, and that the closer that connection (e.g. monozygotic twins) in general the greater the similarities.

15.1 Introduction

The old sayings of 'like mother, like daughter' and 'like father, like son' have been quoted for generations, but until recently for intergenerational patterns of reproductive behaviours and reproductive outcomes these have been largely a subjective impression. In the last few decades, family studies focussed on key events during a woman's reproductive career have generally lent weight to this familiar saying for females, but this has not been the case for males. This chapter will explore the way in which such family-based studies have contributed to our understanding of the life course epidemiology of reproductive health.

Whilst reproductive health is clearly of importance to males and females, both as potential parents and as offspring, the vast majority of the research in this area is focused on females, and therefore much of this chapter will also relate to females' reproductive health. For females the beginning of their reproductive potential is signalled by menarche, whereas in males the marker for achieving sexual maturity is less clearly indicated. Similarly in females the end-point is marked by menopause, whereas for males it is poorly defined, if indeed it ever occurs. This chapter will take a life-course approach to the availability and usefulness of family studies to inform our understanding of the various stages throughout a woman's reproductive life course beginning with the sentinel event of menarche and progressing through till age at menopause. It will consider the availability and usefulness of studies relating to both fertility and infertility, although perhaps unsurprisingly family studies have less to contribute to the latter. Where information is available for males it will be discussed, but the contribution from family studies that informs our understanding of male reproductive outcomes across the life course tends to be sparse.

Furthermore, the extent to which family studies considering reproductive events have added to our understanding of health at other points in the life course will be considered briefly. The chapter will conclude with a brief analysis of the overall usefulness of these studies for understanding reproductive health across the life course, and identify issues that require further attention.

15.2 Age at menarche

There is a great deal of evidence available to support the contention that there has been a gradual decline in the age at menarche across developed populations in the last century at least. The most favoured mechanism for this quite rapid downward trend is that is largely environmental and it has been the result of improved social conditions and nutrition in early and middle childhood in particular.[1] Alongside this secular population trend it is also the case that intergenerational studies consistently report a positive association in the age at menarche between mothers and daughters. One recent study of 4,500 mothers and their daughters in Finland suggested that whilst the age of menarche in the daughters was slightly lower on average than for the mothers generation (a median of 13 years versus 14 years as the secular trend would predict), there was nevertheless a positive correlation between age at menarche across generations (exemplified by a Spearman coefficient of just over 0.2).[2] This degree of correlation is consistent with that found in most familial studies of mothers' and daughters' age at menarche. It is generally argued that this correlation is largely indicative of the level of heritability of age at menarche within families. Reports from the Fels longitudinal study, which collected prospective data over many decades on multiple pairings of female relatives (e.g. mother-daughter, full and half female siblings, aunt and niece, grandmother and granddaughter and so on spanning 1st degree to 9th degree female relatives), estimated that approximately half the phenotypic variation amongst girls from developed nations in the timing of menarche was due to genetic factors.[3]

Despite the consistency seen across studies there are problems that commonly occur when familial studies are utilised to consider continuities in reproductive outcomes across and within generations. These are illustrated for the sentinel event of menarche but extend to nearly all facets of reproductive lives and histories within families. Importantly, some of the potential sources of bias arise because of the way in which the data is collected. If the timing of an event is recalled retrospectively some years after the key event, rather than recorded prospectively (in 'real time') it may be inaccurate and result in biased estimates of the extent of familial clustering and of the relative contributions of genetic and shared environmental characteristics to this clustering. Validation studies have suggested that correlation of the recalled timing with the real time measure can be as low as 0.60 in the case age of menarche (with the increasing length of time between the actual event and the time of recall contributing to the lowered correlation).[3] If this measurement error were non-differential (i.e. in intergenerational studies it did not relate to the same (real time assessed) measure in the other generation) the expectation would be for true intergenerational associations to be underestimated, though in reality the bias could be in either direction. More importantly, it is plausible that the measurement error will be related to measures in the other generation (i.e. there will be recall bias). This might happen, for example, if discussion between a mother and daughter about age at menarche might cause either of them to unwittingly 'remember' age at menarche closer to that of her kin. This sort of bias might be equally applicable to recall of other reproductive events, such as gestation lengths, birth weights or lactation duration.

In addition to measurement error, there have been major secular changes in the environmental determinants of age at menarche and other reproductive characteristics (for example, family size and age at which pregnancies occur, among others). Since heritability, defined in Chapters 2, 3, 4, 10 and 11, is a measure of the relative contribution of genetic variation to variation in a phenotype such as age at menarche, any change in environmental (non-genetic) determinants of a phenotype in a population will inevitably affect the heritability estimate. Even with prospectively collected data timing of the 'natural' occurrence of reproductive characteristics could have measurement error that varies by generation due to exogenous variation in reproductive behaviours.

15.3 Age at first pregnancy (including early motherhood)

Whilst there is usually a considerable lag time in developed populations between age at menarche and age at first pregnancy, this tends to be the next reproductive event which receives most attention from a life course perspective. Much has been written about continuity or otherwise in maternal age at first pregnancy across generations, since this measure tends to signify the beginning of fertility or 'success' in reproductive terms. Like age at menarche most studies have demonstrated a significant positive correlation in age at first pregnancy between females across generations.[4] In particular if a mother had her first pregnancy as a teenager then studies have repeatedly shown that there is an increased chance that her own daughters will also reproduce early, although the relationship is by no means universal.[5] Certainly in developed countries today, whilst daughters of teenage mothers are two to three times more likely to become teenage mothers than their peers whose mothers were older than 20 at the time of their first pregnancy, the majority of daughters of teenage mothers in these countries do not reproduce early.[6] Estimates of this continuity in teenage pregnancy across generations have traditionally been obtained from studies that have considered this association only between pairs of mothers and their first-born daughters. However more recently a study considered the continuity in the timing of parenthood for mothers and sons in a 30 year study in the United States.[4] The authors reported that whilst overall it was less likely that sons (first born or otherwise) would become teenage fathers than their female siblings, there were nevertheless continuities in age at first parenthood between mothers and their sons.

Often the familial continuities in age at first parenthood across generations are considered in a largely biomedical context with a less adequate assessment of the social context in which these behaviours are occurring. This is in part due to the methods used to obtain the data for these analyses which are often retrieved from health records which tend to contain less contextual social and behavioural data. Nevertheless this tendency to repeat reproductive behaviours across generations has occurred during a time of significant changes in the social patterning of marriage and age at marriage, with a concomitant profound uncoupling of marriage and parenthood in particular, in addition to increasingly accessible methods of controlling fertility in both developed and developing nations.

The ongoing concern over the degree of continuity in early parenthood tends to reflect the social adversity that often accompanies teenage pregnancy, and there are some indications that this adversity has increased in more recent generations. For example in a recent study from Baltimore, which was predominantly made up of Black American women, daughters of teenage mothers who also had a teenage pregnancy a generation later tended to be more socially vulnerable and have less resources available to them to escape from economic dependency and poverty than was the case for their mothers generation, especially in terms of education and income.[6] This increasing adversity associated with early motherhood is no doubt also influenced by access to appropriate reproductive health services.[7] Whilst in developed countries there tends to be greater access to such services than in previous generations, it is likely that access remains more limited for the most socially disadvantaged.

15.4 Total family size across generations (fertility rate)

Most family studies have considered patterns in maternal age at pregnancy, but have only compared age at first birth across generations. There is much more limited data to support intergenerational continuity in the area of age of second and later pregnancies across and within generations, although there is some evidence to support the notion that total family size may show some continuity across generations.[8, 2]

A consideration of continuities in the timing of familial pregnancies other than the first raises the issue of pregnancy spacing, which is subject to many social as well as biological pressures which will vary between individuals and within and across families.[9] Furthermore, consideration of intergenerational continuity in family size requires the ascertainment of the total reproductive histories for at least two generations. It is the lack of availability of this complete family reproductive history that tends to limit the analyses that are possible in this area. One study that has been able to accumulate sufficient information across two generations of mothers and daughters is the intergenerational cohort built on the *Aberdeen Children of the 1950s* (ACONF) Study.[10] As described in Chapters 2 and 10, the index participants in that study were women born in Aberdeen in the 1950s and are defined at generation 1 (G1); their mothers are defined as G0 and their offspring as G2. The overall total mean number of live-births per woman was greater in the older (G0) compared to more contemporary (G1) generation with mean family size of 3.7 versus 2.8 children. This is despite the fact that the G1 mothers were between the ages of 44 and 50 when the linkages were made, so had largely completed their families, while the G0 mothers were younger when the cohort was established so may have continued to grow their families after the original study was completed. Although this is a probable underestimate of the absolute family size difference across generations in the ACONF study, the smaller total family size in the more recent generation is likely to reflect social trends in childbearing that have lead to family downsizing and a reduction in total pregnancy number throughout the developed world, including but not limited to changes in contraceptive and pregnancy termination availability and access. This trend was also seen in a recent analysis of intergenerational patterns of reproduction for mothers and their daughters in Finland.[2]

Despite this difference in total family size across generations there was nevertheless a positive correlation between the total completed family size for the two generations. In the ACONF study the chances of a daughter (G1) having only one or two live-born children were almost doubled if her own mother (G0) had only one or two children as opposed to three or more.[8] Similarly, from the Finnish study the total parity of daughters was associated with the parity of their mothers at the time of their own birth.[2] So while there is some evidence to suggest that total family size is repeated across generations, information about this area is sparse due to the data required to address the association fully in more than one generation.

15.5 Continuities in pregnancy specific maternal conditions

The continuity noted in family size across generations probably reflects a complex mix of shared biological, social and behavioural factors within families, illustrated by factors like levels of achieved maternal education. Interestingly the Finnish study[2] reported a consistent inverse association between educational level and total parity in both the mothers and daughters generation, with higher maternal educational levels associated with the lowest overall fertility rates, including the greatest proportion of nulliparity. While social conditions have influenced marriage and reproductive behaviours, the effects of education on reproductive behaviours have remained very consistent over time despite the wider social changes female education has engendered in society as a whole over the same period. Other possible factors relevant to the continuities seen in relative total family size in particular may relate to similar pregnancy experiences, especially if maternal disease complicates pregnancies in both generations.

15.5.1 Continuity in maternal gestational hypertension

The most commonly recognised maternal complication arising in the course of pregnancy is gestational hypertension, with up to 10% of all pregnancies being affected by this condition across populations in Northern Europe.[11] The ACONF Study[10] examines intergenerational continuities in clinically defined hypertensive disorders of pregnancy. In this cohort of several thousand mothers and daughters, the daughters' (G1) risk of having a hypertensive pregnancy directly related to the extent of hypertension complicating her mothers' (G0) pregnancy during her own intrauterine development. Chapter 10 provides a detailed discussion of the appropriate statistical methods for assessing intergenerational continuities and uses the intergenerational continuity of hypertensive disorders of pregnancy in participants in the ACONF Study as an illustration. The risk of a daughter having any hypertension (pre-eclampsia or 'other hypertension') in her own pregnancy was increased 1.5 fold if her mother had pre-eclampsia and by the same amount if her mother had 'other hypertension' during the daughters own intrauterine development. Her risk of specifically developing pre-eclampsia increased 1.8 fold if her own mother's pregnancy was also complicated by pre-eclampsia and 1.6 fold if her mother's pregnancy was complicated only by 'other hypertension.'[8] The similarity in intergenerational risk of either pre-eclampsia or hypertension in pregnancy, suggests there may be a common mechanism linking these two disease processes rather than the pathogenesis of each condition being distinct. The mechanism underlying transmission may well be genetic,[12] or it may reflect a shared environment across two generations, or more probably some combination of the two.

As well as intergenerational continuities of hypertensive disorders of pregnancy, studies have found associations within sisters. Intragenerational familial clustering of hypertensive disorders in pregnancy has been recognized for several decades,[13, 14] with siblings of women who have had pregnancies affected by hypertension being at increased risk of also developing gestational hypertension. Also, a paper published in 1997 using information from the 1958 British Birth cohort provided evidence that a woman's own reduced intrauterine growth was associated with an increased risk of developing hypertension in her own adult pregnancies.[15] A publication by Klebanoff et al used record linkage for a Danish birth cohort born between 1959 and 1961 and confirmed the increased risk of pregnancy hypertension in women born small for gestational age at birth, which is known to be a consequence of maternal high blood pressure in pregnancy.[16]

15.5.2 Continuity in maternal gestational diabetes

Gestational diabetes mellitus (GDM) affects approximately 7%[17] of pregnancies in the developed world, following gestational hypertension as the second most common pregnancy complication. In parallel with the increasing incidence of type 2 diabetes mellitus among young women,[18] the prevalence of GDM may also be on the rise.[19] However, inconsistently applied and shifting standards for the diagnosis of GDM as well as increased access to prenatal screening complicate the evaluation of trends in gestational diabetes prevalence.[20]

Gestational diabetes is not only an important cause of complications for the neonates, but it is also a powerful predictor of future chronic disease risk in both mother and child. Women with gestational diabetes are at elevated risk of later type 2 diabetes[21–23] and offspring of diabetic pregnancies are at heightened risk of developing obesity, glucose intolerance, type 2 diabetes and metabolic syndrome throughout their lives.[24–31] Some,[24, 28] but not all[31] family studies looking at this association have found that the increased metabolic risk only occurs amongst macrosomic offspring of diabetic pregnancies, suggesting that maternal glycemic control in pregnancy may be driving future risks amongst offspring.

Several family studies have also shown that the metabolic syndrome symptoms are more prevalent in children of diabetic mothers than children of diabetic fathers,[25, 30] lending support to the proposition that the intrauterine environment contributes significantly to an offspring's life course metabolic risk profile. A classic series of family studies in the Pima Indians of Arizona, which are also described in Chapter 13, has enabled researchers to tease apart the role of the intrauterine diabetic environment from that of purely genetic predisposition.[25, 26] The comparison of siblings born before and after their mother was diagnosed with diabetes provides unusual insights into the importance of the intrauterine environment for risk of later chronic disease. For example, children born after the mother developed diabetes had nearly four times the risk of type 2 diabetes compared with their older siblings born before the diabetes diagnosis.[25] Systolic blood pressure and mean BMI were also higher in offspring of diabetic pregnancies than in siblings born of pre-diabetic pregnancies.[25, 27] These family studies have been important in establishing the particular risk of a diabetic *in utero* environment above and beyond the risk attributable exclusively to genetic factors.

Unfortunately, there are no published data to gauge the intrafamilial aggregation of GDM. However, women whose mother or father had a history of type 2 diabetes are twice as likely to develop GDM as women without a parental history.[32] Women with a diabetic sibling are also known to be eight times more likely to develop gestational diabetes than those without.[32] Given these strong associations, it would be surprising if GDM in a mother or sister was not a strong risk factor for GDM in an index pregnancy. However, this has not yet been established in family studies.

Whilst maternal pregnancy-specific gestational hypertension and gestational diabetes do appear to contribute to the continuity in familial reproductive outcomes, because of the way they are defined by an artificial dichotomisation of continuous parameters they are only clinically recognised in a minority of pregnancies in each generation. By contrast intergenerational continuities seen in reproductive outcomes, whether they be age at delivery, total family size or indeed other reproductive outcomes, tend to exist for the majority of women. Whilst it is possible that intergenerational continuities in absolute blood pressure and glycemic control *per se* may contribute further to the continuities in reproductive outcomes seen across the population, these measures are not readily available in intergenerational studies to assess this in more detail.

15.6 Continuity in pregnancy outcomes

By far the greatest available body of literature from family studies relating to reproductive outcomes is in regard to continuity across and within generations in measures of size at birth and early life growth. In particular there are now many studies that have demonstrated that a mother's own intrauterine development and her early life growth and environment appear to directly influence her own capacity to reproduce in adult life. Evidence in support of this originated over 70 years ago in a study by Kermack *et al.* in the United Kingdom[33] at a time when there was increasing concern over high infant mortality rates. By looking at death rates in adulthood alongside infant mortality statistics around the time of the adults' birth they determined that the health of the adult population was largely determined by their health status as children, leading to speculation that infant mortality might only be expected to fall when maternal health improved.

After this relatively novel investigation, many studies followed, notably first by Baird and his colleagues in Scotland.[34–39] They considered the perinatal outcomes of infants born in Aberdeen, largely between 1948 and 1972 in relation to the childhood environments of their mothers.[34–39] Baird illustrates their collective findings in his 1949 paper where he states that:

> Efficient child-bearing is influenced by many factors, but none so much as the mother herself. The mother is the product of heredity and environment, and therefore as far as possible the whole woman should be studied ... to discover what psychological, social and physical influences affect reproductive performance.[34]

After these early studies which were concerned with the generic health status of mothers in relation to their children's heath in infancy, associations began to emerge linking more specific reproductive outcomes across generations. In 1968 Ounsted and Ounsted compared the birth weight distributions for selected groups of mothers of infants who were either small for dates, appropriate or large for dates.[40] They described the positive association between the birth weight distributions of the mothers according to the birth weight groups of their infants. There are a growing number of major intergenerational studies considering continuities in these measures of size at birth across generations which are summarized in Table 15.1. Whilst the over-arching objective of all these studies has been to understand the nature of the intergenerational association in measures of size and maturity at birth across generations, there has been considerable variation in the type of family data available and the method of analysis over time. In particular most of the studies used record linkage to collect the required data across generations, but the generation that has been used as the reference generation (that is data collected firstly about the mothers or offspring) has varied and the completeness of the reproductive histories depending on the index generation has also been highly variable. Furthermore, in some studies the intergenerational associations have been considered across the full range of birth weight, and occasionally gestation, but in others the focus has only been on at risk groups such as low birth weight or pre-term infants (see Table 15.1).

Nevertheless these diverse intergenerational studies from many populations have repeatedly demonstrated reasonably stable associations between maternal size at birth and numerous infant outcomes, including low birth weight, preterm delivery, relative intrauterine growth retardation as well as early outcome measures such as perinatal mortality, infant mortality and respiratory distress syndrome.[41–45] Less often positive associations between paternal birth weight and offspring size at birth have also been described.[46–48] However in studies where both maternal and paternal measures were available for each individual infant the paternal measures had a much weaker influence on infant size at birth than the maternal measures.[49]

15.6.1 Intergenerational continuities in birth weight

Overall studies that have been carried out in developed countries have found the intergenerational association between maternal and infant size at birth to be positive with an average increase of between 10 and 20g of infant birth weight for every 100g increase in maternal birth weight (see Table 15.1). One recent study considered intergenerational effects on birth weight and birth length in Guatemala, a developing country, for 215 intergenerational mother-infant pairs and found that infant birth weight increased by 29g on average for every 100g increase in maternal birth weight.[50] Additionally there was a positive significant effect of maternal birth weight on infant birth length (0.2 cm per 100g of maternal weight) in this population. This suggests that the intergenerational relationship in the early life growth measures may be stronger in less-developed countries where maternal growth to adulthood may be restricted by poor environmental conditions throughout infancy and childhood. Thus, the correlation between

Table 15.1 Summary of relevant intergenerational associations in maternal and offspring size at birth (restricted to singletons)

Reference (Year) (Ref. Number)	Study population*				Information source					Intergenerational associations – Estimate of offspring effect per same maternal unit measure**		
	Source	N (pairs)	Mothers year of birth	Infants year of birth	Mothers		Infants			Birth weight (grams)	Gestational age (weeks)	Fetal growth measure
					Birth weight	Gestation at delivery	Birth weight	Gestation at delivery				
Correlation Analysis												
Hackman et al (1983) (41)	US	748	After 1948	1977–79*	Birth certificates	—	Obstetric records	Obstetric records		0.11 (adjusted)	—	—
Carr-Hill et al (1987) (47)	Scotland	505	1950–56*	1968–1981 (First born females)	Obstetric records	Obstetric records	Obstetric records	Obstetric records		0.14–0.18 (adjusted)	—	—
Ounsted et al (1988) (89)	UK	986	Not stated	1964–75*	Recall	—	Birth records	—		0.10–0.30 (crude)	—	—
Magnus et al (1993) (44)	Norway	11092	1967–69*	1986–89	Birth records	Birth records	Birth records	Birth records		0.24 (crude)	0.09 (crude)	Not reported
Multivariate Regression												
Langhoff-Roos et al (1987) (90)	Sweden	276	Not fixed	Term, normal bwt*	Recall	—	Obstetric records	Obstetric records		0.19 (adjusted)	—	—
Little (1987) (49)	U.S.	377	Not stated.	Not stated, 12 month period*	Recall	—	Obstetric records	—		0.11–0.17 (adjusted)	—	—
Emanuel et al (1992) (91)	U.K.	880	3–9 March 1958*	Before 1982-most recent birth	Obstetric records	Obstetric records	Recall	—		0.12–0.19 (crude)	—	—
Alberman et al (1992) (48)	U.K.	1151	3–9 March 1958*	Before 1982-most recent birth	Obstetric records	Obstetric records	Recall	—		0.18 (adjusted)	—	—

Study	Country	N									
Coutinho et al (1997) (92)	U.S.	>100,000	1956–1975 Illinois born	1989–91 All Illinois infants*	Birth certs	—	—	Birth certs	—	0.24 – 0.27 (crude)	—	—
Hennessy et al (1998) (52)	U.K.	2356–2578	3–9 March 1958*	Term infants before 1991 (mothers <33 years)	Obstetric records	Obstet records	—	Recall	Recall	0.27 (adjusted)	Not reported	0.26 (adjusted)
Hennessy et al (1998) (53)	U.K.	3229	3–9 March 1958*	Term infants before 1991 (mothers <33 years)	Obstetric records	Obstet records	—	Recall	Recall	Not reported	0.07 (adjusted)	0.01/per SD (adjusted)
Ramakrishnan et al (1999) (50)	Guatemala	215	1969–77	1991–96* term births	Records	Recall	Recall	Clinical Estimate	—	0.20–0.32 (adjusted)	—	—
Risk ratios												
Klebanoff et al (1984) (42)	U.S.	1348	1930–45	1959–66*	Recall	—	—	Records - prospective	Records - prospective	3.5 LBW (adjusted)	—	—
Klebanoff et al (1984) (93)	U.S.	1335	1930–45	1959–66*	Recall	—	—	Records - prospective	Records - prospective	1.2 LBW (adjusted)	—	—
Klebanoff et al (1987) (43)	U.S.	43,891	1959–66 in State	1979–84*	Birth certificate	—	—	Birth certificates	—	3.0 LBW (crude)	—	—
Klebanoff et al (1989) (54)	Sweden	1154	1955–65	1972–83*	Birth registry	Birth registry	Birth registry	Birth registry	—	Not reported	0.7 Preterm (adjusted) NS	2.0 SGA (adjusted)
Magnus et al (1993) (44)	Norway	11092	1967–69*	1986–89	Birth records	Birth records	Birth records	Birth records	Birth records	3.0 LBW (cf weight over 4000g)	1.46 Preterm NS	Not reported
Sanderson et al (1995) (94)	U.S.	8248	Not stated	1988*	Birth Certificate Recall	Birth Certificate Recall	—	Birth Certificate Recall	Birth Certificate Recall	2.5–2.8 LBW (adjusted)	—	—

Continued

Table 15.1 (continued) Summary of relevant intergenerational associations in maternal and offspring size at birth (restricted to singletons)

Reference (Year) (Ref. Number)	Study population* Source	N (pairs)	Mothers year of birth	Infants year of birth	Information source Mothers Birth weight	Gestation at delivery	Infants Birth weight	Gestation at delivery	Intergenerational associations – Estimate of offspring effect per same maternal unit measure** Birth weight (grams)	Gestational age (weeks)	Fetal growth measure
Klebanoff et al (1997) (55)	Denmark	2103	1959–61*	Up to 1989	Birth registry	Birth registry	Birth registry	Birth registry	Not reported	1.5 Preterm (adjusted)	2.0 SGA (adjusted)
Winkvist et al (1998) (56)	Sweden	4746	1955–72*	1973–90	Birth registry	Birth registry	Birth registry	Birth registry	Not reported	1.1 Preterm (adjusted) NS	1.5 SGA (adjusted) NS
Emanuel et al (1999) (57)	U.S.	38 513	In state after 1949	1987–95*	Birth certificate	—	Obstetric records	Obstetric records	2.3 LBW (adjusted)	—	—
Collins et al (2002) (95)	U.S.	>100,000	1956–1975 Illinois born	1989–91 All Illinois infants*	Birth certificate	—	Birth certificates	—	Compares RRs in different ethnic groups		
ANOVA											
Ounsted et al (1973) (96)	U.K.	315	Not stated	1958*	Recall	—	Records	—	700grams (adjusted)	—	—
Lumey (1992) (97)	Netherlands	575	1944–46*	1960–85	Obstetric records	—	Obstetric records	—	—	—	—

Notes:
*Denotes the origin generation for the study, that is which generation data was collected first.
** Summary results are presented according to the analysis type. They refer to the association between the same measures of maternal and offspring size at birth only. If the results are not for the entire range of size at birth then the groups being compared are provided (e.g. LBW or SGA in both generations). Estimates of are for the effect on offspring size according to 1 unit of maternal measure (e.g. 1 gram or 1 week or 1SD of fetal growth).
NS = not significant at p <0.05 level, otherwise all results significant.
Adjusted = refers to adjustment for contemporary maternal characteristics, notably age parity, height and weight for studies where applicable.
Not reported = Data may have been available to calculate but results not reported by authors whereas '–' refers to data unavailable.

maternal and infant birth weight may be stronger where the environment is consistent across generations, compared with regions that have undergone rapid developmental transition over the last century. It will be of interest to observe whether or not maternal-infant birth weight correlations are weakened as developing nations undergo nutritional transitions in the near future and over what time period.[95]

15.6.2 Intergenerational continuities in length of gestation

As birth weight is a product of gestation length and fetal growth rate, it would be interesting to determine specifically the extent to which gestation length and fetal growth rate are passed between generations. However, until relatively recently when ultrasound assessment became the norm in pregnancy, gestation length tended to be recorded poorly, if at all. Additionally a further complication in considering gestational length is that delivery is not always spontaneous, but may be shortened iatrogenically, either because of medical concerns about the welfare of an infant or increasingly for non-medical or social reasons. This increase in delivery prior to term gestation is more prevalent in the later-born (usually offspring generation) infants who were generally delivered at a time of greater provision of neonatal care facilities in all countries where studies were conducted.[51] This questionable gestation length data provides challenges for assessing intergenerational correlations in gestation length *per se* and fetal growth rate, which is usually measured as birth weight adjusted for gestation length. Studies in which gestational age information has been available for the second generation, but not the first, have concluded that maternal low birth weight is associated with an increased risk of both preterm delivery (that is shortened gestation) and reduced fetal growth of her infants in addition to a reduction in absolute birth weight. However these studies were not able to determine whether the intergenerational continuity seen in size at birth acted through similarities in intrauterine growth rates or control of length of gestation, or perhaps both.

The studies that have considered intergenerational associations in gestation length in the United Kingdom have largely relied on recall to obtain one of the generation's gestational age.[52, 53] Recall data was used for intergenerational information collected by interview from the original members of the 1958 British Perinatal Survey (98% of all births in England, Wales and Scotland during the week of 3–9 March 1958) who had become parents themselves by the mid-1990s. Gestational age was obtained from obstetric records for the index participants (i.e. those born in 1958), whereas the gestational age of their offspring was retrospectively reported at interview. Furthermore, whilst the index participants (first generation) were a random sample of all births at a particular point in time (irrespective of parity of the mother or gestational age), the second generation infants were limited to first-born, term deliveries.[53] Whilst results need to be interpreted along side these generational differences, the authors found a small, but statistically significant relationship between parental gestational age and non-preterm gestational age of infants of 0.067 week per 1 week increase in maternal gestational age and 0.045 week per 1 week increase in paternal gestational age (unfortunately maternal and paternal data were not available together for the same infants). Prior to this study there had been inconsistent results in the intergenerational association in gestational age at delivery (Table 15.1).

15.6.3 Intergenerational continuity in fetal growth

Other studies have attempted to examine whether fetal growth—birth weight adjusted for gestational age—is correlated across generations. In the studies by Klebanoff *et al.* in Sweden and Denmark,[54, 55] Magnus *et al.* in Norway[46] and Winkvist *et al.* also in Sweden[56] internal record linkage was used to provide birth weight and gestational age data for a large number of mother-infant pairs. These studies confirmed that mothers born small for gestational age themselves were up to three times as likely to deliver small for gestational age infants as appropriate or large for gestational age mothers were.[46, 54–56]

The generally weak/modest intergenerational continuities of gestational age (see Section 15.6.2) taken together with the stronger associations of fetal growth have led some authors to conclude that the mechanisms by which infant birth weight was related to maternal birth weight was through correlated fetal growth rate rather than correlated gestation length. However, gestational age is subject to much greater imprecision and measurement error than absolute birth weight which tends to weaken the chance of finding a significant relationship overall.[57]

15.6.4 Summary of studies findings on intergenerational continuity in size at birth

In general there is a great deal of evidence from family studies to support the notion that fetal growth is positively correlated across generations, and that fetal growth is more closely related to maternal than paternal birth weight. However most of the studies which contribute to this now vast body of evidence rely on record linkage at two distinct time periods to gather the data from which these analyses are generated. They tend to take an approach that is temporally flat by only comparing two distinct pregnancies rather than a life course approach which would be more concerned with the life time growth and development of the mother (or father) in relation to their offspring's early life growth and development, and also, where feasible, would consider her entire reproductive history. There are at least two notable exceptions to the temporally flat approach that is standard in intergenerational data gathering: The first is the ACONF study,[8] and the second is the more recent analysis from the 1958 British national birth cohort.[58] Both these datasets contain information on three generations and both conclude that it is not only maternal growth *in utero* that is linked to the growth of her offspring, but also her early childhood growth which contributes additionally to that intrauterine influence. These studies in particular have reinforced the importance of a mother's early life growth for her future reproductive success in adulthood. This information is essential to inform policies directed toward improving pregnancy outcomes in any one generation because they strongly suggest that population-based interventions that wait until pregnancy to intervene will likely be too little, too late (if 'success' is measured by offspring size at least).

15.7 Intragenerational (within family) continuity in reproductive outcomes

Few family studies have looked at serial data for births to the same mother, which is important to analyse reproductive outcomes across the entire life course. Again this tends to be due to the investment in time and resources required to reliably collect this type of data. While these are difficult to find, record linkage studies and 'pregnancy' as opposed to 'birth' cohorts that enrol participants over several years can provide this type of data, and they may be found among Scandinavian record linkage studies and some cohorts such as ACONF. A mother's own intrauterine development, her childhood growth and attained adult height remain fixed throughout all her pregnancies as do her childhood education and early life socioeconomic conditions, all of which are strong determinants of her health and socioeconomic position in adulthood.[59] Therefore when examining differences in consecutive birth outcomes for the same mother any differences in birth outcomes should be largely independent of these variables (see Chapter 3 for further discussion of the use of sibling studies for controlling for the potential confounding by unmeasured fixed maternal/familial characteristics). Studies that have managed to accumulate this type of data, such as the study of nearly 7,000 married women in Aberdeen by Billewicz in the early 1970s, which considered the determinants of birth weights in consecutive pregnancies concluded that individual women had a significant tendency to have pregnancies of similar gestation length and offspring of similar size.[60] He estimated the full-sibling coefficient of correlation between consecutive birth weights to be greater than 0.5, which he suggested could not be explained on the grounds of maternal size alone. This figure was in line with estimates from earlier studies by Karn et al.[61] and Morton[62] in the 1950s who calculated correlation coefficients for siblings' birth weights of 0.4 and 0.5 respectively. They also found the now commonly accepted relationship that birth weights in consecutive pregnancies to the same mother tend to increase (that is with increasing parity). In 1995 the OPCS Longitudinal Study produced a representative sample of over 10,000 women from England and Wales,[63] and a record linkage study of over 330,000 Scottish women[64] confirmed the tendency for mothers to repeat birth weight and gestational age in consecutive pregnancies. Additionally, the data from the Scottish record linkage demonstrated that if there was growth retardation of a fetus, or if an infant was born prematurely to a mother in one pregnancy, the risk of the same outcome occurring in the mother's subsequent delivery was increased 5–6 fold. These findings were reproduced in a Swedish study[56] of familial patterns in birth characteristics where the risk of small for gestational age (SGA) delivery increased progressively with the number of previous SGA deliveries. The authors also described some wider familial patterns which extended to similarities in birth outcomes for siblings, in that if one sister had previously delivered a pre-term infant (that is with a gestational duration of less than 37 weeks) her sisters chance of a preterm delivery was increased by 80%. A more recent study using data from the Swedish Medical Birth Registry demonstrated a similar relationship between mothers, daughters and siblings for risk of prolonged pregnancy (defined as a gestational length of 42 completed weeks or more), although the current likelihood that delivery will be induced in prolonged pregnancy makes this more difficult to assess rigorously over time.[65]

The tendency for women to repeat similar birth weight and gestational age within a generation may reinforce the importance of her own early life development, in addition to concurrent pregnancy specific factors, for her reproductive success.[66]

15.8 The contribution of genetics to continuity in reproductive outcomes

The familial continuities in reproductive outcomes within and across generations, especially in terms of measures of size at birth, have been interpreted by some authors as an example of the genetic inheritance of birth weight (see Chapter 2 for a detailed discussion of how to correctly interpret such studies).[44] In 1954 Penrose first used sibling studies of birth weight to apportion 38% of the variation between siblings to genetic differences between them.[67] By contrast, using a number of inter- and intragenerational associations Newton Morton in 1955 concluded that familial clustering of birth weight was largely explained by shared environmental factors[62] (See Chapter 2 for a full discussion of this study and presentation of its results). Ounsted also concluded that the clustering of birth weight in siblings was largely determined by non-genetic factors.[40] A later Aberdeen study, specifically considering whether birth weight was genetically determined, compared the birth weight of 505 intergenerational pairs of young mothers and their first born infant, and also concluded that genetic factors play only a minor role in determining birth weight, contributing less than 20% to the outcome.[47] More recently, a very large study using data from the Norwegian Birth Registry suggested that fetal genetic factors explained almost one-third of the variation in offspring size at birth as compared to around 20% of the variation being explained by maternal genes,[68] and a study considering the offspring of twins also confirmed that heritability of fetal growth ranges somewhere from 25% to 40%.[69] As noted in Chapter 2, estimates of the heritability of birth weight (i.e. the proportion of total variability due to genetic variability) over the last six decades have varied between 0-70%.[70] However, trying to disentangle what is distinctly genetic from what is purely environmental, and what relates to fetal as opposed to maternal genetic influence, may be creating a false dichotomy in what is really a complex, interdependent relationship.[59, 70] The common theme from the family data seems to be that it is difficult to attribute all of the correlation between intergenerational birth size to a common genome when environmental conditions that may affect biological measures are also shared within and across generations. Whilst there have been continuing attempts to disentangle the causal relationships between parent characteristics and child outcomes into genetic or environmental components using children of twins designs,[72] in reality the partitioning is unlikely to be distinct, and epigenetic mechanisms also now need to be considered as affording additional explanatory value as well as added complexity in this area.[73]

15.9 Familial studies and reduced fertility

To date the emphasis in this chapter has been to consider the impact of knowledge gained from family-based studies on age at menarche and pregnancy related outcomes. It is also of interest to consider what family studies are able to tell us regarding sub-fertility or indeed infertility. There is considerably less evidence from family studies able to assist our understanding in this area as much of the examination of reproductive health within and across families requires at least one successful reproductive outcome (usually in the form of recorded birth), particularly when the majority of studies are based on record linkage rather than a prospective collection of data from within families over several decades irrespective of reproductive events.

However, one condition that has been investigated to some degree in family studies is Polycystic Ovarian Syndrome (PCOS). This syndrome is a heterogeneous disorder estimated to affect between 5 and 10% of women of reproductive age. It is characterised by a lack of ovulation and excessive levels of androgens, and women with this disorder tend to be at increased risk of developing relatively early glucose intolerance, gestational diabetes and later overt diabetes.[74] Family studies, including twin studies, have demonstrated that PCOS tends to occur in clusters within families which has lead several authors to suggest that there must be a substantive genetic component to the syndrome.[75] However a recent study, including a small number of families, failed to find any consistent genetic markers for the manifestations of the syndrome between different affected families,[74, 76] suggesting that it may be inherited as a complex genetic trait. Given that PCOS is both inherited and associated with reduced ovulation and less predictable menstrual cycling it has often been regarded as a contributor to infertility, whether relative or absolute. However a 2006 study of family size in women with PCOS did not find any difference in the number of siblings that they had compared to normal controls.[77] It is potentially becoming increasingly difficult to evaluate the importance of these conditions for continuities in familial sub-fertility as the recent improvements in treating infertility together with increasing access to fertility services inevitably mean that familial correlations in infertility and its causes may be increasingly perturbed. Similarly, as more women attempt to conceive at older ages as their fertility begins to naturally wane, correlations between family members that might have been obvious at age 25 may be obscured if a sister or daughter delays attempts at conception until she is over the age of 35 years or even over 40.

Other conditions which are associated with poorer reproductive outcomes have also been assessed in family studies. For example endometriosis has been considered in studies of first degree female relatives and it has been shown that there is a tendency for familial aggregation of this condition.[78] Where familial clustering has been observed the conclusion that is almost invariably reached by authors is that this is indicative of a genetic basis for the condition. It is interesting to speculate about how much research effort is directed towards understanding familial continuities in conditions which are believed to be almost entirely environmentally mediated. For example there is a paucity of familial studies that specifically consider continuities in tubal infertility, estimated to cause approximately 20% of female fertility problems. Perhaps this is because the causes of tubal infertility are widely thought to be environmental, namely that they tend to occur as the result of specific contraceptive behaviours, including the use of an IUD (intra-uterine device) or via the transmission of clinically silent sexually transmitted infections, such as Chlamydia.

However, while not all the conditions in females which are associated with sub-fertility have been examined in family studies, there is comparatively far less evidence available relating to sub-fertility in males.[79] This is despite the fact that it has been estimated that for a couple experiencing difficulties in conceiving a child up to 50% of the sub-fertility may be attributable to the male partner, with the vast majority of the causes thought to relate to reduced sperm quality.[80] Unlike the conditions that in females are associated with poor reproductive outcomes, the majority of the aetiology of impaired spermatogenesis tends to be unknown. However two recent studies which considered the underlying causes of male infertility, one in male twins[80] and one in male siblings,[79] both concluded that the causes were more likely to be environmental rather than the result of a shared genes.

In general though when family studies are utilized to examine the associations in specific disease states within and across generations this is often to determine whether the underlying cause is likely to be genetic.[81] Increasingly it seems that adverse reproductive outcomes do seem to cluster in families, however the mechanisms underlying this clustering are rarely easily identified and in reality may represent a complex dynamic interaction between genes and environments for individuals who share both these components, and it is possible that given differences in timing of oogenesis and spermatogenesis that the relative influences of these may differ between males and females.

15.10 Age at menopause

Regardless of fertility or infertility (by choice or otherwise) the end of a woman's reproductive capacity is signalled by menopause (essentially the cessation of menstruation). As is the case for almost all other sentinel events throughout her reproductive period, family studies have been used to understand better the predictors of this end-point, both natural[82–84] and iatrogenic via hysterectomy in a study using twins.[84] Both twin studies and family history studies have provided evidence that genetic factors contribute to the variability in natural age at menopause, and more recently an intergenerational family study of mother-daughter, sister-sister and aunt-niece pairs suggested that up to 50% of the inter-individual variability in menopausal age could be attributed to genetic effects.[83] A study of age at natural menopause using the Australian Twin Registry also demonstrated that age at menarche was socially patterned, with more socially advantaged twin pairs having a later age at menopause, and related to age at menarche and reproductive events throughout a woman's reproductive life course, in particular that median age at menopause was earlier in smokers and nulliparous women.[82]

15.11 Reproductive indicators of later health

Recently there has been a focus on how reproductive events may act as early markers of later adult health problems. Interest in this area arose primarily as a result of the fetal origins of adult disease hypothesis,[85] which describes the inverse association between size at birth and chronic adult diseases, especially cardiovascular disease, several decades later within one generation. Family studies have been used to examine whether complications of pregnancy or parameters of offspring size at birth might be also related to parental mortality some decades later.[66] These studies across generations have demonstrated that measures of offspring size at birth (both weight and length) are inversely related to mothers' overall risk of mortality in later life (all cause and cardiovascular).[86] The associations were in the same direction for fathers but tended to be weaker overall (See Chapters 2 and 13 for more detailed discussion of these studies).[86,87]

15.12 Limitation of family studies to contribute to our understanding of life course reproductive outcomes

It is clear that there have been a considerable number of family studies that have made contributions to knowledge in the area of reproductive outcomes across the life course. However, by far the majority have dealt with issues that are relevant to reproductive outcomes in females rather than those relevant to males. Whilst the studies, either within or across generations, have confirmed that there tends to be a high degree of continuity in each of the female reproductive outcomes throughout the life course, rarely has any one study actually taken a life course approach to these issues. Rather our knowledge gained from family studies with respect to reproductive outcomes across the life course tends to comes from piecing together the temporally distinct pieces of information to construct a pseudo life course picture. This has particularly significant implications for seeking interventions to improve reproductive outcomes, because without information that looks at the relative importance of different periods of the life course it is difficult to determine at which points to most effectively intervene. It is also interesting to note that much of the literature in the area of familial continuity in reproductive outcomes is concerned with what proportion of this continuity might be attributable to shared genetics. Perhaps because of this there tends to be a large volume of information in this area from twin studies, which fall under the classification of within family or sibling studies. Many of these twin studies attempt to disentangle the environmental from the genetic influences on a particular reproductive outcome. This may be very useful from an aetiological perspective but may be less useful in understanding the full impact of all life course influences on reproductive outcomes. This is particularly relevant to our understanding of how an individual's genetic potential is continuously subject to dynamic modification by interactions with the environment that exists and changes across the life course, as these influences may be easily manipulated to improve reproductive outcomes.

15.13 Future directions for family studies in the area of reproductive outcomes

The family studies which have contributed to our knowledge about reproductive outcomes across the life course have largely been conducted at a time when reproductive behaviours are undergoing a great deal of transition. In particular maternal age at first pregnancy has increased and total family size has decreased over the last three decades throughout all OECD countries.[88] These changes have occurred in conjunction with changing gender roles for women, and a greater perception and availability of contraceptive options and fertility treatments for today's generation of young women in comparison to their mothers and grandmothers before them. The secular trends in other maternal characteristics, such as rising rates of obesity will also impact on reproductive outcomes for the current generation of women in a way that may not have been the case for previous generations. These changes are largely environmentally mediated at the level of the individual woman, the family and society more generally. Where possible it is important that family studies seeking to better understand the determinants of reproductive outcomes do so within the wider context of these influences which affect reproductive decisions and outcomes, although this is increasingly difficult as trends change so rapidly, and as they differ across generations.

One aspect of evolving reproductive options is the increasing use of artificial reproductive technologies to achieve pregnancies in couples who some decades ago may never have been able to achieve a successful reproductive outcome without this assistance. This in particular deserves attention as the children born as a result of these technologies reach the age of reproductive capacity. Based on some relatively scant evidence to date about intergenerational continuity in 'poor reproductive outcomes' we may in fact see an amplification of need for assistance as these children seek to also become parents themselves.

15.14 Conclusion

Perhaps the most important contribution of family studies is confirmation that the outcomes of reproductive events, especially pregnancy outcomes, are not just subject to the conditions that exist at the time of the pregnancy. They represent the cumulative growth and development of mothers and the influence of the environments in which they have grown until a given point in their reproductive career. This is especially pertinent to public health approaches to improving reproductive outcomes at a population level. It supports the notion that attention to the entire life course development of mothers is required to ensure the health of the next generation, exactly as Baird postulated some 60 years ago.[34]

References

1 **Demerath EW, Towne B, Chumlea WC, Sun SS, Remsberg KE.** Recent decline in age at menarche: the Fels Longitudinal Study. *American Journal of Human Biology* 2004; **16**: 453–7.

2 **Pouta A, Jarvelin MR, Hemminki E, Sovio U, Hartikainen-Sori AL.** Mothers and daughters: intergenerational patterns of reproduction. *European Journal of Public Health* 2005; **15**(2): 195–9.

3 **Towne B, Czerwinski SA, Demerath EW, Blangero J, Roche AF, Siervogel RM.** Heritability of age at menarche in girls From the Fels Longitudinal Study. *American Journal of Physical Anthropology* 2005; **128**: 210–19.

4 **Hardy JB, Astone NM, Brooks-Gunn J, Shapiro S, Miller TL.** Like Mother, Like Child: Intergenerational patterns of age at first birth and associations with childhood and adolescent characteristics and adult Outcomes in the second generation. *Developmental Psychology* 1998; **34**(6): 1220–32.

5 **Kahn JR, Anderson KE.** Intergenerational patterns of teenage fertility. *Demography* 1992; **29**(1): 39–57.

6 **Furstenberg FF, Levine JA, Brooks-Gunn J.** The children of teenage mothers: patterns of early childbearing in two generations. *Family Planning Perspectives* 1990; **22**(2): 54–61.

7 **Benzies K, Tough S, Tofflemire K, Frick C, Faber A, Newburn-Cook C.** Factors influencing women's decisions about timing of motherhood. *Journal of Gynecological, Obstetric and Neonatal Nursing* 2006; **35**(5): 625–33.

8 **Morton SMB.** *Lifecourse Determinants of Offspring Size at Birth: An intergenerational study of Aberdeen women*. PhD thesis, University of London, 2002.

9 **Erickson JD, Bjerkedal T.** Interpregnancy interval: association with birth weight, stillbirth and neonatal death. *Journal of Epidemiology and Community Health* 1978; **32**: 124–30.

10 **Batty GD, Morton SMB, Campbell D, Clark H, Davey Smith G, Hall M *et al*.** The Aberdeen 'Children of the 1950s' cohort study: Background, methods and follow-up information on a new resource for the study of life-course and intergenerational effects on health. *Paediatric and Perinatal Epidemiology* 2004; **18**: 221–39.

11 Wilson BJ, Watson MS, Prescott G, Campbell DM, Hannaford P, Smith WCS. Cardiovascular disease in women in Scotland: long term implications of hypertension in pregnancy (Abstract). *Journal of Epidemiology and Community Health* 2000; **54**: 11.

12 Lie RT, Rasmussen S, Brunborg H, Gjessing HK, Lie Nielsen E, Irgens LM. Fetal and maternal contributions to risk of pre-eclampsia: population based study. *British Medical Journal* 1998; **316**: 1343–7.

13 Mogren I, Högberg U, Winkvist A, Stenlund H. Familial occurrence of Pre-eclampsia. *Epidemiology* 1999; **10**: 518–22.

14 Zhang J, Zeisler J, Hatch MC, Berkowitz GS. Epidemiology of Pregnancy-induced Hypertension. *Epidemiology Reviews* 1997; **19**: 218–32.

15 Hennessy E, Alberman E. The Effects of Own Fetal Growth on Reported Hypertension in Parous Women Aged 33. *International Journal of Epidemiology* 1997; **26**(3): 562–3.

16 Klebanoff MA, Secher NJ, Mednick BR, Schulsinger C. Maternal Size at Birth and the Development of Hypertension During Pregnancy. *Archives of Internal Medicine* 1999; **159**: 1607–12.

17 American Diabetes Association. Gestational Diabetes Mellitus. *Diabetes Care* 2003; **26**: S103–S105.

18 Harris MI, Flegal KM, Cowie CC. Prevalence of diabetes, impaired fasting glucose, and impaired glucose tolerance in U.S. adults: the Third National Health and Nutrition Examination Survey, 1988-1994. *Diabetes Care* 1998; **21**: 518–24.

19 Ferrara A, Kahn HS, Quesenberry CP, Riley C, Hedderson MM. An increase in the incidence of gestational diabetes mellitus: Northern California 1991–2000. *Obstetrics and Gynecology* 2004; **103**: 526–33.

20 Wen SW, Levitt C, Liu S, Kramer MS, Joseph KS, Marcoux S *et al.* Impact of prenatal glucose screening on the diagnosis of gestational diabetes and on pregnancy outcomes. *American Journal of Epidemiology* 2000; **152**: 1009–14.

21 Mestman JH, Anderson GV, Guadalupe V. Follow-up study of 360 subjects with abnormal carbohydrate metabolism during pregnancy. *Obstetrics and Gynecology* 1972; **39**: 421–5.

22 Dornhorst A, Rossi M. Risk and prevention of type 2 diabetes in women with gestational diabetes. *Diabetes Care* 1998; **21**[Suppl 2]: B43–B49.

23 Coustan DR, Carpenter MW, O'Sullivan PS. Gestational diabetes: Prediction of subsequent disordered glucose metabolism. *American Journal of Obstetrics and Gynecology* 1993; **168**: 1139–45.

24 Boney CM, Verma A, Tucker R, Vohr BR. Metabolic syndrome in childhood: association with birth weight, maternal obesity, and gestational diabetes mellitus. *Pediatrics* 2004; **115**[3], 290–6.

25 Dabelea D, Hanson RL, Lindsay RS, Pettitt DJ, Imperatore G, Gabir MM *et al.* Intrauterine exposure to diabetes conveys risks for type 2 diabetes and obesity: a study of discordant sibships. *Diabetes* 2000; **49**: 2208–11.

26 Pettitt DJ, Aleck KA, Baird HR, Carraher MJ, Bennett PH, Knowler WC. Congenital susceptibility to NIDDM. Role of intrauterine environment. *Diabetes* 1988; **37**: 622–8.

27 Bunt JC, Tataranni A, Salbe AD. Intrauterine Exposure to Diabetes is a Determinant of Hemoglobin A_1c and Systolic Blood Pressure in Pima Indian Children. *Clinical Endocrinology and Metabolism* 2005; **90**: 3225–9.

28 Vohr BR, McGarvey ST, Tucker R. Effects of maternal gestational diabetes on offspring adiposity at 4-7 years of age. *Diabetes Care* 1999; **22**: 1284–91.

29 Gillman MW, Rifas-Shiman SF, Berkey CS, Field AE, Colditz GA. Maternal gestational diabetes, birth weight, and adolescent obesity. *Pediatrics* 2003; **111**: e221–e226.

30 Krishnaveni GV, Hill JC, Leary SD, Veena SR, Saperia J, Saroja A *et al.* Anthropometry, glucose tolerance, and insulin concentrations in Indian children. *Diabetes Care* 2005; **28**: 2919–25.

31 Silverman BL, Metzger BE, Cho NH, Loeb CA. Impaired glucose tolerance in adolescent offspring of diabetic mothers. Relationship to fetal hyperinsulinism. *Diabetes Care* 1995; **18**: 611–17.

32 Williams MA, Qiu C, Dempsey JC, Luthy DA. Familial aggregation of type 2 diabetes and chronic hypertension in women with gestational diabetes mellitus. *Journal of Reproductive Medicine* 2003; **48**: 955–62.

33 Kermack WO, McKendrick AG, McKinlay PL. Death rates in Great Britain and Sweden. Some general regularities and their significance. *Lancet* 1934; **226**: 698–703.

34 Baird D. Social factors in obstetrics. *Lancet* 1949; **1**: 1079–83.

35 Baird D. Preventive medicine in obstetrics. *New England Journal of Medicine* 1952; **246**(15): 561–8.

36 Baird D. The epidemiology of low birth weight: changes in incidence in Aberdeen, 1948–72. *Journal of Biosocial Science* 1974; **6**: 323–41.

37 Baird D. Epidemiologic Patterns Over Time. In: Reed D, Stanley FJ, eds. *The Epidemiology of Prematurity*. Baltimore: Urban & Schwarzenberg, pp. 5–15, 1977.

38 Illsley R. Social class selection and class differences in relation to stillbirths and infant deaths. *British Medical Journal* 1955; **2**: 1520–4.

39 Illsley R. Early prediction of perinatal risk. *Proceedings of the Royal Society of Medicine* 1966; **59**(3): 181–4.

40 Ounsted M, Ounsted C. Maternal regulation of intra-uterine growth. *Nature* 1966; **212**: 995–7.

41 Hackman E, Emanuel I, van Belle G, Daling J. Maternal birth weight and subsequent pregnancy outcome. *Journal of the American Medical Association* 1983; **250**: 2016–19.

42 Klebanoff MA, Graubard BI, Kessel SS, Berendes HW. Low birth weight across generations. *Journal of the American Medical Association* 1984; **252**: 2423–7.

43 Klebanoff MA, Yip R. Influence of maternal birth weight on rate of fetal growth and duration of gestation. *Journal of Pediatrics* 1987; **111**: 287–92.

44 Magnus P, Bakketeig LS, Skjaerven R. Correlations of birth weight and gestational age across generations. *Annals of Human Biology* 1993; **20**: 231–8.

45 Skjaerven R, Wilcox A, Øyen N, Magnus P. Mother's birth weight and survival of their offspring: population based study. *British Medical Journal* 1997; **314**: 1376–80.

46 Magnus P, Berg K, Bjerkedal T, Nance WE. Parental determinants of birth weight. *Clinical Genetics* 1984; **26**: 397–405.

47 Carr-Hill R, Campbell DM, Hall MH, Meredith A. Is birth weight determined genetically? *British Medical Journal* 1987; **295**: 687–9.

48 Alberman E, Emanuel I, Filakti H, Evans SJW. The contrasting effects of parental birth weight and gestational age on the birth weight of offspring. *Paediatric and Perinatal Epidemiology* 1992; **6**: 134–44.

49 Little RE. Mother's and father's birth weight as predictors of infant birth weight. *Paediatric and Perinatal Epidemiology* 1987; **1**: 19–31.

50 Ramakrishnan U, Martorell R, Schroeder DG, Flores R. Role of intergenerational effects on linear growth. *Journal of Nutrition* 1999; **129**(2S Suppl), 544S–549S.

51 Klebanoff MA, Mednick BR, Schulsinger C, Secher NJ, Teasdale TW, Baker RL et al. Second generation follow-up of the Danish perinatal study women: Study design and factors affecting response. *Paedratric and Perinatal Epidemiology* 1993; **7**: 9–22.

52 Hennessy E, Alberman E. Intergenerational influences affecting birth outcome. I. Birth weight for gestational age in the children of the 1958 British birth cohort. *Paediatric and Perinatal Epidemiology* 1998; **12** Suppl 1: 45–60.

53 Hennessy E, Alberman E. Intergenerational influences affecting birth outcome. II. Preterm delivery and gestational age in the children of the 1958 British birth cohort. *Paediatric and Perinatal Epidemiology* 1998; **12** Suppl 1: 61–75.

54 Klebanoff MA, Meirik O, Berendes HW. Second-generation consequence of small-for-dates birth. *Pediatrics* 1989; **84**: 386–401.

55 Klebanoff MA, Schulsinger C, Mednick BR, Secher NJ. Preterm and small-for-gestational age birth across generations. *American Journal of Obstetrics and Gynecology* 1997; **176**: 521–6.

56 Winkvist A, Mogren I, Hogberg U. Familial patterns in birth characteristics: impact on individual and population risks. *International Journal of Epidemiology* 1998; **27**(2): 248–54.

57 Emanuel I, Leisenring W, Williams MA, Kimpo C, Estee S, O'Brien W et al. The Washington State Intergenerational Study of Birth Outcomes: methodology and some comparisons of maternal birth weight and infant birth weight and gestation in four ethnic groups. *Paediatric and Perinatal Epidemiology* 1999; **13**(3): 352–69.

58 Hypponen E, Power C, Davey Smith G. Parental growth at different life stages and offspring birth weight: an intergenerational cohort study. *Paediatric and Perinatal Epidemiology* 2004; **18**: 168–77.

59 Kline J, Stein Z, Susser M. Conception to birth: Epidemiology of prenatal development. *Monographs in Epidemiology and Biostatistics* Volume 14. New York: Oxford University Press,1989.

60 Billewicz WZ, Thomson AM. Birth weights in consecutive pregnancies. *Journal of Obstetrics and Gynaecology of the British Commonwealth* 1973; **80**: 491–8.

61 Karn MN, Lang-Brown H, MacKenzie H, Penrose LS. Birth weight, gestation time and survival in sibs. *Annals of Eugenics* 1951; **15**: 306–17.

62 Morton NE. The inheritance of human birth weight. *Annal of Human Genetics* 1955; **20**: 125–34.

63 Macran S, Leon DA. Patterns and determinants of birth weight in consecutive live births: results from the OPCS Longitudinal Study 1980–88. LS Working Paper 74. London: Social Statistics Research Unit, City University, 1995.

64 Maconochie N. Abnormal Fetal Growth: A Longitudinal Analysis of Women and their Pregnancies. London: University of London, 1995.

65 Morgen I, Stenlund H, Hogberg U. Recurrence of prolonged pregnancy. *International Journal of Epidemiology* 1999; **28**: 253–7.

66 Rich-Edwards J. A life-course approach to women's reproductive health. In: Kuh D, Hardy R, eds. A Life-course Approach to Women's Health. Oxford: Oxford University Press, 2002.

67 Penrose LS. Some recent trends in human genetics. *Caryologia* 1954; **6** (supplement): 521–30.

68 Lunde A, Melve KK, Gjessing HK, Skjaerven R, Irgens LM. Genetic and environmental influences on birth weight, birth length, head circumference, and gestational age by use of population-based parent-offspring data. *American Journal of Epidemiology* 2007; **165**: 734–41.

69 Clausson B, Lichtenstein P, Cnattingius S. Genetic influences on birth weight and gestational length determined by studies in offspring of twins. *British Journal of Obstetrics and Gynecology* 2000; **107**: 375–81.

70 Gjessing HK, Lie RT. Biometrical modelling in genetics: are complex traits too complex? *Statistical Methods in Medical Research*; doi:10.1177/0962280207081241), 2007.

71 Khoury MJ, Beaty TH, Liang KY. Can familial aggregation of disease be explained by familial aggregation of environmental risk factors ? *American Journal of Epidemiology* 1988; **127**: 674–83.

72 D'Onofrio BM, Turkheimer EN, Eaves LJ, Corey LA, Berg K, Solaas MH et al. The role of the Children of Twins design in elucidating causal relations between parent characteristics and child outcomes. *Journal of Child Psychology and Psychiatry* 2003; **44**(8): 1130–44.

73 Allegrucci C, Thurston A, Lucas E, Young L. Epigenetics and the germline. *Reproduction* 2005; **129**(2): 137–49.

74 Sanders EB, Aston CE, Ferrell RE, Witchell SF. Inter- and intrafamilial variability in premature pubarche and polycistic ovarian syndrome. *Fertility and Sterility* 2002; **78**(3): 473–8.

75 Vink JM, Sadrzadeh S, Lambalk CB, Boomsma DI. Heretability of polycystic ovary syndrome (PCOS) in a Dutch twin-family study. *Journal of Clinical Endocrinology and Metabolism* 2005; **90**(11): 6014–21.

76 Amato P, Simpson JL. The genetics of polycystic ovary syndrome. *Best Practice and Research Clinical Obstetrics and Gynaecology* 2004; **18**(5): 707–18.

77 Pall M, Stephens K, Azziz R. Family size in women with polycystic ovary syndrome. *Fertility and Sterility* 2006; **85**(6): 1837–9.

78 Kennedy S, Mardon H, Barlow D. Familial Endometriosis. *Journal of Assisted Reproduction and Genetics* 1995; **12**(1): 32–4.

79 Cloonan YK, Holt VL, Goldberg J. Male factor infertility: a twin study. *Paediatric and Perinatal Epidemiology* 2007; **21**: 229–34.

80 Gianotten J, Westerveld GH, Leschot NJ, Tanck MWT, Lilford RJ, Lombardi MP *et al*. Familial clustering of impaired spermatogenesis: no evidence for a common genetic inheritance pattern. *Human Reproduction* 2004; **19**(1): 71–6.

81 Byrne J, Carolan S. Adverse reproductive outcomes among pregnancies of aunts and (spouses of) uncles in Irish families with neural tube defects. *American Journal of Medical Genetics* 2005; **140A**: 52–61.

82 Do KA, Treloar SA, Pandeya N, Purdie D, Green AC, Martin NG. Predictive factors of age at menopause in a large Australian twin study. *Human Biology* 1998; **70**(6): 1073–91.

83 Murabito JM, Yang Q, Fox C, Wilson PWF, Cupples LA. Heritability of age at natural menopause in the Framingham Heart Study. *Clinical Endocrinology and Metabolism* 2005; **90**(6): 3427–30.

84 Sneider H, MacGregor AJ, Spector TD. Genes control the cessation of a woman's reproductive life: a twin study of hysterectomy and age at menopause. *Journal of Clinical Endocrinology and Metabolism*, 1998; **83**: 1875–80.

85 Barker DJP. Fetal and infant origins of adult disease. London. *British Medical Journal Publishing* 1992;

86 Davey Smith G, Sterne JAC, Tynelius P, Lawlor DA, Rasmussen F. Birth weight of offspring and subsequent cardiovascular mortality of the parents. *Epidemiology* 2005; **16**(4): 563–9.

87 Nybo Andersen A, Osler M. Birth dimensions, parental mortality, and mortality in early adult age: a cohort study of Danish men born in 1953. *International Journal of Epidemiology* 2004; **33**: 92–9.

88 d'Addio AC, d'Ercole MM. Trends and determinants of fertility rates in OECD countries: the role of policies. OECD Social, *Employment and Migration Working Papers*. Paris 2004; **27**: 12–43.

89 Ounsted M, Scott A, Moar VA. Constrained and unconstrained fetal growth: associations with some biological and pathological factors. *Annals of Human Biology* 1988; **15**: 119–29.

90 Langhoff Roos J, Lindmark G, Gustavson KH, Gebre Medhin M, Meirik O. Relative effect of parental birth weight on infant birth weight at term. *Clinical Genetics* 1987; **32**: 240–8.

91 Emanuel I, Filakti H, Alberman E, Evans SJW. Intergenerational studies of human birthweight from the 1958 birth cohort I. Evidence of a multigenerational effect. *British Journal of Obstetrics and Gynaecology* 1992; **99**: 67–74.

92 Coutinho R, David RJ, Collins JW Jr. Relation of parental birth weights to infant birth weight among African Americans and whites in Illinois: a transgenerational study. *American Journal of Epidemiology* 1997; **146**: 804–9.

93 Klebanoff MA, Graubard BI, Kessel SS, Berendes HW. Low birth weight across generations. *Journal of the American Medical Association* 1984; **252**: 2423–7.

94 Sanderson M, Emanuel I, Holt VL. The intergenerational relationship between mother's birthweight, infant birthweight and infant mortality in black and white mothers. *Paediatric and Perinatal Epidemiology* 1995; **9**: 391–405.

95 Collins JW Jr, Wu SY, David RJ. Differing intergenerational birth weights among the descendents of US-born and foreign-born whites and African Americans in Illinois. *American Journal of Epidemiology* 2002; **155**: 210–17.

96 Ounsted M, Ounsted C. *On Fetal Growth Rate. Its Variations and Consequences. Clinics in Developmental Medicine, No. 46*, London, Heineman, 1973.

97 Lumey LH. Decreased birthweights in infants after maternal in utero exposure to the Dutch famine of 1944–1945. *Paediatric and Perinatal Epidemiology* 1992; **6**: 240–53.

Chapter 16

Discussant chapter—using family-based designs in life course epidemiology

John Lynch and Seungmi Yang

Abstract

The three chapters in this section offer different but complementary conceptualizations of 'family'. Morton and Rich Edwards used 'family' to document inter-generational concordance of reproductive outcomes, Hatch and Mishra documented how 'family' could be characterized as a risk exposure for later poor mental health, and Lawlor and Leon used 'family' as a means to control for unmeasured confounding by family characteristics to better understand causal mechanisms relating fetal growth to later disease. Lawlor and Leon's approach is similar to that used in studies examining the possible intrauterine origins of birth weight and cognitive ability and we briefly explore that literature. Families surely matter for better understanding individual and population patterns of ill-health. If we know how families transmit different diseases across generations then it may elucidate novel or under-exploited avenues for prevention.

16.1 Introduction

Family history has long been recognized as increasing the risk of a variety of illnesses. Family history of heart disease in parents, for instance, has been associated with 1.2–2.0 fold increased risk of disease onset, after adjustment for known risk factors in the offspring.[1] The big question is—why—what are the mechanisms? Why do we need to have information on previous generations to better understand disease risk in current generations? This is of course a question at the very heart of life course epidemiology. Having a particular illness history in a family means that potentially there is a complex interplay of genetic, epigenetic, social, and behavioural factors that influence transmission of risk across generations. The exact mix of these influences will depend on the particular health outcome. So families are a natural focus of study for anyone wanting to understand disease causation, especially when one adopts an inter-generational life course perspective.

The three chapters in this section provide contrasting and complementary examples of how to conceptualize and examine continuity of risk across generations and how family studies have and can be used to better understand disease causation. The chapter by Morton and Rich Edwards lays out the evidence for how various aspects of reproductive health, mainly in women, have concordance across generations. There is fairly consistent evidence that age at menarche, age at first pregnancy, family size, specific maternal conditions such as gestational hypertension and diabetes, pregnancy outcomes (birth weight, gestational age), infertility and age at menopause all show continuity across generations. For instance, mother's age at menarche is correlated r = 0.2 with her daughters age at menarche, while every 100 gram increase in mother's birth weight is associated with a 10–20 gram increase in offspring birth weight, and birth weights of siblings are correlated r = 0.4–0.5. The sibling concordance in birth weight is of similar magnitude with sociological studies showing correlations of 0.5–0.6 for sibling educational attainment.[2] One particularly interesting epidemiological observation in this chapter is how Morton and Rich Edwards point out that inter-generational continuity in a range of reproductive outcomes persists even though there are large secular changes in family size, age at menarche, and age at first birth. This is a perfect example of inter-generational life course thinking. How do early life exposures play out within a particular birth cohort in regard to reproductive outcomes, how does this work across generations and then how does this fit with secular shifts in the exposures and outcomes of interest at the population level? This sort of 'triangulation' across levels and over time is important if links observed in individual level studies are to make sense in regard to observed trends at the population level.[3] In this case, the inter-generational links remain despite large shifts in the population levels of family size, age at menarche and age at first birth (and the factors that influence such shifts) suggesting something rather bio-socially fundamental about inter-generational transmission of many reproductive characteristics. Morton and Rich Edwards see major developments in the life course epidemiology of reproductive outcomes coming from more information on males, attention to the full life course history across generations rather than having to piece together discrete time windows from different studies, and through greater attention to the proximal and distal social context in which reproductive decisions are made.

The main thrust of the chapter by Hatch and Mishra is to demonstrate how various aspects of families (including grandparents, parents and siblings) are associated with the onset, timing and course of poor mental health, such as anxiety, depression, antisocial behaviour, and substance use. In this chapter, we are introduced to various examples of how 'family' is seen as an exposure both in early and later life that can be characterized in various ways, in regard to family structure, parenting behaviour, and socioeconomic position. It is clear from their necessarily selective review of this literature that family effects on subsequent mental health are inconsistent. Hatch and Mishra put some of this down to the lack of consistency across studies in measuring different aspects of families as exposures and different measurement of relevant outcomes. They argue that the life course epidemiology of mental health needs more prospective, multi-generational studies with consistent measurement protocols over time and extended follow-up, and collection of more paternal information, and better typologies of family types.

Lawlor and Leon bring a somewhat different approach to their discussion of family studies in the context of observed links between fetal and early life factors, especially markers of intrauterine and later growth, and cardiovascular diseases (CVD). The reproducibility of associations between markers of fetal and post-natal growth, and CVD suggests there is something real to be explained.[4] In this context Lawlor and Leon show how different study designs using twins, siblings, paternal vs maternal characteristics, and inter-generational (parental and grandparental) studies have been used to explore the mechanisms that might link aspects of fetal growth with later CVD.

So while Morton and Rich Edwards used 'family' to document inter-generational concordance of reproductive outcomes, and Hatch and Mishra documented how 'family' could be characterized as a risk exposure for later poor mental health, Lawlor and Leon use 'family' as a means to understand causal mechanisms relating fetal growth to later disease. Their underlying causal diagram might look something like Figure 16.1. The question they pose is how family studies might help

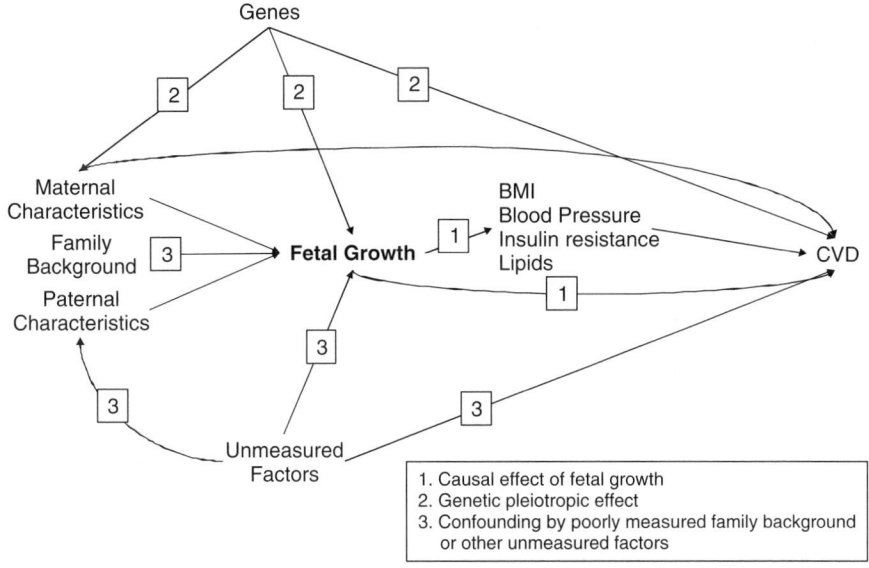

Fig. 16.1 One possible causal diagram underlying the association between fetal growth and CVD.

disentangle which mechanisms are operating—1) a truly causal effect (direct or indirect) of fetal growth, 2) a pleiotropic effect of genes, or 3) an effect driven by confounding from family background characteristics or unmeasured factors. While the diagram relates to CVD, one could easily imagine a similar structure for a causal diagram concerned with reproductive outcomes, mental health, respiratory or infectious diseases, or indeed any outcome that has a putative intrauterine developmental origin.

The ingenious way Lawlor and Leon describe how different analytical strategies in the stable of 'family-based designs' can be used could be equally well applied to other areas of epidemiology that relate to family continuities and hypothesized mechanisms of an intrauterine or social developmental origin such as in infectious diseases,[5] diabetes[6] and respiratory conditions.[7] Indeed similar ideas have been used in studies examining links between birth weight and cognitive ability.[8–10]

16.2 What have we learned from family studies on links between birth weight and cognitive ability?

Epidemiologic studies have shown that birth weight is positively associated with cognitive ability in childhood, across the full distribution of both birth weight and cognitive ability after adjustment for potential confounding factors including family socioeconomic position and parenting practices. These findings, like those for birth weight and CVD, at least provide some basis for suggesting a potential intrauterine developmental origin of cognitive development. However, as is also the case for birth weight and CVD, few studies have been able to adjust for the full range of potential confounding factors from across the life course that may explain the association. And even those studies that do control for a large number of factors may end up still being left with residual confounding due to poor measurement of socioeconomic position, maternal behavior and health, parental cognitive ability, and education that all have plausible effects on both birth weight and offspring cognitive ability. Family studies with twins and siblings who share maternal and family characteristics provide opportunities to better understand the mechanisms behind the association of birth weight with cognitive development.

16.2.1 Twin studies of birth weight and cognitive ability

Three within twin-pair studies have attempted to determine whether the relationship between birth weight and intelligence is primarily driven by genetic or environmental factors. In the largest twin study to date, there was no association within monozygotic twin-pairs (N = 81), leading the authors to suggest that genetic factors explained the association.[11] However, two other smaller studies of 25[12] and 27[13] monozygotic twin pairs found that within twin pairs birth weight differences were positively associated with cognitive ability. The small sample sizes of these studies mean that all estimates were imprecise but most point estimates suggested modest positive effects within monozygotic twins. Moreover, as suggested elsewhere twin studies of this sort are subject to the largely unquantifiable bias that results from it being difficult to be certain that the correct birth weight in same-sex twins is associated with each twin in childhood or adult life.

As discussed in the context of cardiovascular diseases in Chapter 13, twin-singleton comparison studies, both within families (i.e. comparison of the twins with non-twin siblings) and between families (i.e. comparison of a population of twins with a population of singletons or the general population, most of whom will be singleton) can inform us whether there is an intrauterine origin of cognitive ability as twins experience more intrauterine growth restriction and have lower average birth weights than singletons. Thus, if twins have a lower cognitive ability than singletons, the intrauterine origin hypothesis is apparently supported. Numerous studies comparing twins and singletons from different families have shown that twins have lower cognitive ability than singletons from ages as early as 8 months to 11 years,[14–17] suggesting that the intrauterine growth restriction experienced by twins is associated with a deficit in cognitive development.

However, within family twin-singleton comparison studies, where twins are compared to their own non-twin siblings and that, therefore, better control for maternal and family characteristics, show contradictory results. For example, Ronalds *et al.*[18] found that twins had lower cognitive ability than their singleton siblings at ages 7 and 9. This difference was not explained by sex, maternal age, birth order, and father's social class, suggesting that the cognitive ability difference is not due to differences across families. They further showed that adjustment for birth weight and gestational age halved the difference in mean cognitive ability suggesting that cognitive ability differences could be due to the intrauterine growth specific to a particular birth in the same family. On the other hand, data from the Twins Early Development Study, a within family study of twins born in England Wales in 1994–1995, found no cognitive ability differences between twins and their singleton siblings at ages 2 and 3.[19]

Potential explanations for such contradictory findings across twin-singleton studies may be related to improvements in obstetric and pediatric practice over time. For example, studies that found significant differences in average cognitive ability between twins and singletons were from children born in the 1920s–1950s while studies showing no difference were based on those born in the 1980s–1990s. Alternatively, these findings may indicate that the difference in cognitive ability among twins and singletons decreases substantially as children age irrespective of birth weight, so that there are no substantial differences in cognitive ability after adolescence.[17] It is possible that part of this effect may be due to quantitative and qualitative differences in post-natal parenting and education between twins and singletons within the same family. Thus, even though there seems cognitive deficit related to growth restriction in twins compared to singletons born to the same mother, twins apparently show 'catch-up' in their cognitive ability as they grow.

In contrast to the findings in twins of an apparent association between intrauterine growth restriction and cognitive ability, in Chapter 13 Lawlor and Leon suggest that there is no evidence that twins when compared either to singletons from different families or those from their own family, have increased CVD risk. They point out though, that the nature of growth restriction among twins is qualitatively different than growth restriction among singletons and so this may be an uncertain model upon which to base our tests of the intrauterine developmental origin of CVD or for that matter in regard to cognitive ability. Even if the biology of growth restriction is different for twins than singletons, it does not help resolve the apparent effects of growth restriction on cognitive ability but not on CVD.

16.2.2 Non-twin sibling studies of birth weight and cognitive ability

Lawlor and Leon in Chapter 13 describe how within and between sibship comparisons have been used to examine whether the association of birth weight with CVD risk can be explained by fixed familial characteristics, such as socioeconomic background and maternal growth and health up to the time of her first pregnancy. Similar studies have also been used to understand the association of birth size with cognitive ability. In the earliest study, Record et al.[8] showed that differences in cognitive ability between children aged 11 from different families were greater than that of 2,521 sibling pairs within families. They concluded that the observed difference seen between children from different families (and thus in previous general population studies) was largely due to confounding by socioeconomic position. Lawlor and colleagues[9] also found that though birth weight was positively associated with cognitive ability in children at ages 7–11, it was not related to cognitive test scores within 1,645 sibling pairs when the association was separated into between- and within-families. There are, however, three studies that have found positive within sibling associations, suggesting that the association is not fully explained by family characteristics and so supporting the intrauterine developmental origin hypothesis.[20–22] By far the largest sibling study to date included only men, and found similar within and between birth weight associations with low cognitive ability at ages 17–19 in a sample of 96,187 individuals from 51,723 families.[22] One possible reason for the inconsistency across family-based studies could be because the nature of any intrauterine developmental origin of cognitive ability varies with age. However, Yang et al.[10] have recently shown that there was a very weak positive association between birth weight and cognitive ability within siblings from more than 1,000 families at ages 5–12 and that the pattern of association did not vary by age.

In sum, family studies demonstrate inconsistent results on the association between birth weight and cognitive ability even using clever twin and sibling designs. These contradictory findings prevent us from drawing a firm conclusion on whether there is an intrauterine developmental origin of cognitive development or that the association is due to residual confounding by family characteristics. There also remain unresolved issues such as differences in birth cohort, age, geography, and differential measurement across studies. All of this mirrors the literature on links between fetal growth and CVD where it has proven difficult to come to a definitive conclusion about exactly which mechanisms are operating and their relative contribution to CVD.

So what can we conclude from such inconsistent results? While we may not be able to disentangle the precise mechanisms that drive associations between birth weight and cognitive ability, the twin and sibling studies do help us understand that any causal effect of birth weight on cognitive development is likely small relative to maternal and family characteristics. For instance Yang et al.[10] showed that while a 100g increase in birth weight was associated with an improvement of a standard deviation score of 0.07 in cognitive ability, one year of additional education of the mother was associated with 0.2–0.3 standard deviation score among children aged 5–12.

In other words, one year longer in school for the mother had three to four times the impact on cognitive ability in the child than increasing birth weight by a plausible 100g. These findings take us back to the concept of family used in Chapter 15 by Hatch and Mishra in which the direct effects of family members and their relationships to each other are seen to have potentially important health consequences on individuals within the family.

16.3 Where do we go from here?

Families surely matter for better understanding individual and population patterns of ill-health, but as we suggested at the outset, the goal is to find out why. If we know why or perhaps more importantly how families transmit different diseases across generations then it may highlight novel or under-exploited avenues for prevention. These chapters provided different perspectives on that prevention goal and highlight the need for family-based studies to be applied to other health outcomes. To move us closer to the goal of being better able to successfully intervene the authors of all three chapters in this section called for more and better data with longer follow-up across generations and larger numbers of study participants. This is surely an important goal and is embodied in efforts in many countries to collect myriad long term data on birth and inter-generational cohorts. But it is also true that we face limits in our ability to collect such data (participant burden is high and attrition over long periods of time may generate bias) as detailed in Chapter 6, and to appropriately statistically handle and make sense of it, if and when we get those data.[23, 24] It is interesting that Lawlor and Leon also see some of the advances in understanding the mechanisms linking fetal growth to CVD involving contrasts among twins and singletons with growth impairment and singletons without growth restriction, and better understanding of the biological mechanisms that control such processes. At least in the short term, it seems much of this sort of work will have to be undertaken in basic and experimental biology. The role for epidemiology is less clear.

It is clear that epidemiology alone cannot get to the bottom of some of these important questions. In some cases, our tools are simply too blunt. As the short review on birth weight and cognitive ability showed, even using clever twin and sibling designs, the evidence is still mixed, making definitive conclusions rather difficult. Will the same inconclusive patterns be seen when applying such approaches to CVD or infectious or respiratory diseases?

These chapters nevertheless demonstrate how useful a 'family' orientation can be in life course epidemiology and the approaches utilized here should be more widely applied in other areas of epidemiologic research. The potential of life course epidemiology is only enhanced by using family-based study designs to better understand inter-generational continuity of disease risk and to get at the mechanisms that cause such inter-generational links. But because the ultimate goal is to provide knowledge for intervention then we must also balance a desire to understand the fascinating biology that underlies social and biological developmental plasticity against an assessment of public health importance, in terms of the size of any causal effect (in both relative and absolute terms) and our capacity to intervene on that cause. For instance it might be useful to have a stratification of adult CVD risk by gestational age adjusted birth weight to examine the added absolute risk associated with growth restriction over and above having one or more of the big four CVD risk factors (hypertension, dyslipidemia, smoking, and diabetes) in adulthood. Of course such comparisons are themselves tricky to interpret if intrauterine growth restriction is a major influence on the development of the conventional CVD risk factors. There is evidence from individual level studies that birth weight is associated with blood pressure,[25] diabetes,[26] and perhaps smoking but little effect on cholesterol.[27] However, such effects need to be 'triangulated' against longer term population trends of falling blood pressure probably since the turn of the

20th century,[28, 29] cholesterol,[30] and smoking since mid 20th century,[31] and rising levels of insulin resistance and diabetes since the 1980s.[32]

On the association between fetal growth and chronic disease Kramer asked, 'Is it causal?' 'Is it important?'[33] We will do well to keep both those questions in mind regardless of our particular topic of investigation on the life course processes that influence disease risk.

References

1. O'Donnell CJ. Family history, subclinical atherosclerosis, and coronary heart disease risk: barriers and opportunities for the use of family history information in risk prediction and prevention. *Circulation* 2004; **110**: 2074–6.
2. Conley D, Pfeiffer KM, Velez M. Explaining sibling differences in achievement and behavioral outcomes: The importance of within- and between-family factors. *Social Science Research* 2007; **36**: 1087–1104.
3. Lynch J, Davey Smith G. A life course approach to chronic disease epidemiology. *Annual Review of Public Health* 2005; **26**: 1–35.
4. Lawlor DA. The developmental origins of health and disease: where do we go from here? *Epidemiology* 2008; **19**: 206–8.
5. Hall AJ, Yee LJ, Thomas SL. Life course epidemiology and infectious diseases. *International Journal of Epidemiology* 2002; **31**: 300–1.
6. Bergvall N, Lindam A, Pawitan Y, Lichtenstein P, Cnattingius S, Iliadou A. Importance of familial factors in associations between offspring birth weight and parental risk of type-2 diabetes. *International Journal of Epidemiology* 2008; **37**: 185–92.
7. Upton MN, Davey Smith G, McConnachie A, Hart CL, Watt GCM. Maternal and personal cigarette smoking synergize to increase airflow limitation in adults. *American Journal of Respiratory and Critical Care Medicine* 2004; **169**: 479–87.
8. Record RG, McKeown T, Edwards JH. The relation of measured intelligence to birth weight and duration of gestation. *Annals Human Genetics* 1969; **33**: 71–9.
9. Lawlor DA, Clark H, Davey Smith G, Leon DA. Intrauterine growth and intelligence within sibling pairs: findings from the Aberdeen children of the 1950s cohort. *Pediatrics* 2006; **117**: e894–e902.
10. Yang S, Lynch J, Susser E, Lawlor DA. Birthweight and cognitive ability in childhood among siblings and non-siblings. *Pediatrics* 2008: **122**(2): e350–e358.
11. Boomsma DI, van Beijsterveldt CE Rietveld MJ Bartels M van Baal GC. Genetics mediate relation of birth weight to childhood IQ. *British Medical Journal* 2001; **323**: 1426–7.
12. Willerman L, Churchill JA. Intelligence and birth weight in identical twins. *Child Development* 1967; **38**: 623–9.
13. Scarr, S. Effects of birth weight on later intelligence. *Social Biology* 1969; **16**: 249–56.
14. Strauss RS. Adult Functional Outcome of those born small for gestational age: twenty-six-year follow-up of the 1970 British birth cohort. *JAMA: The Journal of the American Medical Association* 2000; **283**: 625–32.
15. Richards M, Hardy R, Kuh D, Wadsworth MEJ. Birth weight and cognitive function in the British 1946 birth cohort: longitudinal population based study. *British Medical Journal* 2001; **322**: 199–203.
16. Power CJ. The Influence of birth weight and socioeconomic position on cognitive development: does the early home and learning environment modify their effects? *Journal of Pediatrics* 2006; **148**: 54–61.
17. Christensen K, Petersen I, Skythe A, Herskind AM, McGue M, Bingley P. Comparison of academic performance of twins and singletons in adolescence: follow-up study. *British Medical Journal* 2006; **333**: 1095.
18. Ronalds GA, De Stavola BL, Leon DA. The cognitive cost of being a twin: evidence from comparisons within families in the Aberdeen children of the 1950s cohort study. *British Medical Journal* 2005; **331**: 1306.

19 Koeppen-Schomerus G, Spinath FM, Plomin R. Twins and non-twin siblings: different estimates of shared environmental influence in early childhood. *Twin Research* 2003; **6**: 97–105.

20 Matte TD, Bresnahan M, Begg MD, Susser E. Influence of variation in birth weight within normal range and within sibships on IQ at age 7 years: cohort study. *British Medical Journal* 2001; **323**: 310–4.

21 Lawlor DA, Bor W, O'Callaghan MJ, Williams GM, Najman JM. Intrauterine growth and intelligence within sibling pairs: findings from the Mater-University study of pregnancy and its outcomes. *Journal of Epidemiology and Community Health* 2005; **59**: 279–82.

22 Bergvall N, Iliadou A, Tuvemo T, Cnattingius S. Birth characteristics and risk of low intellectual performance in early adulthood: are the associations confounded by socioeconomic factors in adolescence or familial effects? *Pediatrics* 2006; **117**: 714–21.

23 Hallqvist J, Lynch JW, Blane D, Bartley M, Lange T. Critical period, accumulation and social trajectory: Can we empirically distinguish lifecourse processes? *Social Science and Medicine* 2004; **58**: 1555–62.

24 Glymour MM. Commentary: Selected samples and nebulous measures: some methodological difficulties in life-course epidemiology. *International Journal of Epidemiology* 2007; **36**: 566–8.

25 Gamborg M, Byberg L, Rasmussen F, Andersen PK, Baker JL, Bengtsson C, *et al.*, on behalf of the NordNet Study. Birth weight and systolic blood pressure in adolescence and adulthood: meta-regression analysis of sex- and age-specific results from 20 Nordic studies. *American Journal of Epidemiology* 2007; **166**: 634–45.

26 Harder T, Rodekamp E, Schellong K, Dudenhausen JW, Plagemann A. Birth weight and subsequent risk of type 2 diabetes: a meta-analysis. *American Journal of Epidemiology* 2007; **165**: 849–57.

27 Huxley R, Owen CG, Whincup PH, Cook DG, Colman S, Collins R. Birth weight and subsequent cholesterol levels: exploration of the 'fetal origins' hypothesis. *JAMA: The Journal of the American Medical Association* 2004; **292**: 2755–64.

28 Goff DC, Howard G, Russell GB, Labarthe DR. Birth cohort evidence of population influences on blood pressure in the United States, 1887-1994. *Annals of Epidemiology* 2001; **11**: 271–9.

29 McCarron P, Davey Smith G, Okasha M. Secular changes in blood pressure in childhood, adolescence and young adulthood: systematic review of trends from 1948 to 1998. *Journal of Human Hypertension* 2002; **16**: 677–89.

30 Arnett DK, Jacobs DR, Jr., Luepker RV, Blackburn H, Armstrong C, Claas SA. Twenty-year trends in serum cholesterol, hypercholesterolemia, and cholesterol medication use: the Minnesota Heart Survey, 1980–1982 to 2000–2002. *Circulation* 2005; **112**: 3884–91.

31 Burns DM, Lee L, Shen LZ, Gilpin E, Tolley HD, Vaughn J, Shanks TG. Cigarette smoking behavior in the United States. In: Burns DM, Garfinkel L, Samet JM editors. *Smoking and Tobacco Control Monograph 8: Changes in Cigarette-Related Disease Risks and Their Implications for Prevention and Control*, US Dept. of Health and Human Services, National Cancer Institute, Bethesda, MD. pp. 13–42, 1997.

32 Ford ES, Giles WH, Mokdad AH. Increasing prevalence of the metabolic syndrome among U.S. adults. *Diabetes Care* 2004; **27**: 2444–9.

33 Kramer MS. Invited commentary: association between restricted fetal growth and adult chronic disease: is it causal? Is it important? *American Journal of Epidemiology* 2000; **152**: 605–8.

Chapter 17

The future of family-based studies in life course epidemiology: challenges and opportunities

Gita D Mishra and Debbie A Lawlor

Abstract

Family-based studies can provide a more comprehensive view of life course epidemiology than studies that do not engage with family effects. They can establish intergenerational associations, help to understand the influence that one family member can have on the health and wellbeing of another family member and they can help to unravel the mechanisms behind the relationships of genetic, social, and environmental factors that impact on health at different life stages. In this chapter we summarise the common threads across the previous chapters and highlight the key methodological challenges and opportunities of using family study designs in life course epidemiology. We discuss a number of points, including some that receive less attention in the preceding chapters, that we feel are important for the future direction of research using family-based studies in life course epidemiology.

17.1 Introduction

The previous chapters demonstrate the burgeoning field of family-based studies in life course epidemiology. As noted in Chapters 1 and 6, an increasing recognition over recent decades for the critical role of early life exposures in shaping development, and hence later health and wellbeing, has resulted in support for existing birth cohorts and the initiation of a number of new and very large birth cohorts. By definition birth cohorts are family-based studies, including at least two generations (parents and children), but overall the full potential of family-based studies—intergenerational, sibling, and twin studies—to unravel the complex relationships between genetic, social, and environmental factors that impact on health at different life stages has not been fully realised in life course epidemiology. The preceding chapters are a salutary reminder of the crucial importance of conducting, analysing, and interpreting family-based studies appropriately.

While many associations are well established in life course epidemiology, such as low birth weight with the risk of cardiovascular disease (CVD), the mechanisms remain unclear (Chapter 13). The direction of association for some exposures with outcomes in adulthood, such as birth weight and gestational age, is obvious, but in other life course examples this is not the case. For instance, the association between parental depression and offspring mental disorder may mean that parental mental health directly affects the offspring or visa versa that offspring behaviour leads to poor parental mental health (Chapter 14). Or is it the influence of their shared environment, such as poor housing conditions, which link the two? These and many other examples illustrate some of the key questions in life course epidemiology today:

- Are the associations causal?
- What are the mechanisms?
- How do observed associations operate across generations?
- How do different risk factors interact across the life course?

The aim of the book is to provide the knowledge and skills to design, analyse, and interpret family-based studies in life course epidemiology. Family-based studies offer the possibility to address some of these questions by helping to unravel the complex interplay of genetic, social, and behavioural factors. They provide an opportunity to test specific causal mechanisms and life course models[1] and can help understand whether the timing of risk factors (critical and sensitive periods) are important (Chapter 1). Family-based studies not only have the potential to provide a more comprehensive view of life course epidemiology (taking account of a broader range of exposures, including across generations, that studies based only on individuals can), in the absence of randomised trials, they hold the promise of developing causal models from observational studies. This can be achieved in several ways: by comparing within and between sibling and twin associations where tight control for fixed factors within twin-pairs and sibling groups is possible (Chapters 3, 4, 13); by comparing parental-offspring associations to test causality for intrauterine exposures (Chapters 2, 13); and by using maternal genetic variants as instrumental variables for testing causality of intrauterine modifiable risk factors (Chapters 2, 13). In a selection that is illustrative rather than exhaustive, the series of topics presented in Part IV describes how family-based studies have been used in life course epidemiology. In this final chapter, we provide a brief summary of the key methodological challenges and opportunities of using family-based studies in life course epidemiology.

17.2 Methodological challenges

This section provides a summary of some key points to guide researchers undertaking family-based studies in life course epidemiology, together with cross references to chapters where there is greater detail on how to deal with these challenges.

17.2.1 Representativeness and generalizability

As with all research it is important to consider the representativeness of the study sample with respect to the target population. An additional feature of family-based life course studies are how representative these studies are in time and place. One difficulty of life course epidemiology in general is that we frequently want to examine the effect of exposures at key developmental periods (intrauterine, infancy, and childhood) on common complex disease outcomes, such as CVD and cancer, in later life (Chapter 9). By definition, cohorts with information on these disease outcomes will be in their 60s, 70s, or older, and their exposures during their early life development will have been very different to exposures of pregnant women, infants, and children nowadays to whom we would want to make causal inference. Specific to family-based studies, the nature of families and how they relate to each other has changed markedly over the last century (Chapters 2, 4, 6, 9, 10, 12). This includes changes to social norms and technology that have resulted in increases in single-parent families, same-sex parents, multiple step-parents and siblings, and increases in multiple births resulting from infertility treatment, and the greater potential for preterm and small for gestational age infants (more common in multiple births) to survive. These changes have implications for defining who belongs to a life course cohort study (Chapter 6), how associations are defined between family members, as well as how we interpret results of studies from previous generations for relevance to contemporary populations.

Furthermore, findings from one family-based study may not be generalizable to different populations defined by geography or ethnicity. For instance, the assumption that siblings have the same fixed familial socioeconomic position may break down in countries/cultures/populations where one child is 'favoured' over others, such as in their diet or for further education, based on their gender, birth order, early signs of promise, or other characteristics. Finally, in twin studies, there is the question of how representative twins and their families are of the general population to which we want to make causal inference (Chapter 4).

These issues of representativeness highlight the importance of examining associations and testing hypotheses in different populations, but in doing so having a clear understanding at the start of the study about how populations differ and therefore whether one would anticipate similarities or differences in associations (Chapter 7). For example, the inverse association between birth weight and CVD is similar in magnitude in birth cohorts from the 1950s in the UK, when infant mortality and living conditions had improved compared to pre-war years, to that found in UK birth cohorts from the 1900s.[2] This finding provides some evidence that the factors driving the inverse association between birth weight and CVD may be relevant to contemporary populations. With respect to changes over time, it would be ideal to examine whether the magnitudes of associations between generations of the same families change over time. For example, is the association of birth weight between parents and children similar for a group of great-great-great grand parents and great-great grand parents as it is for their contemporary offspring (the parents and children)? To our knowledge, and perhaps not surprisingly given the changes in research priorities and data collected over time, no such studies have been conducted. Nonetheless if we consider today's birth cohorts as having the potential to be truly multigenerational and to provide research resources for future generations of researchers, we need to ensure that links between generations and details of how characteristics have been measured are very clearly documented (Chapter 6 and Section 17.2.4 below).

17.2.2 Sample size and statistical power

For the main part this book has discussed the potential of family-based studies to test causal hypotheses or disentangle causal pathways. When family-based studies are used in this way they frequently involve comparing magnitudes of associations within and between different family structures. For example, comparing maternal-offspring associations to paternal-offspring associations, as described in Chapter 2, or comparing within and between sibling or twin associations (Chapters 3 and 4). Such studies require considerably greater sample sizes than studies concerned with a single association. In particular type 2 errors can be misleading when comparing associations. If we take a completely hypothetical example of a sibling study in which we are interested in comparing the within and between sibling association of body mass index at puberty with future blood pressure at age 60 in order to examine the extent to which fixed family characteristics, in particular childhood social class and parental education, might have confounded any association. One interpretation of a p-value of 0.05 used to test the null hypothesis that there is no difference in this association within and between siblings, would be that the association is not confounded by fixed familial characteristics, since it is the same within siblings as between (non-) siblings (Chapter 2). However, if the mean differences (95% Confidence Intervals) were, for example, 10mmHg (95%CI: 2, 18) for the between (non-) siblings association and 5mmHg (95%CI: 0.5, 10) for the within sibling association, we would surely question the interpretation of no difference and realize that the study is too small to provide evidence of a difference with a high level of certainty. At the other extreme very large studies might show statistically significant (low p-value) differences between regression coefficients, but the magnitude of this difference might be too small as to indicate strong confounding influences.

Chapters 2 and 13 describe the combination of Mendelian randomization studies (using genetic variants that are known to be robustly associated with a non-genetic risk factor of interest as an instrumental variable for that risk factor) with a family-based study. In these examples, maternal genotype is used as an instrumental variable for an intrauterine exposure. These studies also require very large sample sizes to provide precise estimates that are useful in translating research into public health or clinical practice.[3]

One consequence of the requirement for large sample sizes has been that family-based studies in life course epidemiology have largely used continuously measured outcomes, such as blood pressure, body mass index, intelligence quotient.[4–8] The use of continuously measured outcomes also reflects the fact that statistical methods for binary or time to events outcomes are sometimes more complex than those for continuous outcomes (Chapters 10, 11, 12). However, we frequently want to understand the role of developmental and degenerative processes on disease events rather than continuous traits. Thus, there is a need for large studies but also large collaborative efforts that allow datasets to be combined, where this is appropriate, in order to realize the full potential of family-based studies in life course epidemiology.

17.2.3 Missing data and attrition

All prospective studies have to face the challenge of loss to follow-up, which can affect statistical power and cause bias (Chapters 10, 12). Furthermore, in life course studies where we aim to collect very large amounts of data for current and future research priorities (Chapter 6), it is likely that there will be missing data at each data collection sweep as well as considerable attrition of the cohort due to loss to follow-up. For family-based life course epidemiology studies these issues are amplified since missing data may occur not just in the main participant but also in any of the family members (Chapters 8, 10). When family structure and/or interrelationships are central to a particular analysis, missing data from one family member might mean that available data from other family members cannot be used. In Chapter 6 it is suggested that participants being recruited for a birth cohort are made aware of the life-long commitment that it expected of them and that only those prepared to accept this commitment are recruited (even at the expense of reducing generalizablity). In Chapter 8 the possibility (and indeed frequently the need) of using proxy informants to obtain information for different family members is discussed. Chapter 8 also highlights the need for more work in determining the validity of such proxies for life course epidemiology. What is apparent throughout this book and increasingly in epidemiology in general is the importance of acknowledging and describing patterns of missing data in any study and considering methods for imputing missing data, with appropriate understanding of the assumptions underlying any imputation method.

17.2.4 Measuring exposures and outcomes

All epidemiological studies have to strike a balance between a gold standard measure (for example, histology from a liver biopsy in the case of non-alcoholic fatty liver disease) and what is feasible, but reasonably accurate, in large-scale studies of healthy volunteers (imaging or biomarkers for non-alcoholic fatty liver disease). In family-based life course epidemiology studies there are added complexities because of interests in measuring trajectories over the life course in order to understand normal and abnormal development and degeneration and the processes that influence these. For many characteristics, the methods that can be used to assess them at different ages will have to be different. At certain life stages proxy informants may be required (Chapter 8). We believe that further work is required to understand the extent to which measurement instruments used at different life stages that aim to assess the same characteristics really do so. Furthermore, the 'best' biomarker, or method for measuring a characteristic in epidemiological studies, will change over time with technological advances. Inevitably researchers will want to use the 'best' at any particular time, but this could then be problematic for comparing measures of the same characteristic at different ages, within an individual or across different generations, when different methods for measuring the characteristic have been used. Clear documentation of how all characteristics have been measured in a study, together with the rationale for using a particular method are essential (Chapter 6). It would also be valuable, where possible, to compare different methods within subgroups of the study population to determine the extent to which they agree.

17.2.5 Analytical strategy

As with all research it is essential to be clear about the underlying assumptions of any family-based life course epidemiology study (Chapters 2, 3, 4, 5) and to use the most appropriate statistical methods (Chapters 10, 11, 12). Analytical protocols should be specified before starting analyses and changes to these once analyses have begun clearly reported and justified. Ideally, several different family-based approaches, with appropriate statistical methods, should be used to address the same hypothesis (Chapter 2). Consistency in the results from different methods will strengthen the belief in these results. Where there is inconsistency a clear understanding of the underlying assumptions of each method might help to further causal understanding.

An important challenge to analytical strategies in life course epidemiology is to develop testable theoretical causal models that elucidate the risk and protective factors at each life stage, and the underlying biological, behavioural, and psychosocial pathways that link family members, over one and several generations. So far few family-based studies have mapped out a conceptual framework that encapsulates such hypothesized mechanisms. The use of directed acyclic graphs (DAGs) can be particularly useful, and more compelling than a verbal description for these complex interrelated hypotheses, since they force one to be explicit about the direction of proposed associations and challenge one to be clear about what variables to include in statistical models as potential confounders or mediators.[9]

17.3 The way forward for family-based epidemiological studies

17.3.1 The potential of new large family-based studies

Over recent years and in various countries, many large scale family-based studies have been initiated or are already underway (Chapters 6, 7 and 9).[10] For instance, both Denmark and Norway have recently established birth/prenatal cohort studies with around 100,000 participants (mother-offspring pairs) and with information on both mothers and offpring.[11, 12] The United States is intending to have a national project of similar scale that commences from birth (Chapter 6). By contrast, the *Generation Scotland* study will recruit adults over a 6-year period, to form a total of 50,000 individuals that comprise of siblings and parent-offspring groups.[13] In addition to providing DNA, study members will have their health tracked via linkage to existing electronic health databases in a project that aims primarily to study the degenerative process of chronic disease. However, this study will also incorporate the potential for family-based studies of the developmental processes involved in chronic complex disease, since it plans to target participants from an existing birth cohort—the Aberdeen Children of the 1950s—who already have detailed perinatal, infant and childhood information, including on siblings and across generations.[14]

Furthermore, for any participant in *Generation Scotland* who was born since 1948 in Aberdeen, it will be possible to link them to detailed perinatal data available in the Aberdeen Maternal and Neonatal Databank. We are aware of one new and very large family-based study that is currently planned for a low and middle income country. The *China Children and Families Cohort Study* intends to recruit 300,000 families with enrolment occurring prior to conception for some couples.[10]

Many of the examples described above intend to use linkage of participants to information held on them in national registers to enhance direct data collection (Chapter 6). There are also examples of family-based life course studies that have relied solely on record linkage between existing databases.[5, 15–18] For example, record linkage of the Swedish birth registry, conscription examination data, and mortality records have been used to compare within and between sibling associations of both gestational age and birth weight with blood pressure,[5] and the association of offspring body mass index (as an instrumental variable for own (parent's) body mass index) with parental mortality.[15] In another example, the Utah family genealogy records, collected for religious purposes by the Church of Jesus Christ of the Latter-day Saints, were linked in the 1970s with the Utah Cancer Registry[16] and have become the Utah Population Data Base. More recently extensive medical records, with detailed information on medication and treatment response, have been linked for a large sub-sample of the Utah Population Data Base. Hence the study has emerged progressively out of disparate components as an invaluable resource spanning several generations for investigating both the heritable contribution and lifestyle factors to cancer and other phenotypes.[16–18]

These new and very large family/birth cohort studies and the potential of linking between existing datasets to generate family-based studies demonstrate the future potential for extending life course epidemiology through family-based designs. Our hope is that this book will stimulate investigators involved with these studies to collect and clearly document information on a broad range of family members, on methods of linking different family members, including in complex family structures, and to use the methods described in this book.

17.3.2 Extending family-based studies to different populations

As well as a need for more studies in low and middle income countries (Chapter 7), studies of different ethnic groups within any given geographical population, amongst whom there may be distinct family patterns and behaviours, as well as distinct genetic variants, are likely to enhance our understanding of developmental and degenerative influences on future disease. Comparisons across studies from different geographical, ethnic, and cultural backgrounds can determine whether associations are robust despite differences between these groups (and therefore likely to involve mechanisms that are similar across disparate populations) or what differences between populations explain differences of associations across these populations.

Migration studies have been used for many decades to try and understand the extent to which genetic or non-genetic factors might explain differences in disease prevalence between populations, but relatively few studies have formally examined differences between ethnic groups in family-based associations. There are some existing and new studies that do focus on life course epidemiology in different ethnic groups. For example, the new *Born in Bradford Study* aims specifically to compare and contrast characteristics and associations across the life course in families of European and South Asian origin who reside in the UK, in order to understand the key determinants of health and wellbeing in both populations (Chapter 6). The Strong Heart Study of American Indians has detailed the genetic and shared familial environmental influences on CVD in this group[19] and the studies of intergenerational and sibling associations in the Pima Indians, which are described in Chapter 13, have contributed important understanding to the intergenerational transfer of obesity and diabetes. However, greater collaboration and comparisons between these studies and a stronger appreciation of how family structures can be applied in these studies would be useful.

17.3.3 Extending family-based and life course epidemiology studies to different disease areas

Previous books in the life course series have highlighted the importance of life course epidemiology to understanding the determinants of chronic complex diseases and demonstrate that most of the research has addressed these important outcomes, in particular cancer, cardiovascular disease, diabetes, mental ill-health, musculoskeletal diseases, and respiratory disease. The use of family-based studies in life course epidemiology has focused largely on a narrower range of outcomes, mostly diabetes and cardiovascular disease, mental health, and reproductive health. The final section of this book illustrates how family-based studies have enhanced understanding of life course epidemiology in these areas, and we hope that these examples will serve as a stimulus to extend these approaches to the study of the developmental and degenerative influences on other chronic complex diseases. In addition, we believe that family-based studies could provide an invaluable opportunity to study mechanisms across the life course that influence the acquisition and transmission of infectious diseases, such as HIV,[20, 21] hepatitis-B,[22] and H-pylori infection.[23]

17.4 Conclusion

In many ways the future of family-based studies represent new territory in scientific terms, for instance by using observational studies to establish causal pathways rather than just associations. As noted in Chapter 6 it is important to see data collected in our new and existing large cohort studies as resources to be used widely by researchers from different disciplines both today and into the future. Funding bodies around the world increasingly recognize this need and rightly provide funding on the basis that data collected will be shared widely in the scientific community. However, as pointed out in Chapter 9, there has to be some appreciation and reward for the efforts of those involved in coordinating, collecting and documenting all of the data in these studies.

In the same way that family studies have emerged out of collaborations between researchers from genetics to epidemiology and sociology, it is also likely that these will incorporate new interests in others fields, such as the role of the built environment in public health and the implications of climate change, over coming decades. Family-based studies should not be the preserve of rich nations and there is a need for collaboration across all geographical boundaries in order to fully understand life course influences on health and support appropriate development of global public health infrastructure at a time of rapid geopolitical and economic change. The requirements for large sample sizes and comparisons between associations in different populations described in this final chapter and throughout the book highlight the need for greater collaboration between study investigators. The key message from this book must be that we should all work together more closely in order to share knowledge, skills, and study resources. In an increasingly multi-cultural society, family-based studies may themselves provide significant impetus for researchers of all backgrounds and nationalities to seek to work across boundaries and beyond traditional academic restrictions.

References

1 **Kuh D, Ben Shlomo Y, Lynch J, Hallqvist J, Power C.** Life course epidemiology. *J Epidemiol Community Health* 2003; **57**: 778–83.

2. Lawlor DA, Ronalds G, Clark H, Davey Smith G, Leon DA. Birthweight is inversely associated with incident coronary heart disease and stroke among individuals born in the 1950s: findings from *the Aberdeen Children of the 1950s* prospective cohort study. *Circulation* 2005; **112**:1416–20.

3. Lawlor DA, Harbord RM, Sterne JAC, Timpson NJ, Davey Smith G. Mendelian randomization and instrumental variables. *Statistics in Medicine* 2008; **27**:1133–63.

4. McNeill G, Tuya C, Smith WC. The role of genetic and environmental factors in the association between birthweight and blood pressure: evidence from meta-analysis of twin studies. *Int J Epidemiol* 2004; **33**: 995–1001.

5. Lawlor DA, Hubinette A, Tynelius P, Leon DA, Davey Smith G, Rasmussen F. Associations of gestational age and intrauterine growth with systolic blood pressure in a family-based study of 386,485 men in 331,089 families. *Circulation* 2007; **115**: 562–8.

6. Yang S, Lynch J, Susser E, Lawlor DA. Birthweight and cognitive ability in childhood among siblings and non-siblings. *Pediatrics* 2008; **122**(2): e350–e358.

7. Lawlor DA, Clark H, Davey Smith G, Leon DA. Childhood intelligence, educational attainment and adult body mass index: findings from a prospective cohort and within sibling-pairs analysis. *International Journal of Obesity* 2006; **30**: 1758–65.

8. Lawlor DA, Timpson N, Harbord R, Leary S, Ness A, McCarthy MI, Frayling TM, Hattersley AT, Davey Smith G. Exploring the developmental overnutrition hypothesis using parental-offspring associations and the *FTO* gene as an instrumental variable for maternal adiposity: findings from the Avon Longitudinal Study of Parents and Children (ALSPAC). *PLoS Medicine* 2008; **5**: e33.

9. Hernan MA, Hernandez-Diaz S, Werler MM, Mitchell AA. Causal knowledge as a prerequisite for confounding evaluation: an application to birth defects epidemiology. *American Journal of Epidemiology* 2002; **155**: 176–84.

10. Brown RC, Dwyer T, Kasten C, Krotoski D, Li Z, Linet MS *et al.* Cohort profile: the International Childhood Cancer Cohort Consortium (I4C). *Int J Epidemiol* 2007; **36**: 724–30.

11. Magnus P, Irgens LM, Haug K, Nystad W, Skjaerven R, Stoltenberg C. Cohort profile: the Norwegian Mother and Child Cohort Study (MoBa). *Int J Epidemiol* 2006; **35**: 1146–50.

12. Olsen J, Melbye M, Olsen SF, Sorensen TI, Aaby P, Andersen AM *et al.* The Danish National Birth Cohort—its background, structure and aim. *Scand J Public Health* 2001; **29**: 300–7.

13. Smith BH, Campbell H, Blackwood D, Connell J, Connor M, Deary IJ *et al.* Generation Scotland: the Scottish Family Health Study; a new resource for researching genes and heritability. *BMC Med Genet* 2006; **7**: 74–82.

14. Leon DA, Lawlor DA, Clark H, Macintyre S. Cohort profile: The Aberdeen Children of the 1950s study. *International Journal of Epidemiology* 2006; **35**: 549–52

15. Davey Smith G, Sterne JAC, Tynelius P, Lawlor DA, Rasmussen F. Use of offspring body mass index as an instrumental variable suggests that the causal effect of increased body mass index on mortality is underestimated in conventional observational studies. *Journal of Epidemiology and Community Medicine* 2006; **60**: A25.

16. Cannon Albright LA. Utah family-based analysis: past, present and future. *Hum Hered* 2008; **65**: 209–20.

17. Daniels M, Merrill RM, Lyon JL, Stanford JB, White GL, Jr. Associations between breast cancer risk factors and religious practices in Utah. *Prev Med* 2004; **38**: 28–38.

18. Miki Y, Swensen J, Shattuck-Eidens D, Futreal PA, Harshman K, Tavtigian S *et al.* A strong candidate for the breast and ovarian cancer susceptibility gene BRCA1. *Science* 1994; **266**: 66–71.

19. North KE, Howard BV, Welty TK, Best LG, Lee ET, Yeh JL *et al.* Genetic and environmental contributions to cardiovascular disease risk in American Indians: the strong heart family study. *Am J Epidemiol* 2003; **157**: 303–14.

20. Kourtis AP, Lee FK, Abrams EJ, Jamieson DJ, Bulterys M. Mother-to-child transmission of HIV-1: timing and implications for prevention. *Lancet Infect Dis* 2006; **6**: 726–32.

21 **Venkatesh KK, Prasad L, Mayer KH, Kumarasamy N.** HIV transmission transcends three generations: can we prevent secondary transmission in India? *Int J of STD & AIDS* 2008; **19**: 418–20.
22 **Norris S, Siddiqi K, Mohsen A.** Hepatitis B (prevention). *Clin Evid* 2006; **15**: 1049–60.
23 **Kivi M, Tindberg Y.** Helicobacter pylori occurrence and transmission: A family affair? *Scand J Infect Dis* 2006; **38**: 407–17.

Index

Please note: page numbers in bold refer to material in tables or boxes.

Aberdeen Children of the 1950s (ACONF) 100, 102, 113, 210–11, 298–9, 306
ACDE model 254
ACE model 230, 252–4
ADE model 253–4
adiposity 23, 256–7, 273
adolescence 118, 130
adoption studies 47–8, 87, 152
adult disease, developmental origins 22–8
adult health outcomes 182–3
  birth weight 87–8, 108, 300–1
  childhood obesity 3
  sibling studies 41–3
  twin studies 68–70, 71–2, 72–3
  see also later life outcomes
adult height, twin correlations 59
age adjustment 234–5
age at first parenthood 297–8
age at menopause 309
age-at-onset data
  frailty models 238–41
  genetic inputs 50–1
  mental disorder 280–3, 286–7
age at placement, adoption studies bias 47–8
alcohol abuse 279, 282
alcohol consumption
  maternal 42–3, 106–7, 108, 283–4
  proxy reporting 153–5, 157–62, 173
  shared familial behaviour 5
ALSPAC (Avon Longitudinal Study of Parents and Children) 101, 114, 115
analysis of variance (ANOVA) 64–6, 232–5
analytical strategy 329
angina risk 267–8
anonymous data 121
antenatal clinics 109–10, 114
anthropometric measurements, proxy reporting 153–5
anxiety disorders 283
Asia, low birthweights in 21
associations, intergenerational 31–2
assortive mating 201, 204
attrition matters 116–19, 141, 328
Avon Longitudinal Study of Parents and Children (ALSPAC) 101, 114, 115

Bayesian formulation 207
Bayesian Markov Chain Monte Carlo estimation 232, 240
Bayesian multivariate frailty models 240–1
behavioural characteristics 13–14, 59
behavioural difficulties 89
behavioural genetic (BG) research 40, 46–52, 90
Belarus Promotion of Breastfeeding Intervention Trial (PROBIT) 133, 135, 137

bi-ethnic birth cohort 116–17
bi-variate logistic regression 208
bias
  recall bias 296, 305
  selection bias 75–6
  unobserved bias 40–5
binary data
  with GLMM 237, **248–9**
  multilevel models 206
  tetrachoric correlation analysis 207–9
birth cohort studies 106–21
  diversity 103–4
  documentation 104
  family-based designs in 186
  intergenerational 131–3
  proxy reports 152
  standardisation 99–104
birth length 20–1, 301–5
birth order 89–90, 91
birth size 264–9, 306
birth weight
  adult height 69–70
  body composition 140
  causal factors 108
  cognitive ability 319–23
  family correlations 14–22, 31–2, 33
  genetics 307–8
  heritability 50
  intergenerational continuities 300–5
  later life outcomes
    blood pressure 70–1
    continuity in 300–1
    CVD risk factor 41, 264–9
  maternal height 213–15
  maternal obesity 87–8, 256–7
  parental later life outcomes 29–31, 269–71
  parental smoking 22–4
  socioeconomic issues 44–5, 210–15
  twin studies 57, 62–70
block design test scores 231–8, **246–9**, plates 1–4
blood pressure
  maternal 267
  offspring as adult 70–1, 264
  paternal 268–9
  see also gestational hypertension
body mass index (BMI) 22–8, 51
  see also obesity
Book Ends, Tony Harrison 1–2
Bradford *Born in Bradford* study 116–17, 330
Brazil Birth Cohort Studies 133, 134, 136, 142, 143
breast feeding 5, 22
  replacements for 139
British 1958 birth cohort 100, 111, 306
British 1946 birth cohort (MRC NSHD) 187–8

cancer (childhood) 104
cardiovascular disease (CVD)
  birth weight 264–8, 268–9
  early life factors 263–74
  fetal growth 318–19
  parental outcomes 29–31
  world-wide impact 130
causal associations 25–8, 40–3, 325–6
characteristics, intergenerational transfer 14–22
CHD (coronary heart disease) 3
Child Health and Development Study (CHDS) 100
childhood intelligence (IQ) *see* cognitive ability
children, proxy reporting 154, 172
chorionicity (MZ twins) 62–3, 72–3, 91
chronic disease epidemiology 130–1, 133–8, 182, 299–300
classical twin studies 58–62, 73–4
clustering in families 203–7
cognitive ability
  birth weight and 319–23
  breast feeding and 5
  IQ data 23–4, 43, 50–1, 108, 109
  perinatal factors 23–4, 182–3
cognitive function decline 231–40, **245, 246–9**
combining study methods 27–8
communicable diseases 130
community support 116–17
composition of exposures 139
conceptual considerations, in studies 141–4
conduct disorder 282–3
confidentiality 119–21
confounding factors 3–4, 23–4, 40–4, 99–103
  see also residual confounding
confounding structure 139–40
contraceptive options 298, 309, 310
coronary heart disease (CHD) 3
cousins 16–18
  intergenerational studies 87
covariance modelling 59–60
covariates 216–18, 234–5
cross-sectional random effects model 234, **245–6**
cultural behavioural characteristics 21–2
CVD *see* cardiovascular disease (CVD)

Danish Metropolit Cohort 100, 102, 113
Danish National Birth Cohort 106, 114–15, 118, 119
data
  availability 107–9
  consistency 102–3
  contamination 156
  missing 116, 216–18
  sharing 120–1, 122
  sources 106, 114
dedication 121–2, 141
degenerative model 2–3
dementia onset modelling 239–40, **242**
dementia studies 154
demographic characteristics 162
depression
  incidence 130, 279–82
  parental 31, 89
  twin studies 286–7
developmental origins of disease 2–3, 22–8, 181–4

developmental overnutrition hypothesis 27–8
deviation from normal 14
diabetes
  maternal 256–7, 267, 270–1, 273
  offspring risk 88, 273
diet, children 172
diethyl-stilbestrol (DES) 4, 19
direction of association 325–6
disclosure of medical results 120
disease
  areas in future aims 331
  genetic linkage studies 50–1, 52
  models of causation 2–3
diversity, in studies 103–9, 121–2
divorce or parental separation 284
dizygotic (DZ) twins 48, 59, 91
  birth weights 266–8
  chorionicity 62–3
documentation 122
dummy variables 205–6

early adulthood 118, 130
early life exposures
  adult health risks 41–3, 263–74
  mental health and 282–4
  sibling FE models 44–5
  unobserved 43
early motherhood 297–8
economic transition 138–9, 140
education 209, 298–9
egg donation 18–19, 87
endometriosis 308–9
energy expenditure, across countries 139
environment and genes 46–7
environmental correlations
  assumptions 252–3
  height modelling 205–7
  shared *vs.* non-shared 254–5
environmental exposures
  across generations 13–14
  age at menarche 296–7
  assumption in twin studies 59–61
  birth weight 50
  intergenerational transfer 15, 49
  phenotypic variation 46
  post-natal DZ twins 48
  sibling studies 39–40
environmental pollution 139
environmental variance, in traits 60, 199–201
epigenetic effects 49, 86
equal environment assumption (EEA) 252–3
ethical issues
  in cohort studies 103, 119–21
  in longitudinal studies 188
  see also confidentiality; incentives
ethnic groups, in future aims 330–1
ethnicity, and birth size 21–2
evidence base, reliability 155–63
exposure-disease associations 140
exposures
  composition 139
  measurement 328–9
  outcomes in offspring 22–8

see also early life exposures; environmental exposures; parental exposures; prenatal exposures

families 1–2, 4–6
  concept of 144
  membership 110–11, 113, 285–6
family-based birth cohort studies, in LMIC 138–44
family-based studies 4, 6–7, 85–93, 317–23
  challenges 325–31
  clustering in 203–7
  developmental origins 181–4
  future aims 322–3, 329–31
  high income countries 130–1
  in LMICs 129–30, 131–3
  mental health 279–88
  and new birth cohort studies 186–8
  reproductive health 295–311
  special situations 163–73
  statistical analysis 203–7, 251–8
  types of 92–3
family discord 280, 284
family environment, for twins 59
family events 39–40
family income fluctuations 42–3
family-led characteristics, in siblings 42–3
family-level confounders 44–5
family-level phenotypic variation 46
family medical history 317–19
family members, as proxies 151–2
family relationships, mental health and 285–6
family size 89–90, 298
fathers
  in cohort studies 111–12
  see also non-paternity; paternal
favouritism, among siblings 327
FE model *see* fixed effects (FE) model
fertility problems 308–9
fertility rate 298
fetal genes 20, 68–70, 307–8
fetal growth 305–6
  adult health and 100, 318–19
  growth restriction 29, 75, 264–8, 307
  intergenerational studies 210, **212**, 256–7
  maternal behaviour and 4–5
  twin studies 75
fetal insulin hypothesis 256–7, 267
fetal origins hypothesis 68–74
fetal overnutrition hypothesis 273
fetal programming hypothesis 73–4, 269
fetoplacental environment 57, 68–70
fixed effects (FE) model 40–5, 89
folate supplementation 25–6
follow-up questionnaires 115
forestry metaphors 103, 104, 105, 121
frailty models 238–41, **242**
functional ability assessment **168–71**
funding issues
  birth cohort studies 106
  longitudinal studies 143, 183, 187
  proxy reporting **154**
  research agenda 107–9
future aims

cohort studies 99–103, 188–9
family-based studies 310–11, 322–3, 325–31

gene-environment interactions 46–7, 49
  cohort studies 99–103, 287
    mental health 287
  family-based studies 86
  statistical analysis 202–3
generalized linear mixed models (GLMM) 236–8, **248–9**
genes
  fetal 68–70
  inherited by siblings 39–40
genetic correlations
  assumptions 253
  birth weight 31–2, 33, 50
  height modelling 205–7
  lipid levels 5
  non-paternity 215–16, **217**
genetic data, ethics and 120
genetic linkage studies 40, 52, 90–1
genetic modelling 59–60
genetic variation
  disease outcomes 25–6
  individual-level differences 46
  in intergenerational studies 14
  unobserved 43
genetics literature 50–2
genotype, for offspring 195–6
gestation length 305
gestational diabetes mellitus (GDM) 299–300
gestational hypertension 299, 300
global relative recurrence odds ratio 208–9
grandparents 15–16, 184–5
growth restriction, fetal 75, 307
Guatemala Human Capital Study 133, 134, 136

half siblings 31–2, 33, 285–6
health databases 118–19
health registers 106, 115
health-related behaviours
  future studies 322–3
  maternal 267–9
  proxy reporting 157–62, **164**
health status **166–8**
height
  adult 69–70
  childhood 199–201, **222**
  heritability 60
height modelling 204–7
heritability 46
  adoption studies 47–8
  adult height 59, 204–7
  age at menarche 296–7
  assortative mating and 201
  birth weight 31–2, 33
  gene-environment interactions 49
  sibling studies 46–7
  statistical analysis 204–7, 252–3
    simple linear regression 195–6, **222**
    variance components model 199, **201**, **222–4**
  twin studies 48
high income countries 130–1

hostility, sibling relationships 285–6
hygeine hypothesis 90
hypertension
  gestational 299, 300
  see also blood pressure

incentives for retention 115, 117–18, 142, 188
index participants
  availability of 163
    dual or multiple reports 172
    offspring of 113–14, 185–6
index-proxy agreement **174–6**
India, birth weights 20–1
India South Delhi Cohort 133, 134
individual-level characteristics 42–3, 46
individual's rights 119–21
instrumental variable (IV) analysis 26
insulin resistance, maternal 267, 269
intelligence quotient (IQ) 23–4, 43, 50–1, 108, 109
inter-pair twin differences 70–2, 74
intercept analysis 203, 204, 235, 238
intergenerational associations
  cohort size 113–14
  continuity in 306
  data collection in LMIC 142–3
  health outcomes 269–71
  mechanisms of 31–2
  see also nature and nurture
intergenerational exposures, outcomes in offspring 22–8
intergenerational studies 13–14
  design features 197–8
  latent variable models 257
  in LMICs 133–8
  more than two generations 210–15
  overview 87–9
  prenatal growth retardation 75
  proxy reporting 7, 151–2
  statistical analysis 195–8, 256–7
  transfer of characteristics 14–22
International Childhood Cancer Cohort Consortium 104
intra-pair twin differences 66–8, 71–2, 74
intrauterine environment
  and birth weight 18–19, 20, 31–2, 33
  birth weight and cognitive ability 183, 319, 320
  developmental effects 22–5, 26
  gestational diabetes 299–300
  growth retardation 29, 75, 264–8, 307
  maternal obesity 27–8
  shared by twins 59, 70–2

latent variable models 257
later life exposures, unobserved 43
later life outcomes 309–11, 328–9
life course approach 1–4, 92, 131
life course epidemiology, defined 3, 181–2
life time health 255–6
lifestyle
  maternal 15
  parental 19, 23, 24
  twins 61
linear regression analysis 195–6
linear regression models 211–13, **225**

lipid levels 5, 264, 319
literature review
  behavioural genetics 50–2
  evidence base 155–62
  FE models 44–5
  life course epidemiology 50–2
  proxy reporting 155–62
  statistical analysis models 251–8
long-term studies
  birth cohort 99–103
    forestry metaphors 103, 104, 105, 121
    in LMIC 141–4
  funding issues 183
  intergenerational 195
  latent variable models 257
  repeated measurements 210
  statistical analysis 231–40, **245, 246–9**
longitudinal models, statistical analysis issues 255–6
low and middle-income countries (LMIC) 129–30
  existing birth cohorts 131–8
  management of study 138–44

male infertility 309
male sexual maturity/menopause 295
Markov chain Monte Carlo (MCMC) methods 240, **249–50**
Mater University Study of Pregnancy 131, **134, 154**
maternal age 45, 297–8
maternal behaviours 4–5, 102
maternal birth weight, intergenerational transfer 14–22
maternal conditions, pregnancy-specific 298–300
maternal cousins 17
maternal education 298–9
maternal effects, statistical analysis 25–8, 201–2, **222–4**
maternal genes, reproductive outcomes 307–8
maternal grandparents 17, 19–21
maternal health outcomes, offspring birth weight 29–31, 268
maternal height 199–201, 213–15, **222**
maternal MTHFR variant 26
maternal obesity 27–8, 88, 256–7
maternal smoking 4, 5, 6, 22–4, 88
materno-fetal nutrient supply 91
measurements, repeated 235–6
measuring outcomes 328–9
mechanisms of association 31–2
medical databases 118–19, 330
medical history 119–21
menarche, age at 60, 295, 296–7
Mendelian laws, inheritance of traits 195–6
Mendelian randomization studies 25–8, 27–8
menopause, age at 309
mental health 279–88
  early life exposures 282–4
  family history 318
  gene-environment interaction 287
  index-proxy agreement **174–6**
  parent/offspring association 325–6
  proxy reporting 162
  sibling and twin studies 285–7
  statistical analysis 197
metabolic health, maternal 268
metabolic syndrome 300

methodological considerations 141–4, 326–9
migration in studies
   in future aims 330
   intergenerational 21–2
   missing data 217–18
   statistical analysis 197
miscarriage 107, 109
missing data 216–18, 242, 328
mobility *see* migration
monozygotic (MZ) twins 59, 91
   BG studies 48
   birth weights 266–8
   chorionicity and zygosity 61–3
mortality determinants 154, 185, 186
mortality rates, dementia and 239
mortality records 330
mortality risks, age-specific 182
mortality studies, proxy informants 173
mothers
   as participants in studies 111
   proxy reporting 142, 151–2
   see also maternal
Mplus software 207, 215
MRC National Survey of Health and Development 187–8
multilevel models 203–7
multivariate frailty model 238–40
multivariate linear regression models 211–13, **225**

national registers 330
nature and nurture 39–40
   BG research 46–52
   family-based studies 85–6
   twin studies 58–62, 229
neural tube defects (NTDs) 25–6
non-biological fathers 111–12
non-communicable diseases
   family history 317–19
   rates 129–31, 138–41
non-paternity 24–5, 30, 31, 270
   statistical analysis 215–16, **217, 227–8**
Norwegian MoBa study 101, 114–15

obesity
   childhood 3, 87–8
   lifestyle and 23
   maternal 17–28, 267
observable characteristics 46
occupational exposures 138, 139, 140
offspring
   of cohort members 113
   height 199–201
   obesity 23, 27–8
   outcomes of parental exposures 14, 22–31, 31
   size 138
   see also birth weight
optimal phenotypic states 130
ordinary least squares (OLS) regression model 41–2, 44
outcomes, later life 309–11, 328–9
ovum donation 50

parents 184–5, 269–71
parent of origin effect 199, 202, **222–4**
parent-offspring associations 22–5, 27–8
parental behaviour, offspring mental health 280–1, 283–4
parental depression, child conduct disorder 282–3
parental exposures, offspring outcomes 29–31, 87, 271–2
parental health, offspring exposures 14, 28–31
parenthood, age at first 297–8
parenting quality 88–9, 286
participants in cohort studies 110–14, 118
paternal
   see also non-paternity
paternal CVD risk 29–31, 268–9
paternal effects, statistical analysis 201–2, **222–4**
paternal grandparents 17, 19–21
paternal height 199–201
paternal intergenerational comparisons 19–21
paternal smoking 5, 6, 22–4
path analysis 213–15, **225–7**
perinatal exposures 182–3, 267
perinatal outcomes 75–6, 182–3, 300–1
personal identification numbers 115
personality, age-specific heritability 50–1
phenotypes
   characteristics 46
   optimal state 130
   twin studies 230–1
phenotypic correlations 204–7
phenotypic variations 46, 49
Philippines Cebu Cohort Study 133, 134, 136
physical activity 107, 157–62, 172
physical health, proxy reporting 162
Pima Indians 273, 300, 330
placentation 62–6, 268, 269
poetry, on family relationships 1–2
political will 140–1
polycystic ovarian syndrome (PCOS) 308
population registers 106
postnatal depression 282, 283
postnatal environment, DZ twins 48
postnatal growth 76
power calculations 74, 101, 114–15
pre-conception recruitment 109–10
pregnancy, age at first parenthood 297–8
pregnancy outcomes 300–1
pregnancy-related disorders 207–9, 298–300
prenatal environment *see* intrauterine environment
prenatal exposures
   siblings 39, 44–5
   unobserved 43
prenatal programming hypothesis 73–4
prospective trials 99–103
proxy-index agreement **164–71, 174–6**
proxy informants 7, 153, **154**, 163, 173
   cohort participants 172–3
   family members 151–2
   mother, for partner 142
   siblings 147
   twins 147
proxy reporting 173
   for children 172
   data contamination 156
   dual or multiple 172
   validity and reliability 155–62

psychiatric illness 130, 133, **174–6**
psychological outcomes 51
public health policy 3, 14, 22, 322–3

questionnaires 115, 142, 153

R codes 234, 237, **245–6, 248–9**
random analysis of variance (rANOVA) 232–5
random coefficients model 204–5
random effect analysis 232–5
random effect models 90, 241–2
random slope effects 204, 235, 237–8, **246–9**
recall bias 296, 305
regression coefficient 200–1
relative recurrence risk 207–9
reliability 153–62
repeated measures 235–6
reproductive health 295–311, 317–18
reproductive indicators, of later health 309–11
reproductive outcomes 306–8, 310–11
research agendas, driving forces 107–9
research ethics 119–21
residual confounding 40–4
resource issues 106, 115, 141
retention matters 103, 116–17, 188
  incentives 115, 117–19, 142, 188
Russia Izhevsk Family Study **154,** 173

sample size 114–15, 327–8
SATSA (Swedish Adoption/Twin Study of Aging) 231–40, **245, 246–9**
schizophrenia 100, 106–7
selection bias, twin studies 75–6
serotonin transporter (5-HTT) gene 287
shared gene assumption 253
siblings 87, 113, 186
  birth weights 16–18, 31–2, 33, 268–9
  favouritism among 327
  reproductive outcomes 306–7
sibling relationships, mental health and 285–6
sibling studies 89–91
  birth weight and cognitive ability 320
  full- and half- comparisons 48
  heritability 46–7
  in LMIC 143–4
  mental health 285–7
  proxy reporting 147, 151–2
  residual confounding 40–4
  theoretical underpinning 39–40
  trait variances 230
simple linear regression
  heritability 195–6, **222**
  parent of origin effect 199, **222–4**
single-parent families 285–6, 326
sisters 87
size matters, in cohort studies 114–15
slope *see* random slope effects
smoking
  familial behaviour 5
  grand-maternal 17
  maternal 4, 5, 88, 265
  or other tobacco use 139
  parental 17, 19, 22–4
  proxy reporting 157–62

social changes 187
  world-wide impact 130, 140–1
social changes 99–103, 326–7
social class 184–5, 209, 210–15, 265
social disadvantage 297–8
socioeconomic data
  age at menarche 296
  birth weight 15, 269
  cognitive development 23–4
  as confounding factor 3
  longitudinal studies 13–14, 15, 183–4
  mental health 283
  obesity in 23
  perinatal conditions 44–5
  proxy reporting 162
  twin studies 255–6
software for statistical analysis 232
South Africa Birth to Twenty Study 133, 135, 137
Southampton Women's Survey 87, 109, 198
spouses 5, 19
Sri Lankan Twin Registry 138
standardisation, cohort studies 102–9
starting points, cohort studies 109–10
Stata codes **222–8**
statistical analysis
  analytical strategy 329
  family-based studies 251–8
  intergenerational studies 195–7
  missing data assessment 116
  twin studies 230–1
statistical models, seven deadly sins of 258
statistical power 114–15, 327–8
steparent families 326
stepfather families 285–6
structural equation modelling 59–60
study clinics 114, 142
sub-fertility 308–9
substance abuse 279, 282
surrogate mothers 18–19, 87
survival data 209
Swedish Adoption/Twin Study of Aging (SATSA) 231–40, **245, 246–9**

Taiwan Birth Cohort Study 133, 135, 137
teenage pregnancy 297–8
teratogenesis 19
tetrachoric correlation 199, 207–9, **224–5**
three generation data collection 142–3
timing, in life course epidemiology 5–6
timing of recruitment, cohort studies 109–10
tobacco use 139, 157–62
  see also smoking
traits
  inheritance 195–7
  similar 199–201
  variances 59–61, 230–1
twins
  birth weights 18, 31–2, 33, 57
  prenatal environments 50
  types of 91
twin studies 48, 91–2, 229, 230–1
  age-at-onset data 238–41, **242**
  birth weights 265–8, 320–1
  classical 58–62, 73–4

health-related behaviours **159**
limitations 74–6
in LMICs 138, 143–4
longitudinal studies 186, 257
mental health 286–7
proxy reporting 147, 151–2
SATSA 231–40, **245, 246–9**
selection bias 75–6
separated twins 62
socioeconomic background 255–6
theoretical underpinning 57–8
within-pair associations 232–5

umbilical cord insertion 64–6, 72, 91
unique exposures 139
unobserved bias 40–5
US National Children's Study 106, 109
US National Childrens' Study 114

validity of proxy reporting
 assessment 153–5
 evidence base 155–62
variables
 confounding structure 139–40
 endogenous and exogenous 213–15
variance
 random effect analysis 232–5
 of a trait 59–61, 230–1
 see also analysis of variance (ANOVA)
variance components model 199, **202,** 203–7, **222–4**
vascular health, maternal 268

WinBUGS software 207, 210, 217, 232, 240, 241, **249–50**

zygosity 62–8, 72–3, 91